Unani Medicine in the Making

Unani Medicine in the Making

Practices and Representations in 21st-Century India

Kira Schmidt Stiedenroth

Routledge
Taylor & Francis Group
LONDON AND NEW YORK

The publication of this book was funded by the DFG (German Research Foundation).

First published in 2020 by Aksant Academic Publishers

Published 2025 by Routledge
4 Park Square, Milton Park, Abingdon, Oxon OX14 4RN
605 Third Avenue, New York, NY 10158

Routledge is an imprint of the Taylor & Francis Group, an informa business

ISBN: 9789463724210 (hbk)
ISBN: 9781041190011 (pbk)
ISBN: 9781003708797 (ebk)
NUR 740

Cover illustration: Shelf with medicines in a private Unani clinic in Hyderabad (2012).

Cover design: Coördesign, Leiden

DOI: 10.5117/9789463724210

Table of Contents

Acknowledgements

The present work was only possible thanks to the kind support and help of numerous persons and institutions, among whom the Unani fraternity in India deserves special mentioning. During fieldwork, I received friendly cooperation from many individuals, including: Dr. Abdullah, Hakim A. Ahmad (Delhi), Hakim A. Ahmad (Lucknow), Mr. K. Ahmad, Dr. M.R. Ahmed, Dr. Z. Ahmad, Dr. M.A. Ali, Hakim S. M.M. Ameen, Prof. R. Ansari, Dr. A.H. Ashraf, Dr. A.J. Ashraf, Mrs. A. Chakraborty, Dr. A.K. Dar, Dr. Farah, Prof. Habeebunnisa, Dr. A. Haleem, Dr. S.S. Hameed, Hakim M. Islahi, Dr. M. Iqbal, Dr. S. Iqbal, Prof. M.A. Jafri, Prof. S. Jamil, Mr. Javed, Hakim A. Kausar, Prof. S. Khalifatullah, Hakim A. Khan, Dr. A.A. Khan, Dr. L.A. Khan, Dr. S.A. Khan, Dr. S. Khatoon, Dr. A. Latif, Dr. Y. Munshi, Dr. Nasirah, Dr. A. Qadeer, Hakim A. Quddus, Dr. A. Rahman, Prof. Dr. R. Rahman, Dr. M. Raza, Dr. S. Rehman, Hakim M.A. Sajjad, Dr. Sajid, Dr. M. Saquib, Prof. M.A. Siddiqui, Dr. S.H. Siddiqui, Prof. M.H.M. Siddiqui, Dr. M. A. Shareef, and Dr. M.A. Waheed. I am particularly thankful to Dr. Amina Ather, Mr. Mohsin Dehlvi, Mr. Mehr-e Alam Khan, Dr. Syed Asad Pasha, and Prof. S. Zillurrahman, whose active assistance allowed me to meet many of the persons mentioned above. I also extend my gratitude to Neshat Quaiser for his advice and to Kiran Bhushi for hosting me in Delhi. My deepest thanks, however, go to those practitioners who allowed me to sit in their clinics and observe their daily interactions with patients.

In Germany, I am thankful for the support and guidance provided by my supervisors. Bo Sax's deep knowledge about Indian society has been a great source of inspiration since my early days as a student of anthropology, his encouragement and advice were instrumental for the present work. Stefan Reichmuth made this project possible in the first place. I am in debt for his enthusiastic interest in my research and for his invaluable suggestions. I am also grateful to my colleagues from the Unani research project in Bochum and to those at the South Asia Institute in Heidelberg. Further, I am thankful to the DFG for funding the position that allowed me to conduct research for this book.

Parts of this book were presented in conferences and colloquiums in Bochum, Edinburgh, Heidelberg, Kiel, Muenster, and Sancheong; I am grateful for the useful questions and comments provided by colleagues and students on these occasions. I am particularly thankful to Fabrizio Speziale and to an anonymous reviewer for their valuable suggestions to improve the original manuscript. I also thank Saskia Gieling from AUP for her editorial support.

Many colleagues and friends helped me further through inspiring conversations, useful recommendations, critical remarks, access to literature, and proof reading of early drafts. Special thanks to: Md. Mujibul Anam, Didem Aydurmuş, Heri Beckmann, Cathrine Bublatzky, Elinor Chisholm, Sina Emde, Nico Henrich, Kai Fürstenberg, Susanne Kurz, Lukas Ley, Francisca Lira, Helena Lohneis, Marcel Lötzsch, Karen McNamara, Swarali Paranjape, Karin Polit, Claudia Preckel, Catherine Scheer, Julia Seibert, Jacky Singh, Roman Sieler, and Till Westermann. My gratitude goes also to all my friends and to my beloved family for their constant love and reassurance. Last but not least, I owe the greatest thanks to my best friend and companion Joerg Hornung, who stood by my side with unconditional support, loving patience and encouraging words through the ups and downs of this research and writing endeavor.

Notwithstanding all the assistance received, I bear sole responsibility for any errors or omissions in this book.

Introduction

In India, Unani medicine is one of the officially recognized indigenous systems of medicine. The term Unani is the anglicized form of the Arabic *yūnānī* ('Greek'), which alludes to its origin in ancient Greece. Graeco-Islamic medicine[1] probably arrived in South Asia around the twelfth century, and it flourished during the Mughal period (Speziale 2010a). After the decay of the Mughal empire, Graeco-Islamic medicine continued to be supported in some Muslim princely states during British rule, but most of its physicians ceased to have the patronage and social status they once enjoyed. During the late Colonial Period, medicine was made a theme for the nationalist struggle for independence and the institutionalization of Unani medicine was consolidated. Currently, Unani's official support is coordinated by the AYUSH Ministry,[2] which is in charge of the development of so-called Indian Systems of Medicine (ISM) or indigenous medical systems of the country. Unani medicine is practiced in public and private (college) hospitals, in government research institutions, as well as by many private practitioners all over the country.

Drawing on analyses of Urdu sources, the work of historians of Graeco-Islamic medicine, and ethnographic details collected during clinical consultations, conversations, and interviews with a myriad of physicians and other actors of the Unani fraternity in India, this book unpacks what Unani medicine is today by attending to its multiplicity, scrutinizing apparent tensions between an understanding of Unani as a unified system of medicine and its multiple enactments as indigenous medicine, Islamic medicine, medical science, and alternative medicine. My research questions and ethnographic analysis have been informed by theoretical works and secondary sources related to the history and anthropology of (traditional forms of) medicine in South Asia and of Graeco-Islamic medicine in particular.

1 Throughout this work, I use the words Unani medicine, Graeco-Islamic medicine, Unani, and *ṭibb* ('medicine') interchangeably. While Unani medicine is the current official denomination in India, the term Graeco-Islamic medicine seems more apt to address this form of medicine before its institutionalization.

2 AYUSH is an acronym for Ayurveda, Yoga, Unani, Siddha and Homeopathy. It was the name of a department of the Ministry of Health and Family Welfare, Government of India, dedicated to improve education and research of these forms of medicine. AYUSH also includes naturopathy and, since 2010, *Sowa-rigpa* (Tibetan medicine). On 9 November 2014, Narendra Modi from the Bharatiya Janata Party (BJP), then newly elected Prime Minister of India, established AYUSH as a separate Ministry, naming Shripad Yesso Naik (BJP) its minister (AYUSH 2015).

Through a focus on enactments of Unani and how these emerged and were reinforced, the present work challenges an assumption commonly reproduced in studies on indigenous medicine[3] in South Asia: that modern science and traditional forms of medicine are incommensurable. While acknowledging the asymmetries involved in legitimating efforts, I question the idea that the modernization of traditional medicine, with the inclusion of new technologies and medical knowledge, invariably leads to the biomedicalization and standardization of traditional forms of medicine. Further, my data presents empirical evidence on the diverse nature of medicine (Berg and Mol 1998) and proposes to rethink the apparent incommensurability[4] between the epistemologies of Unani medicine and that of biomedicine and modern science.

Multiplicity, Practice Ontology, and Looping Effects

Answering the question 'what is Unani medicine?' requires examining the multiplicity of its being: an officially recognized system of medicine, medical knowledge, humoral medicine, traditional medicine, a source of professional recognition, a platform for the articulation of Muslim identity. This list is not exhaustive. It addresses some of the different enactments of Unani medicine that are dealt with in the chapters of this book. Practice ontology provides a framework for understanding how practices produce Unani medicine—not only knowledge about it.

Annemarie Mol examined how a disease, atherosclerosis, was multiple in the sense that it was enacted in different ways in the context of a Dutch hospital. Pathologists, clinicians or the patients did not see atherosclerosis differently. Rather, their practices made, or enacted, different versions of it, while still retaining its integrity as a single disease. Hence, atherosclerosis is not fragmented, but multiple: it is 'more than one and less than many' (Mol

3 I agree with Janes in that 'there is no satisfactory term to refer to non-Western, indigenous medical systems' (1999: 1803). The term 'traditional' medicine is problematic because it implies a lack of change (ibid.). Similarly, as I discuss in Chapter 1, the term 'system of medicine' implies homogeneity and cohesion (Attewell 2007), while practices are often characterized by a lack thereof. Throughout this book I use the terms 'traditional forms of medicine' and 'traditional medicine' interchangeably while acknowledging their limitations and flaws. The same applies for the term 'biomedicine' which implies more cohesion than it actually has (Sieler 2015: 159). I have refrained from using quotation marks when mentioning them.

4 Thomas S. Kuhn defined incommensurability as different standards or definitions of science (2012 [1962]: 147). He explained the incommensurability of competing paradigms as follows: 'Practicing in different worlds, the two groups of scientists see different things when they look from the same point in the same direction' (Kuhn 2012: 149).

2002; Mol and Law 2002: 11). When we consider objects not just as the focus of people's perspectives, but as 'things that are manipulated in practices', then 'reality multiplies' (Mol 2002: 4–5).

For Mol, only a single reality is enacted at a single time. In her study, the enactments of atherosclerosis took place in different rooms and by different persons, all within the same hospital, though. Whenever some of these enactments diverged to the point of contradicting each other, a hierarchy had to be established. This effort, which Mol calls coordination, is necessary for the preservation of unity and is characterized by the 'winning' of one enactment over the others, while incompatible ones are discarded. In this way, while there is manifoldness, there is no pluralism (2002: 84). Mol's idea of multiplicity seems to fit the object of this study, Unani medicine, very well. Like doctors and patients did in the case of atherosclerosis, hakims and researchers seemed all to agree about what Unani is, even though in practice it was enacted in different ways, as the following pages will illustrate. Following Mol, different versions of an object may create frictions which need to be coordinated, and each attempt of coordination is political, because relations of power are decisive when it comes to decide which version is enacted at each time. Authority, then, is crucial in the ethnographic analysis of ontologies of practice. However, its role should not be overestimated, as, in the case of Unani, authorities are multiple, too.

An important consequence of the shift of attention from epistemologies[5] to ontologies in scholarly work is that instead of focusing on the preconditions necessary for acquiring true knowledge and addressing the question if representations of reality are accurate, knowledge about an object 'is not understood as matter of reference, but as one of manipulation' (Mol 2002: 5). It is here that Mol's philosophical questions meet ethnography, because the way in which these manipulations take place, i.e. the ways in which ontological politics are made, correspond to actions that can only be analysed in the making through empirical examples. Only an observation of how coordination takes place and different enactments are reconciled can answer the question of being. This is what Mol calls a 'shift from an epistemological to a praxeographic appreciation of reality' (2002: 53).

Enactments of Unani are done simultaneously in different places: a hakim who is feeling the pulse of a patient during a consultation, a practitioner

5 The usage of the term epistemology requires clarification. Hankinson has pointed out its standard philosophical meaning as 'theory of knowledge' as opposed to its use in social sciences as 'belief-system' (1995: 61). In the case of Unani both are related: the fundamental principles are determined by its theories of knowledge and vice-versa, as discussed in this book.

prescribing a medicine in a government facility, a Unani college student learning about modern research methods for her exam. At the same time, a patient may be visiting a hakim thinking of him as a practitioner of *desi* (indigenous) medicine, while the hakim himself may make claims of authority as a practitioner based on his BUMS (Bachelor in Unani Medicine and Surgery) degree, and recommend cupping as treatment because it is 'prophetic medicine'. Are all these enactments of Unani? What about patients visiting a hakim thinking that he is a vaid (practitioner of Ayurvedic medicine)? And what about BUMS graduates who officially practice Unani but, in reality, clearly use biomedical nosologies and therapies? Mol has addressed this kind of questions using her idea of distributions, through which 'difference isn't necessarily reduced to singularity if different "sites" are kept apart' (2002: 88). Mol sees distribution as spatial metaphor. While the different enactments of Unani in different settings may represent distribution as real, the idea of distribution also applies for the different contexts where Unani is enacted in different ways. Sometimes—within a single consultation, for example—Unani was represented differently without producing any friction at all. In this way, not all enactments are by definition concurrent, on the contrary: they may be even complementary to each other. The contexts set the framework through which simultaneous enactments may be considered to conflict or to complement one another.

While Mol's practice ontology approach helps us to effectively examine multiplicity without fragmentation—and hence to understand how Unani can be a coherent system of medicine while retaining a characteristic multiplicity—, it does not address the historicity of ontological practices and how they create realities on the long term. This is understandable since the context of her study, the hospital, provided a clear and manageable setting to understand the ontologies of a single disease. However, when we ought to analyse the multiplicity of something like Unani medicine in India, new questions arise: why do certain representations prevail above other ones over time? How are dominant enactments perceived as 'more real' than others, being even naturalized to the extent that they are non-negotiable in practice, while others are characterized by more flexibility? It is here that Ian Hacking's concept of looping effects (2002 [1995]) appears to be useful.

Hacking is another philosopher interested in ontology. He focused on the patients of multiple personality disorder and how they come into being as specific kinds of persons, what he called human kinds (ibid.). Human kinds are interactive kinds, they can become aware of how they are classified and they may modify their behaviours accordingly (Hacking 1999: 32). He called this feedback effect 'the looping effect of human kinds' to refer to how 'people classified in a certain way tend to conform or grow into the ways that they are described; but they also evolve in their own ways, so that classifications and descriptions have to be constantly revised' (1995: 21). What Hacking seeks to emphasize through his focus on interaction is that things social are not just constructed unidirectionally, but they also make themselves (1999: 116). Hakims, BUMS students, researchers, government officials, manufacturers of Unani products, and even patients enact Unani in different ways, and these enactments produce the feedback effect that Hacking named 'loopings'. Hacking's idea of 'dynamic nominalism', i.e. 'how our practices of naming interact with the things that we name' (2002: 2) also describes very well a phenomenon explored in this book, namely the role of different denominations in the ontologies of Unani medicine. To understand how this works, a look into the history of Graeco-Islamic medicine is inevitable, even though my focus as an anthropologist rests on current social processes.

The question this book addresses is not only related to 'what counts as knowledge in specific historical circumstances' or 'why particular beliefs and systems of belief arise and are accepted in particular historical circumstances, how they are sustained under relevant social conditions, and how they reflect political and economic interests' (Lynch 2013: 451). Moreover, I seek to understand how Unani medicine, i.e. what is accepted and understood as such today—and, more generally speaking, as traditional medicine—, was made, created, constituted, and naturalized. While '[b]iomedicine informs anthropology on all levels of inquiry, the definition of what we aim to study, to the way in which we write fieldnotes and to the way we stake our claims in arguments with medicine' (Ecks 2008: 85), specific enactments of traditional medicine also influenced the way in which I approached the subject of this study in the first place, namely as a problem of conflicting epistemologies between modern science and humoral-based forms of medicine. Attending to enactments of Unani medicine and the looping effects they generate makes it possible not only to acquire a deeper understanding of Unani medicine in particular and traditional medicine in general, but also to question certain tenets that have been taken for granted even in the academic study thereof.

My aim is not to prove *that* ontologies are historical and context-dependent, but to take a closer look into the processes that shape contemporary Unani medicine in India in order to understand *how* particular ontologies emerge and become established. This book examines the ways in which those involved in the realm of Unani medicine enact different ontologies in practice (Mol 2002) while at the same time producing looping effects (Hacking 2002 [1995]) which lead to the perpetuation specific kinds or ideas, some of which this work seeks to contest.

Unani and Traditional Medicine in South Asia

Graeco-Islamic medicine has been mostly studied by historians of Muslim cultures and societies. There are only a few anthropological or sociological works dealing with Unani in the context of South Asia.[6] If we compare the number of anthropological publications dedicated to Unani with those dedicated to other forms of Asian medicine, the marginality of Unani medicine is striking: to date, there is no single edited volume about Unani medicine, in comparison to volumes and special issues dedicated to the study of Ayurveda (Wujastyk and Smith 2008) or Tibetan medicine (Pordié 2008a; Schrempf 2007).

The dominance of Ayurveda is inescapable in the academic study of Indian medicine. Unani has been commonly mentioned in works about traditional medical systems of South Asia, but when studied more in depth it has been mostly from a comparative perspective, whereby Ayurveda received most of the attention (Bode 2008; Bright 1998; Sheehan 1983). Both Bode's and Bright's works thematized the commoditization of Unani medicine in the context of the modernization of Indian society, engaging in an analysis of how pharmaceutical products adapted to modern demands. While Bright's work was informed by phenomenological theories, as she sought to demonstrate how what she called 'everyday kitchen medicine' was related to 'the body politic of commoditized drug production' (1998: 262), Bode followed 'the social life' of Unani drugs, as proposed by Whyte, van der Geest & Hardon (2002) following Arjun Appadurai's framework to study 'the social life of things' (2013). Bode and Bright concluded that the market shaped Unani medicine, and that Unani pharmaceutical products embodied both tradition and modernity at the same time, dissolving the dichotomy (Bode 2008: 221ff.; Bright 1998: 263). Because these studies explored at length the production and circulation of Unani pharmaceutical products, I only rehearse the topic briefly in this book, even though it is of extreme importance for an understanding of contemporary Unani medicine.

6 For studies on the practice and influence of Graeco-Islamic medicine among Muslim Swahili communities in Kenia and Zanzibar see for example Beckerleg (1994), Parkin (2000; 2007) and Swartz (1997). For a study on the integration of Graeco-Islamic medicine in the Malay peninsula see Laderman (1992).

Only few other publications deal with contemporary practices of Unani medicine (Liebeskind 1996; Reichmuth 2016; Sheehan and Hussain 2002). Historians with intimate knowledge about Graeco-Islamic medicine in South Asia have criticized some of the developments brought about in the postcolonial context, notably modern research efforts aiming at the scientific validation of Unani medicine and its de-Islamization (Speziale 2010a) and the institutionalization of training (Attewell 2005; Speziale 2010a). The term 'medical communalism' was coined to address how Unani representatives in India often blamed the government for lack of support based on communal arguments (Quaiser 2012a). All these topics have crucially informed my research and are discussed in different chapters of this book.

The Biomedicalization of Traditional Medicines

Biomedicine has been described as 'one of the most successful Western exports ever', which makes it 'ideologically, scientifically, financially and politically dominant nearly everywhere, producing asymmetries with other forms of healing' (Naraindas et al. 2014: 6). These asymmetries have been part of recent research agendas proposing the questioning of their 'naturalness' and how they have been created through looping effects involving practices, institutions as well as the politics, power and resistance related to them (ibid.). Although it can be agreed that the dominance of biomedicine characterizes the asymmetries of medical pluralism in the modern world, the assumption that this was always the case is wrong (Baer et al. 1997: 212ff.). Even though traditional medical systems borrow from biomedicine in order to legitimize their professionalized branches, biomedicine's dominance has never been absolute (ibid.). This is an important point, as it reflects one of the perceived paradoxes that guided the initial stages of this research project, based on my reading of the anthropology of Asian medicines.

In the study of what he called 'medical revivalism in modern India', Charles Leslie asserted that the adoption of institutions and concepts from biomedicine in Ayurveda and Unani can be seen as the continuation of a 'tradition of syncretism' of both forms of medicine, which had been influencing each other for a long time and whose practices were by the nineteenth and twentieth centuries already 'radically different from the classical texts' (1976b: 356f.). Leslie termed these 'syncretic traditions' that varied from the classical texts 'traditional culture medicine' and argued that its practitioners knew some of the classical texts but their practices were more influenced by commentaries and oral transmission (1976b: 358f.). He agreed that professionalized Unani (and Ayurvedic) physicians, i.e. those trained in colleges and participating in institutions, practiced mostly a form of 'popular culture medicine' characterized by the combination of concepts such as hot and cold food, vitamins, germ theory, and religion (ibid.) Certainly, Leslie nailed down the common characteristics of Unani medicine as practiced in institutional settings and provided a solid basis for the study of modernization processes related to traditional medicines. While the distinction between 'classic' literate systems and their 'local appearances' was still made in the 1990s (Leslie and Young 1992: 2), the argument was moving away from the idea of corruption through inclusion of exogenous elements towards an understanding of Asian medicine as evolving and constantly transforming itself (ibid.).

Leslie's depiction of the modernization process and its outcomes as ambiguities (1974, 1976b) remains a prevalent view today. His statement that 'Āyurvedic and Yunānī medicine have evolved in an ambiguous para-professional relationship to cosmopolitan medicine [biomedicine]' (1976b: 365) remains as relevant as 40 years ago. This is reflected in policies such as the current National Rural Health Mission (NRHM) programme by the Government of India, which seeks to fill the gaps in health care coverage through the appointment of Unani (and other non-biomedical) practitioners in rural areas where there is a lack of biomedical practitioners.

The official distinction and recognition between MBBS (Bachelor of Medicine and Bachelor of Surgery) doctors, doctors of traditional medicine, and folk practitioners who lack formal training has been discussed in papers that problematize the sanctioning of medical practices in the Indian health care system, pointing out to the hierarchies and ambiguities involved in establishing what counts as legitimate medical practices and what as quackery based on formal training which emulates the biomedical model (Bode and Hariramamurthi 2013; Lambert 2012). For the case of Tibetan medicine, it has been suggested that the different forms of training grant different forms of recognition as medical professionals, depending on the contexts where the medical expertise has to be applied (the so-called 'taskscapes') (Pordié and Blaikie 2014). In this way, training and official recognition have adapted pragmatically, creating different kinds of practitioners of Tibetan medicine, each with a specific task to be fulfilled in a particular environment (ibid.).

The mingling of biomedical knowledge with indigenous medicine has been discussed as the consequence of institutionalized training. Biomedical training in colleges of indigenous medicine often serves primarily the interest of the government to fill gaps in the (biomedical) health coverage. This has impacted the practice of indigenous medicine on a larger scale in what Smith & Wujastyk called 'the biomedicalization of Ayurveda' (2008:

8). Harish Naraindas claimed that the inclusion of biomedical nosologies in Ayurvedic colleges lead to the creation of 'modern doctors of traditional medicine' (2006, 2014a, 2014b). Initially, Naraindas (2006) argued that this form of mixed training in institutionalized settings lead to a conceptual bilingualism used in medical practice, whereby practitioners shift from one language—and their belonging epistemologies—to another, given the case. He referred to the enactment of one among the competing epistemologies, i.e. Ayurvedic or biomedical, as 'nosopolitics' (2014a, 2014b). In a later work, however, Naraindas distanced himself from the idea of conceptual bilingualism, arguing that Creolization is a better term to describe this phenomenon because Ayurvedic practitioners are not fully conversant in both the languages of allopathic and Ayurvedic medicine, but rather they 'speak' a new and simplified language on its own, whereby one language—according to him that of biomedicine—dominates (2014b: 124). Like Naraindas, and in line with Leslie's proposition of syncretic traditions (1976b), Laurent Pordié suggested that new forms of traditional medicine integrating biomedical concepts may be analysed as medical forms on their own (2008b). In his study of Tibetan medicine, Pordié proposed 'neo-traditionalism' as an analytical category that fairly subsumes the social phenomena at stake in producing neo-traditional practitioners (ibid.). The concept refers to forms of practices that arose in a new social, political and economic environment and which can be characterized by the appropriation of ideologies and epistemologies which, at least initially, are considered by the outside scholar to be exogenous (Pordié 2008b: 12f.).

While these works address some of the realities of the contemporary practices of traditional medicines, thus also being useful in the analysis of the Unani case, they do not correspond to all forms of contemporary Unani practice. This is because the inclusion of biomedical notions and techniques in Unani clinical practices, as some examples from the field shall illustrate, did not necessarily effect a substitution or transformation of Unani knowledge. This is precisely one of the ideas that the present work seeks to challenge, a task undertaken in Chapters 3 and 4.

The epistemological gap between traditional forms of medicine and modern science have been discussed as causing tensions. Jean Langford, for example, focused on the disparities between Ayurvedic epistemology and modern science, arguing that the 'anxiety about how to translate *doṣa* [the equivalent to humour in Ayurveda] into scientific facts is sustained in part by the needs to accommodate the somatic imagery of modern diagnostic technologies' (2002: 155). Her discussion of the use of modern diagnostic methods in Ayurvedic practice highlighted their failure to visualize metaphysical elements such as the humours, creating tensions (2002: 159). These 'tensions' between traditional and modern ways of knowing have also been reflected in studies addressing the so-called validation of indigenous knowledge, especially regarding drugs. For the case of Ayurveda, it has been argued that a process of pharmaceuticalization is taking place, whereby Ayurvedic drugs are validated under modern scientific parameters while rendering its underlying epistemic framework superfluous (Banerjee 2004). Other authors have been critical about the use of modern scientific research—whose epistemologies are considered to be incompatible with that of traditional forms of medicine—in order to prove the efficacy[7] of traditional medicine and its therapies (Adams 2002a, 2002b; Adams et al. 2005; Bode 2009, 2015; Bode and Payyappallimana 2013; Janes 2002; Pordié 2010), arguing against a biomedicalization of traditional forms of medicine. Here, biomedicalization means not just the inclusion of biomedical concepts and practices in indigenous medicine, but more generally the use of modern scientific research for the validation of indigenous medical knowledge as well as the pharmaceuticalization of traditional medicine. Through these, and through the use of modern diagnostic methods and other technologies considered to be biomedical, modern science is assumed to impose a biomedical epistemology on indigenous medicines, exercizing thus domination in form of an 'epistemic violence' (Spivak 1988), whereby only the framework accepted by the international scientific community, i.e. that of Western modern science, is accepted as valid (Pordié 2014b: 50).

Two problems (at least) emerge from this critique against biomedicalization: the idea that the epistemologies of indigenous forms of medicine necessarily diverge from (or even oppose) that of modern science, and the notion that the dominance of modern science is absolute. Recent studies have proposed alternatives to the critical views which assume a divide and incompatibility between indigenous and modern scientific or biomedical ways of knowing. Notably, the 'reformulation regime' in the Ayurvedic pharmaceutical industry has been 'characterised by the emergence of a world specializing in the production, the invention, and the marketing of polyherbal therapeutic specialities building on strong continuities, both conceptual and material, with India's traditional medicines' (Pordié and Gaudillière 2014a: 7). This regime, while strongly influenced by the modern market economy and the dominance of modern scientific research, is an

7 I use Bode & Payyappallimana's distinction between 'efficacy' as the 'outcomes of research sanctioned by the international biomedical and pharmacological community' and 'effectiveness' to imply 'the worth of treatments on the ground, i.e. for patients who make use of them' (2013: 2).

example of how Ayurveda adapts to the current global scenario not by simply absorbing modern scientific paradigms and reproducing asymmetries by doing so, but rather by 'reshuffling' existent asymmetries instead (Pordié 2014a: 50). This is done through the creation of forms of an 'alternative modernity' (Chatterjee 1993) resting on 'a dialectic which constantly redefines and displaces the boundaries between the "inside" and the "outside," between what is accepted as modern and what is promoted as tradition' (Pordié and Gaudillière 2014a: 4). While Ayurveda—through the persons involved in activities related to it—, has been recognized as being able to make use of advances related to modernization, industrialization and the global market economy for its own benefit, its relation with modern science and biomedicine continues to be understood largely as generating tensions and an 'uneasy hybridity' (Pordié 2015: 6) between the epistemological basis of traditional forms of medicine, the forms of new knowledge production, appropriation and circulation, as well as their commercialization (Gaudillière 2014a; Pordié and Gaudillière 2014b; Pordié and Hardon 2015) attributed to the current politics of drug discovery, production and distribution.

A close examination of concepts underlying Unani enactments invites us to reconsider the conceptualization of the relationship between Unani medicine and modern science as surrounded by 'tensions' based on diverging epistemologies, in accordance to the critique on binary epistemologies (Pordié and Gaudillière 2014a: 3). Perhaps one of the most important findings of the present work is that Unani medicine is not necessarily incompatible with biomedicine or modern science. Most of those involved in the practice and research of Unani medicine did not consider biomedicine or modern science to present a concurring or dominating epistemological framework against which Unani had to compete. This consideration should not be regarded merely as the product of the current dominance of modern science. Instead, it was rooted in the history of Unani medicine itself and was reflected in some of its clinical practices. While not denying the existence of tensions and an uneasy relationship between Unani medicine and biomedicine or modern science, this book proposes that these are not mainly rooted on diverging epistemologies of healing, but rather on configurations of the political and economic world order instead.

Theory vs. Practice?

For years, scholars of traditional medicines sought in classical canonical texts for the underlying epistemologies that determined physicians' understanding of health and healing and their application in clinical practice. Textual medical traditions were judged superior than so-called folk-healing practices, which were based mostly in vernacular knowledge. Graeco-Islamic medicine was studied by scholars of Oriental and Islamic studies with a background in history and philology (Bürgel 1976; Ullmann 1997 [1978]) before it caught the attention of a few anthropologists. The study of the texts attributed to Graeco-Islamic medicine, hence, preceded the academic engagement with their medical practices. Non-Western textual medical traditions were understood to follow their own—albeit different from the Western—rationale, and thus to be scientific in their own terms. Charles Leslie referred to humoral-based textual forms of medicine as 'great-tradition medicine' (1976a: 2), while vernacular forms of healing were part of what he called 'little traditions', following the classification of civilizations between hierarchic and lay societies laid down by Redfield (1960). As medical anthropologists increasingly studied the practice of textual medical traditions, the variations of the recorded practices vis-à-vis the texts that were considered to form their basis were explained through the influences of colonialism, modernization, the hegemony of biomedicine, and other developments such as technological and scientific advancement as well as professionalization (Leslie 1976a). Leslie was a pioneer in acknowledging these variations in medical practices not as inconsistencies, but as medical forms in their own right. He distinguished, among others, between the Ayurveda and the Unani of the texts, professionalized Ayurveda and Unani, as well as 'popular-culture medicine', the latter being an extension of the syncretic medicine of traditional culture, mingling concepts and practices from the textual and cultural tradition with modern concepts of vitamins, germ theory of disease, popular astrology, and religion (1976b: 358f.). Through this pragmatic approach, the different forms of practice of Ayurveda and Unani medicine were not seen as less authentic than forms of practice closer to the canonical form, but rather as different manifestations or forms of practice, each being worth of academic engagement.

Leslie's approach continued to influence medical anthropological research of Indian medicine for decades. For instance, Langford argued that the ancient texts provide the bases or parameters that guide Ayurvedic practice. She distinguished between 'contemporary Ayurveda' and 'the Ayurveda of the ancient texts', pointing out to the broad plurality of medical practices that may be perceived as Ayurvedic by patients and healers alike (2002: 4). In spite of this separation between Ayurveda as in the texts and Ayurveda in practice, she argued that the idea of illness as the product of changes related to the three *dosas* or humours as known in Ayurveda corresponds to 'one common thread running through these diverse practices' (ibid.).

The humoral aspect, thus, was seen as the essential core of Ayurveda, the shared ground between classical texts and actual practice.

Ibn Sina, perhaps the most authoritative figure in the Unani tradition, understood medicine as science or knowledge (*'ilm*) consisting of the knowledge of the principles underlying its practice (which he called 'theory' or 'knowledge') as well as the knowledge of the modes of practice ('practice'). Unlike the current general understanding, practice here does not refer to the direct application of knowledge, but to knowledge about its application instead (1993: 1f.; Kurz 2014: 15f.). Following Ibn Sina, theory engages with the fundamentals of medicine and shall not be questioned by a physician, as they constitute an area of inquiry for philosophy and physics instead of medicine (1993: 4f.). The 'practice', by contrast, consists of knowledge based on empirical observation and reasoning and which has a practical application. While the fundamental principles underlying Graeco-Islamic medicine have remained largely constant over time, practical aspects concerning diseases and their treatments kept changing for several reasons, including the need to adapt to different environments and diseases due to geographical expansion, trade, varying religious norms, warfare and travel, to mention a few (Pormann and Savage-Smith 2007: 2).

Even though it is represented as a textual tradition, Unani medical knowledge is not only based on textual sources. As Chapter 2 evinces, innovation and originality are still considered important virtues of good hakims. Hence, analyses of concepts of health and healing should take into consideration the dialectic relationship between different entanglements of tacit and exclusive knowledge with textual knowledge and actual practice, including the representations thereof, instead of considering them as separate entities.[8] In the case of textual-based medicine, '[i]t is important to recognize that both texts and practice exist in parallel and, importantly, their forms of interpretation inform one another' (Sieler 2015: 10). The textual sources of the Graeco-Islamic tradition cannot be compared to the actual practices of Unani practitioners because they cannot be separated from each other in the first place. Unani medicine is constituted by its extensive textual tradition, be it as a 'baseline' or 'common thread' influencing practices, as Langford argued for the case of Ayurveda (2002: 4), or as an anchor for intellectual, communal, or even scientific identity, as I discuss in Chapter 1. However, Unani medicine is equally made out of practices and knowledge that is not found in the textual sources, but it is gained through intimate

8 This distinction may make sense in certain cases, however, for analytical purposes, as long as it does not suggest an actual separation between them.

lineages of transmission or own experimentation and experience. It is for this reason that the engagement with Unani textual sources in this book does not seek to compare theory and practice, but rather to understand, to any possible extent, how the multiplicity of Unani medicine is configured out of sources and practices in different contexts through looping effects.

From the Topic to Fieldwork

The present study is the product of my engagement in an interdisciplinary research project on the representations of Graeco-Islamic medicine in South Asia. In March 2012, my colleagues and I hosted a conference in Bochum to which we invited, among others, several scholars of Unani medicine from India and Pakistan, including the owner of a Unani pharmaceutical company.[9] Their presentations ranged from topics related to the history of Graeco-Islamic medicine to pharmacological research on the efficacy of Unani therapies used for the treatment of hepatitis. They talked about the four humours, which they presented as the basis of the Unani system of medicine, and yet they explained the action of Unani remedies on terms of efficacy using modern scientific research. I was puzzled: how could they explain health and disease based humoral theory, while at the same time testing their medicines in the laboratory on rabbit tissue, drifting away from the holistic approach that Unani representatives are so proud about in order to follow standard procedures of a scientific framework that vehemently rejects the existence of the four humours? During the conference, I asked them this question, but none of them seemed to identify a contradiction in accepting both modern science and the humoral paradigm. For our guests, conducting modern research did not equate the rejection of humoralism, on the contrary: in their eyes, proving that the medicines work confirmed that the old hakims who developed Unani medicine were right all the time. I was not convinced by this reasoning. Informed by the literature, I saw their ideas with scepticism, if not with a certain degree of distress. I thought of them as influenced by the hegemony of biomedical science, which imposed its yardstick upon all forms of medicine, making them part of a power game they would never have a chance to win. I thought that modern scientific research on Unani would invariably lead to its biomedicalization, and that

9 The conference 'History, Culture and Science: Asian and European Perspectives on Complementary and Alternative Medicine (CAM)' took place from 12-18 March 2012 at the Ruhr-University Bochum.

the Unani scholars trying to demonstrate the validity of Unani medicine using modern scientific research were falling into an epistemological trap that could end eroding Unani medicine sooner or later.

About six weeks after the conference I left for India. My first meeting was with Mehr-e Alam Khan, the officer in charge of the publications at the CCRUM (Central Council for Research in Unani Medicine) in Janakpuri, New Delhi. Mr. Khan explained that proving Unani medicine scientifically was a priority for the government. After this first meeting, I left with a list of further contacts and permission to visit the Regional Research Institutes of Unani Medicine (RRIUMs) under the CCRUM umbrella in seven cities, from Srinagar to Chennai. In the following three months, I toured the country visiting practitioners, government officials, Unani colleges, and the research institutes under the CCRUM. I observed how Unani physicians made use of modern diagnostic methods and modern concepts of research with the same ease as that they explained to me the humoral theory as the basis of Unani. As an outside observer, I remained intrigued by this apparent incongruity and by how informants remained oblivious to it. I routinely asked them 'how do you reconcile the fundamental principles of Unani medicine with modern scientific research or modern diagnostic methods?' And every time that I asked this question, I was confronted with confused looks. 'What do you mean?', they would ask. Clearly, my informants were not seeing a problem where I saw one. Only later on did I realize that I was asking the wrong question.

The topic of the present work developed with research itself. Initially, I was looking at investigating the institutionalization of Unani medicine and its development as Complementary and Alternative Medicine (CAM). I soon found out that CAM was not a useful category to investigate Unani in India: Unani could be Indian medicine, Islamic medicine, prophetic medicine, humoral medicine, herbal medicine and a system of medicine; 'complementary medicine' was just one among the many enactments of Unani. I originally wanted to integrate non-registered hakims into my study, too, but because I entered the field with valuable official contacts—some of whom I had met at our conference in Bochum—, contacting the informal sector proved to be difficult because my initial contacts were careful to introduce me to practitioners that they considered to be best representatives of Unani medicine. Another aspect that I initially wanted to examine was the role of the textual tradition into the contemporary practices of Unani medicine. But that also became a problematic task: how could I presume to compare a textual corpus I was hardly knowledgeable about with practices that turned out to be multiple themselves?

Conducting Fieldwork

Between 2012 to 2013, I spent a total of nine months conducting multi-sited ethnographic research in India. During my first stay, I focused on institutions and on getting a general picture of Unani medicine in the country, travelling across the country to visit the CCRUM headquarters and several of its regional branch offices, Unani colleges and hospitals, out-patient departments (OPDs) in government facilities, private Unani clinics, hakims, manufacturers of Unani products and their production units, research institutions as well as government officers. I visited numerous Unani *davāk̲h̲ānahs* ('dispensaries') and hospitals. These visits allowed me to have long conversations with Unani physicians and, in some cases, also to observe them attending patients. The core of the clinical observations, however, took place during my second stay, when I sat in the clinics of three hakims practicing Unani medicine and one BUMS graduate who declared to practice biomedicine in Mumbai and Hyderabad. I observed their daily routines and medical consultations and sat with patients and staff in the waiting room, chatting with them. Some of the hakims and their staff invited me to share lunch and dinner with their families, thus I also had the opportunity to observe their interactions outside the professional realm of their clinics, in the intimacy of their homes and in company of their friends and family.

In Mumbai, I first spent several weeks in different clinics of the *Azim Davakhana*, a family enterprise run by Hakim Azim and his brothers. It had several branches in different locations with predominantly Muslim population in and around Mumbai. Hakim Azim had no formal training in Unani medicine, he claimed to be a *k̲h̲āndānī* (family) hakim, i.e. one belonging to a family tradition. His father's life remained obscure to me, all I knew was that his father had opened the *davāk̲h̲ānah* ('dispensary') and that Hakim Azim had been practicing for twenty to 25 years on his own, after having learned from his father since he was thirteen or fourteen years old. Hakim Azim was between forty and fifty years old, he was a big bulky bearded man with incipient baldness, always wearing a shalwar *qamīẓ* ('long, loose shirt') and often a topi. He spoke in a very calmed way and would listen carefully to his patients. He was very fond of *pān* ('betel leaf'), during his shifts in the clinic he would always bring some to chew. His charming smile was reddened because of this habit.

Hakim Azim's brothers held BUMS degrees, they shared different shifts for the consultation hours in the four dispensaries they owned. I visited three dispensaries, but most of the time I observed the practices in one of them located in a northern suburb of Mumbai known for its Muslim population and its history of multiple communal riots in the past. According to Hakim Azim, the clientele was more affluent there. The dispensary had enough space for about six plastic chairs and several benches where patients sat waiting for their turn to come inside the clinic. Sometimes, as I waited —like everyone else— for Hakim Azim to come, I observed clients approaching the counter asking for specific medicines. Most medicines consisted of an assortment of one Ayurvedic and two Unani brands, but Hakim Azim also manufactured his own medicines—albeit on a very small scale—following what according to him were exclusive family recipes.

Next to the counter, a door led to the tiny clinic. Inside, a desk was situated in front of a wall with shelves attached to it. A screen on the desk showed different images from CCTV cameras which recorded different angles of the dispensary: the cash counter, the medicine shelves, the waiting room. Many patients stared at the screen during the consultations. Hakim Azim sat on an office chair next to the desk and the door, in this way he could open and close it to let patients in and out without getting up. There was another chair close to the desk, this is where patients had to sit during the consultation. On the opposite wall there was a large bench which was sometimes used as a doctor's table. Most of the time, the persons accompanying the patients would sit on it. I sat there, too. The cream coloured walls were slightly dirty, two posters showing the anatomy of the human body with English terms were hanging on them. There was a table clock in the room, too, its tic-tac was the only audible sound in the tiny clinic during the silent moments when Hakim Azim read his patients' pulse. The patients were, in their majority, young men with sexual problems: premature ejaculation, night emissions, erectile dysfunction. Hakim Azim told me about their cases each time after the consultations. I could not follow those, as he and his patients whispered in each other's ears. My time with Hakim Azim was brief, as my presence clearly disturbed those intimate consultations with mainly male patients. He gave me the number of a Dr. Hussain and said: 'He practices allopathy, but he is the best physician I know.'

Although not a Unani clinic, the *Fakhar Clinic* run by Dr. Hussain gave me important insights into how a BUMS graduate practiced biomedicine. This small clinic was situated between Kamathipura and Nagpada, now a mostly Muslim neighbourhood known as Mumbai's red light district and infamous for its former mafias. The clinic was located in an inconspicuous small walkway with shops and private residences. Dr. Hussain knew the area since his student times, when he came as a bachelor from Uttar Pradesh (UP) and stayed with a Jewish woman as a paying guest. He obtained his

Unani degree from the former Tibbia College, where he was active as student speaker. He initially wanted to study allopathic medicine but, like many others, he decided to try Unani medicine after he was not admitted to the MBBS course. Practicing allopathic medicine was easier for him since he admittedly lacked deep knowledge about Unani. Having no family background, it would have been very difficult for him to establish himself as a reputed and popular Unani practitioner. He kept learning about biomedicine through his participation in seminars and courses, the certificates of which were displayed in the waiting room of his small clinic. He specialized in venereal diseases including HIV and AIDS.

Dr. Hussain saw his profession as a service, and because infectious diseases were common in the area, he argued that biomedicine could serve his patients better, even though he acknowledged the advantages of Unani therapies on the long term. There was a tiny dispensary attached to the waiting room of his clinic. Imtyaz, a friendly young man, handed out medicines to the patients according to Dr. Hussain's instructions. Both allopathic and Unani medicines were available from this tiny pharmacy, whereby the assortment of the former was by far more numerous. The consultation room was located next to the dispensary, it consisted of Dr. Hussain's desk and a patients table with a curtain. Next to it were shelves with sterilized syringes and antibiotics ready to use. The antibiotics were used frequently, as most of his patients came with different infection complaints. There was also a sink with sterilizing soap where Dr. Hussain washed his hands after examining each patient. The wall in front of the desk had a small opening, through it the doctor could address Imtyaz directly and dictate the prescriptions for him to hand out to the patients through another window of the small pharmacy into the waiting room. I accompanied Dr. Hussain daily during the morning shifts, from 10am to 3pm. After three weeks observing his clinical daily routine, I decided to search for a hakim actually practicing Unani medicine.

Through an Internet search I ended up meeting Hakim Ahmad at the *Ahmad Davakhana*. The Ahmad family run two dispensaries with attached clinics in two Muslim neighbourhoods in Mumbai. The Ahmad family has manufactured branded Unani products under a label funded by Hakim Ahmad's father since the late 1930s. The medicines were sold exclusively in their two clinics. Their family name was well known in Unani circles, Hakim Ahmad's uncles were also involved in the practice and manufacturing of Unani pharmaceutical products which they sold under a different label. At the time of my fieldwork, Hakim Ahmad's father was already retired and two of his sons shared the shifts in both dispensaries. Hakim Ahmad, the second youngest son, allowed me to come to his shifts. Hakim Ahmad's five brothers were all Unani physicians, they belonged to the sixth generation of practitioners of his family. He and his brothers held Unani degrees, as did their father and grandfather. His youngest brother was passing his BUMS practical year when we met in 2013.

The oldest *Ahmad Davakhana* was located in a commercial building surrounded by other shops. From the outside a board advertised its name and the kind of medicines available there. Two men in their fifties worked at the counter, selling medicines over the counter and assisting the hakim with the files of the patients. The counter was a large wooden and glass vitrine, the walls of the dispensary were covered with brown and translucent glass bottles and plastic jars wearing the simple blue and white labels of the house's brand. A large cushioned bench was on the opposite side of the counter, where patients sat waiting for the hakim to come. Hakim Ahmad's father used to sit on it, too, just next to the door leading inside the clinic. Although he was no longer practicing due to his deteriorated health, he was still present and was greeted by patients with utmost respect. He looked fragile and vulnerable, but he was always friendly and kind to all people who came, calling the next patients into the clinic and sometimes giving them additional advice after the consultation with his son. In spite of his old age and related health problems, he would not miss any prayer, which he performed inside the clinic when his son was out in the mosque for the same purpose.

The clinic itself was a small room consisting of a desk, some chairs and a cushioned bench-cum-doctor's table. The name of his father was still on the desk he once occupied. A door led to a neglected back room where newspapers and printed pamphlets were piled beneath a layer of dust. Here, there was a computer I never saw turned on, an old wooden desk and a chair, the door leading to a toilet and a ladder leading to an upper storey where Hakim Ahmad kept some of his medical books. He would climb the ladder to bring down some books for me to read in the clinic or take home. His collection included numerous CCRUM publications in Urdu and English, as well as other books on Unani and biomedicine and copies thereof. The patients coming to see Hakim Ahmad in this clinic were mostly lower middle-class Muslims, men and women alike. A few relatively wealthy families and Hindu laborers occasionally came, too. Although he had a postgraduate degree in *'Ilm al-adviyah* (Unani pharmacology), Hakim Ahmad considered himself a general practitioner.

The other dispensary was slightly different, it had been opened only recently by Hakim Ahmad. It was located close to a train station, next to a bustling bazaar, hidden behind a front building in a dirty dead-end passage next to a shop selling construction tools. It consisted of a squared room, a quarter of its squared area was separated by walls and a slide-door. The counter was run by a man in his late 20s who asked me to call him Khan Bhai. He was a former madrasa teacher from Uttar Pradesh who had been hired for the job because of his Urdu skills, necessary in order to read the labels of the medicines as well as the prescriptions. Two cushioned benches were arranged in the dispensary, patients—mostly Muslims of low and low-middle incomes—would wait there for the hakim while reading the different Urdu and English newspapers lying around. The clinic itself consisted of a desk and a chair where Hakim Ahmad sat, in front of the desk there was a chair where I sat. On the side, there was a cushioned bench-cum-doctor's table where patients were asked to sit down. Coloured posters showing anatomical images of organs such as the heart and the liver with the name of its parts in Urdu were displayed on the walls. An analogue sphygmomanometer, a stethoscope, and a pile of books on Unani and biomedicine in Urdu and English were placed on the hakim's desk, the latter covered by a towel to avoid them getting dusty. A ventilator helped keep mosquitoes away. Unlike the other clinics I conducted fieldwork in, this dispensary was not always full of patients, perhaps because it had recently opened. On some occasions, the whole day would pass with only one or two patients coming. Because of this, he would take longer to see each case, and we spent a great amount of time talking. I learned a lot from Hakim Ahmad, he was very interested in me learning Unani medicine. After I spent nearly two months observing his consultations, I moved to Hyderabad.

I spent three months in the *Shifa Mahal* run by Hakim Sadiq, a self-made hakim who proudly claimed that all his knowledge was the product of his own self-study and experience. His motivation to learn Unani arose when his wife got seriously ill and no doctor could help her. That was, according to him, some 50 years ago. His wife passed away, but in the course of the time Hakim Sadiq had become a well-respected hakim, and even professors from the Nizamia Tibbia College in Hyderabad consulted him, as I could witness. One of his sons, Hakim Sabir, held a BUMS degree and practiced with his father. It was fascinating to see how they learned from each other: Hakim Sadiq would know a lot about Unani medicines, while his son would explain to him biomedical terminology learned in college. In this way, although Hakim Sadiq could be described primarily as a traditional hakim because of his lack of formal training and because he prescribed medicines based on his own recipes, his practice was very much open for modern medical concepts, as I discuss in Chapter 3. The

Shifa Mahal was located in the ground floor of the hakim's residence in a low middle-class Muslim neighbourhood close to the old city in Hyderabad. A framed calligraphy with a Quran verse hung above the threshold leading to the clinic, it read 'And when I am ill, it is he who cures me.'[10] Each of the waiting rooms had a door leading directly to the hakim's desk. The desk faced a wall between the doors, female and male patients would seat each at the left or the right side of the desk, respectively. In this way, the hakims could see a female patient, but other men could not. Early in the morning, I was invited to occupy a small chair next to the hakim's big office chair. Dr. Farzanah was a BUMS graduate who worked in the clinic attending female patients from 9am, she had been working there since one and a half years, for a 'nominal payment'. Her main gain was to learn from Hakim Sadiq and Hakim Sabir, whom she saw as her mentors. Dr. Farzanah wanted to learn as much as she could. Her husband was an MBBS doctor running a clinic not too far from the *Shifa Mahal*, she was hoping to open her own Unani clinic for women and children one day. Another trainee was Sakinah, who claimed to have studied Unani, though according to Hakim Sadiq she was 'unqualified'. Sakinah had been coming every day to the clinic for the past four months in order to learn from the hakim's experience, too.

Behind the desk and the chairs, facing the opposite wall, there was a big table full of plastic containers with pills and powders produced by Hakim Sadiq's staff. Here, around six *davāsāz* ('compounders'), young men and women alike, handed out the medicines to the patients based on the prescription sheets, called *ciṭṭhī* ('paper'). A few patients who came only for medicines would hand their *ciṭṭhīs* directly to the compounders, bypassing the physician who was busy attending patients. Some of the young male compounders wore jeans and shirts, others shalwar *qamīẓ* and topi. The young women working there were always covered in black niqabs, the only flesh they showed was around their eyes and their hands and feet, just as Sakinah did. Dr. Farzanah also wore a dark abaya, but she covered her face and hair with a colourful veil, hiding all of her face except for the eyes, which shone behind rounded glasses. Hakim Sadiq normally wore a white kurta and a checked lungi and chappals, while his son wore Western wardrobe, usually dark jeans or trousers, a dark shirt, and black shoes. The clinic was both the consultation room as well as the dispensary. The corridor was also a therapeutic space: some treatments were carried out by trained members

10 *'Aur jab maiṉ bīmār ho jātā hūṉ to vohī mujhe shifā detā hai'* was the Urdu translation of the original Arabic found in the Quran (26: 80).

of the staff on patients sitting on a bench situated there or lying on a mat on the floor. Unlike in Mumbai, where the private clinics that I observed consisted of a separate room where the door could be closed in order to ensure maximum privacy, here the clinic was an open space. Sitting on an edge of the hakim's desk, a patient would have other waiting patients behind, the different physicians and the anthropologist sitting on the front, plus several compounders standing in front of the medicines table behind the physicians. In spite of this arrangement, intimacy was guaranteed when needed. Hakim Sadiq and his son would take male patients to a private chamber for a private consultation, for instance when the hakim had to examine a male patient's genitals or when he had to explain exercises to a woman who observed strict purdah. Female patients were taken by female staff to another room where the gynaecological examinations and treatments were always carried out by female staff.

Hakim Sadiq's clinic was special because it was a place of convergence and transparency. Every person could see how the physicians conducted the consultations, they could observe different stages of the preparation of medicines and how they were packed in individual doses, and also how the treatments were given. Sometimes patients were not able to walk next to the hakim's desk because their condition did not allow them to do so. In such cases, Hakim Sadiq or his colleagues and apprentices approached the patients in the waiting room. Hence, the clinic was not just reduced to the hakim's desk, but the whole *Shifa Mahal* was part of it.

My role in the field was that of a researcher and more that of an observant than a participant one. It was important to me to establish this role clearly, because I am not a medical practitioner as patients and also informants often thought I was. This was troubling at times. On one occasion, after I asked a clarifying question, a practitioner asked me sincerely, after we had spent several weeks working together: 'why are *you* conducting this research? You are no medical person; how can you understand medicine? Shouldn't a doctor better be doing this?' These questions made me feel insecure as I knew that, in a way, the practitioner was right: having a background in medicine would have facilitated my understanding in many clinical matters enormously. But that would have carried some disadvantages too, as previous medical knowledge could have biased my approach. I learned about the practice of Unani from scratch, and my lack of professional medical knowledge allowed me to approach clinical practices in a very open way. Instead of taking things for granted, I kept asking questions. This may have been irritating for some informants, but it provided invaluable insights which I hope are reflected in this study.

At some point I did become a participant, though. I was seen as part of the staff—although not as a physician—by patients and practitioners in the clinics I spent more time, and the staff also started to treat me as one of them. I was informally assigned to conduct menial jobs like collecting the prescriptions of patients, taking payments, and holding a torch while the physicians examined the nose and throat or the cervix of (female) patients. In the hectic of the clinical daily routines, it seemed natural not to just sit there taking notes. As time passed by, I assisted some practitioners with blood pressure measuring or cleaning blood after *ḥijāmah* ('cupping therapy') sessions with female patients. Even though I was already 'working' in the clinics, I always kept writing my notes, so that everyone could be aware of the actual purpose of my presence. I was not an apprentice, since I made clear that I did not intend to practice medicine. And yet, the two hakims with whom I spent longer time, Hakim Ahmad and Hakim Sadiq, were interested in me learning how they practiced, as they patiently explained some cases and demonstrated how their therapies worked. They told me to write down important information, and one of them even rebuked that my handwriting was too tiny, how would I understand my own notes when I came back home to study them? I explained that I typed them on my computer, religiously, every day, to which he nodded, approvingly, and said: 'Don't defame my name in Germany. You should get everything right.'

Sources and Methods

This work is based on formal and informal conversations, discussions, consultations, and observations, most of which were recorded on paper and not on tape. Writing notes during conversations seemed to me an adequate way to establish my role as a researcher, visibly recording information. This was important during the clinical consultations. My notebooks contained the core of my ethnographic fieldwork. I also taped recorded interviews, mostly during the first fieldwork period. Sometimes people who had seen me recording interviews of others asked me, while talking, 'aren't you going to record this?' I did not tape-record during the clinical consultations, as the hectic routine of the clinic made it impossible to ask each patient for informed consent. Having a recorder would have been probably intimidating to some patients, who often discussed very personal matters with the hakims. While I did not ask explicitly for consent, patients saw me taking notes. A few times, patients wanted to know who I was and what I was doing. The hakims would often answer with a certain degree of pride that I had come from Germany to conduct research on Unani medicine. Most patients nodded approvingly, only on one occasion a patient objected to my taking notes and I dropped the pen. All the names of the patients and of the four Unani physicians have been anonymized. I have only used real names for persons who explicitly asked me to do so or when information was collected in formal exchanges, like recorded interviews. However, I have reserved the right to protect the identity even of informants who gave me their consent to mention them by name when I felt that their statements could compromise them or their colleagues.

The bulk of my ethnographic material was obtained during observations and interactions with numerous practitioners, researchers, students, producers and scholars of Unani medicine. While I initially intended to include the patients' perspective, too, it soon proved to be difficult for practical purposes. In Mumbai, where I commuted up to four hours daily to reach some of the clinics I visited, planning visits to patients at their homes in different parts of the mega-city would have cost me an enormous amount of time, which I preferred to spend observing consultations in the clinics. My interaction with patients was mostly limited to the waiting rooms of the clinics. I maintained contact with only a small number of patients after I left the field. However, most of the time I focused on the Unani professionals. Hence, the present work discusses Unani mainly from their perspective, and not from that of patients.

Apart from direct interactions in the field, I collected press cuttings of relevant news or articles related to Unani medicine, both from Urdu newspapers in the field as well as online when I was back in Germany. I also included different sources related to Unani medicine, ranging from discussions on Facebook to official regulations, from legal frameworks such as the Drugs and Cosmetics Act to advertisements found in newspapers and websites and to official booklets and publications and Unani books in Urdu and English. However, I made no attempt to be inclusive regarding these sources, as there is an enormous amount of material which, for the sake of time, I could not take into consideration even if it was available to me.

1. A System of Medicine?

The most salient way in which Unani was portrayed in contemporary India is as a system of medicine. This form of representation was ubiquitous in government settings as well as among private practitioners and even the media. Sometimes people went as far as to replace the word Unani by the word system, and I found no less practitioners talking about '*hamārā system*' ('our system') when referring to Unani. Yet there seemed to be a tension between efforts to portray Unani as a single system of medicine and the myriad of practices encountered across the country. This chapter addresses this apparent tension, asking if Unani is a system of medicine and, if so, how can it be multiple at the same time.

Scholarly work focusing on diversity and ambiguities takes for granted that systems of medicine have been historically shaped as such, and that forms of medicine actually lack the cohesiveness, homogeneity and continuity that the term system implies (Attewell 2007: 21ff.; Langford 2002: 14ff.). Variations in the practice of medicine have been observed by anthropologists since decades, and nowadays it is accepted that medicine is not a closed and homogeneous system of knowledge and practices as it was the case decades ago. Charles Leslie differentiated between the actual contemporary forms of practice of Unani and Ayurveda—which he termed 'traditional-culture medicine'—from the Unani and Ayurveda described in classical sources, for example (1976b: 358). This 'traditional-culture medicine' was a system of medicine in its own terms, just as the Ayurvedic medicine of the Sanskrit classic texts and the Unani medicine 'of the classic Arabic texts' (ibid.). Notwithstanding the limitations of such a classification—which at that time was not considered problematic—, Leslie's acknowledgment of 'syncretic' forms of medical practice as legitimate forms of medicine was path-breaking in the study of so-called traditional forms of medicine. Divergences between actual practices and the epistemology and theories of classical medical texts were no longer considered as deviations or corrupted forms of medical practice, but as medical practices in their own right, following an own rationale. The concept of medical system, however, was still much in vogue at that time. It was used not only to denote forms of medicine, but also 'pluralistic structures of different kinds of practitioners and institutional norms' (1976a: 9).

Medical anthropological research from the late 1970s presented empirical evidence of the pluralistic character of so-called medical systems (Littlewood 2007). The concept began to be criticized for being too simplistic and for implying a systematization that does not always exist, and social science scholars began questioning the unity of biomedicine. The production of medical knowledge became a topic in medical anthropology, resulting in the emergence of Science and Technology Studies (STS) as a separate field in the 1980s, turning attention to gender, class and race as vectors that, together rather than on their own, accounted for diversity of practices (Martin 2012: 29). The homogeneity of (bio)medicine was questioned on the basis of ethnographic studies and terms such as multiplicity and intersections were coined. Variations in practice and the dissolve of what had been taken for granted as a unit, like for example Western medicine, emerged as a topic of social science research (Mol and Berg 1998: 3ff.). Krause, Alex & Parkin talked about a shift in medical anthropological literature from systems of medicine to latticed practices and multiple bodies (2012: 15). Their paper reviewed the work of anthropologists such as Poll & Parkin (cit. in ibid.) who, from the 1990s, started questioning the concept of system when talking about medicine.

The focus on fragmentation in medical practices by historians and anthropologists provided the basis for a substantial body literature engaged with medicine in different cultural contexts, proving that variations are the norm and not just scattered exceptions, thus questioning the classification of forms of medicine as closed, structured and standardized systems of medicine (Attewell 2007; Langford 2002; Littlewood 2007; Mukharji 2007). The limited coherence in terms of health knowledge and practice was pinpointed and the question 'whose systematization produces the system, the local's or that of the ethnographers?' shifted attention to the role of researchers in portraying forms of medicine as systems (Littlewood 2007: ix). Similarly, it was argued that anthropologists are at risk of portraying forms of thought and practice of others as 'more coherent than they are; of wanting to show order or structure and so constructing it' (Lewis 2007: 33). As patients and practitioners 'often engage with more than one paradigm of meaning', the search for a single logic becomes problematic (Krause et al. 2012: 17). More than deviations, variations in practice seem to be part of the idiosyncrasy of medicine (Alter 2005b; Berg and Mol 1998; Ebrahimnejad 2009b; Mol 2002). But if the variation of practices has been acknowledged by scholars as an intrinsic aspect of medicine itself, why was Unani still represented as a unified system of medicine?

This chapter seeks to understand how and when Unani is a system of medicine. What holds Unani medicine together, in spite of a great variety of practices? Rather than starting from the multiplicity of practices, I begin unfolding unification efforts. Official representations have resulted in looping effects, whereby the classification of Unani as a system of medicine actually made Unani a system of medicine, as it is reflected in clinical practices and other enactments in Unani circles and even the media in spite of the variations and fragmentations of its history and its current practice.

Official Representations of Unani Medicine

Government Institutions and Official Publications

Walking through the corridors of different branches of the CCRUM (Central Council for Research in Unani Medicine) all over India, I observed the portrays of eminent physicians such as Hippocrates and Hakim Ajmal Khan and charts illustrating successful research projects which were hanging on the mostly green walls of the premises. The similarity of the places and the resulting photographs was such that back from the field it was difficult for me to discern which photograph belonged to which place. Most of the CCRUM dependent institutes had interiors with green walls and similar images hanging on their walls. The CCRUM headquarters in Janakpuri, New Delhi, were no exception. The portraits and charts were standardized, some of them were exactly the same pictures. They evoked the past and present of Unani medicine, reminding observers like me about the textual tradition of Unani, its Greek origin, and the scientific character of research conducted by the institutions, conveying a sense of unity and uniformity.

The CCRUM, with its branch offices all over India, is the biggest Unani institution in the country. Its role is to formulate patterns of, and to conduct and coordinate research in Unani medicine. The council and its branches not only have laboratories where pharmacological research is conducted following the OECD principles of good laboratory practice, it also runs Unani OPDs (out-patient departments) and IPDs (in-patient departments) where new Unani formulations are clinically tested. As the standardization of Unani medicines is one of its priorities, the CCRUM publishes the National Formulary of Unani Medicine (NFUM), the standard for classic Unani formulations for industrial producers.[11] The council is also the main

11 The term classical formulations refers to compound medications found in classical texts bearing the same name, with occasional variations in the ingredients and preparation, as opposed to proprietary medicines which were developed by producers. Classical formulations need to display the text source in the label. For example, the package of the *Kẖamīrah Ābresham Ḥakīm Arshadvālā* produced by Delhvi Remedies read: '(Classical Unani Medicine) Prepared as per "Bayaz-e-Kabir" Vol II.' Proprietary medicines do not mention any classical source.

institution promoting Unani. For this purpose, it publishes two Unani medical journals: *The Hippocratic Journal of Unani Medicine* (quarterly, in English) and the *Jahāṉ-i Ṭibb* ('World of Medicine', an Urdu annual), as well as translations of classical texts, commentaries thereof and other materials such as a handbook of Unani home remedies (CCRUM 2001 [1979]) in Urdu or the *Standard Unani Medical Terminology* (CCRUM 2012) for practitioners, students as well as the general public, the latter published in collaboration with the World Health Organization Country Office for India.

Through its research and publishing efforts, the CCRUM's influence on Unani representations is tremendous. Its books are probably found in every Unani college library as well as in the private collections of endless practitioners. Because it publishes both in Urdu and English—apart from the reprints of rare books in original Arabic or Persian—its publications reach a great number of readers. In the Karol Bagh Tibbiya College, for example, the library has various copies of an Urdu translation of Abu Bakar Muhammad Zakaryah Razi's *Kitāb al-Hāvī*, published 2004 by the CCRUM. Although the reading of this book was not compulsory for BUMS students, it is considered a classic of the Unani literature. The CCRUM is not the only publisher of Unani medical texts—another well-known and influential publisher for Unani medical books is the Aijaz Publishing House in Darya Ganj, Old Delhi—, but the CCRUM network extending all over India facilitated the dissemination of its own translations and editions, making them widely available. A look at the bibliographies of published research papers on Unani reveals that CCRUM publications are often quoted. This is explained in part because the CCRUM is the only translator of certain books, and because those conducting natural science research searching for information in the classic sources often do not engage in analyses of the originals due to a lack of sufficient knowledge in Arabic or Persian.

The authority of the CCRUM through its widespread English and Urdu translations is a relatively recent development which will require further study in the future. This is particularly important in the realm of classical texts, where the actual meaning of terminology had been adapted to modern understandings, leading to mistranslations or to adaptations. The problem of translation was addressed in the CCRUM publication dedicated to medical terminology mentioned above, which explicitly offers not an English translation, but a 'possible English equivalent' of each Unani term it lists (CCRUM 2012). This makes clear that we are not dealing with a one-to-one translation, and interpretation as such remains possible, especially by BUMS students and graduates whose training has been much influenced by biomedical concepts and terminology. This ambiguity, some critics fear, could threaten the very existence of Unani medicine.

The CCRUM was established in 1979 as a separate research institution dedicated exclusively to Unani medicine. Before, there was the Central Council for Research in Indian Medicine and Homeopathy (CCRIMH). This council was established in 1969, it was an autonomous institution under the Ministry of Health and Family Welfare. Although a few institutions dedicated exclusively to research on Unani medicine were established in this period, it was not until the separation of this council in four separate ones (Ayurveda and Siddha, Naturopathy and Yoga, Homeopathy, and Unani) that the CCRUM expanded with regional institutes all over the country. This split up was undertaken in order to 'further develop these systems in consonance with the basic philosophies of the respective systems' (CCRUM 2015b). Therefore, the different epistemological bases of each form of medicine were considered a hindrance for the achievement of common goals. Medical plurality, thus, contributed to the systematization of forms of medicine, and the boundaries between systems were clearly established in government settings such as the Karol Bagh college hospital, where Ayurvedic and Unani OPDs were strictly separated from each other.

I visited the Ayurvedic and Unani Tibbiya College in Karol Bagh for the first time on a hot morning of May in 2012. Joint families, elderly people, women with small children, and young men were sitting all around the college hospital facility, either waiting for their turn to get into the OPDs or queuing to receive medication from the two separate dispensaries: one for Unani and the other, across the yard, for Ayurvedic medicines. The history of the college goes back to 1889, when Hakim Abdulmajid Khan, a member of the prominent Sharifi family of Unani physicians, founded the Madrassa Tibbiya in Delhi (Quaiser 2001: 335). In 1903, his younger brother Hakim Ajmal Khan took over the institution and reformed Unani education through the inclusion of Ayurveda and Western medical knowledge in the curriculum, following reformist aims prevalent at that time (Quaiser 2010: 529f.). The college has been affiliated to the University of Delhi since 1973 and currently hosts 28 departments: fourteen for Unani and fourteen for Ayurveda. According to its official website, the IPD has a capacity of 150 beds (Delhi Government 2015).

This college combines, as its name reveals, both Unani and Ayurvedic training, yet this combining does not mean a mixed form of Unani and Ayurvedic practice. Instead, the Karol Bagh College hosts two distinct colleges in one campus, each Ayurvedic and Unani college having its own staff, following its own curricula and granting its own degree. Although it is a college and hospital for both Ayurveda and Unani, the divisions between both forms of medicine are manifest everywhere, from the separate OPDs and IPDs to the queues for the dispensaries. The arrangement of the OPDs was made according to the diseases treated and the form of medicine used. For example, the OPD two was 'Unani orthopaedic', whereas the OPD three was 'Ayurveda orthopaedic'. Several practitioners of Unani and Ayurveda sit in each OPD respectively, and students of the same are there too, filling the registers and assisting the appointed practitioners as part of the clinical year of the BUMS and BAMS course. The separations are necessary, a student from the college told me, because students of either Ayurveda or Unani medicine had to be trained in their own system. The other reason, he went on, is for patients to choose what system they want to use for their treatment. What this tells us is that the concept of systems of medicine in an institutionalized setting such as the Karol Bagh college hospital primarily addresses differentiation between different forms of medicine. A clear separation between the OPDs ensures, thus, that the students are only exposed to the form of medicine they are pursuing studies in. Additionally, this makes it possible to place the patients at the centre of their own health-seeking choices. These differentiations are required in a context of medical pluralism that distinguishes between medical systems as separate entities, where students were trained in either one or another form of medicine.

The Karol Bagh college is not the only facility combining training and health care delivery in Unani and other forms of medicine on the same campus. Other examples include the Anna Government Hospital for Indian Medicine in Chennai and the Dr. Ram Manohar Lohia Hospital in New Delhi. Shared premises make it easier for patients to come to one place and then decide where to seek treatment from. This decision is often based on practicalities, like the OPD with the shortest queue, as a patient in the *Hindustani Davakhanah* ('Indian Dispensary')—a primary health care facility in Bali Maran, Old Delhi, which belonged to the Sharifi family and now is part of the Ayurvedic and Unani Tibbiya College—explained. Although the government institutions distinguish between systems, and often these systems are associated with Hindus or Muslims, the choices between the systems are not based on religious affiliation (Bode 2006; Speziale 2010a). In these 'mixed' facilities, it is up to the patients alone to choose for one of the two medical systems. The structural divisions of the OPDs and hospital wards in Ayurveda and Unani and even of the dispensaries give no space for an integrative approach; this is not the aim pursued by the Government of India. The only spaces of convergence for patients visiting the Ayurvedic and Unani Tibbiya College are the waiting room, the dressing room ('OPD Nr. 13') and, interestingly, the various rooms allocated for different, modern diagnostic techniques such as X-ray, blood tests, and the like. Following the strict separation between systems of medicine, as it was widely done in government institutions, it may seem ironic that the only bridges between Ayurveda and Unani in a college which 'marked defiance to the medical epistemological absolutism with a key element of the logic of the colonial relations of domination' (Quaiser 2012b: 129) were the rooms for the modern diagnostic procedures. Some Unani physicians even prescribed biomedical drugs, instructing patients to buy them outside the hospital. However, they would not prescribe Ayurvedic medicines. The structure of government institutions such as the Karol Bagh Tibbiya College or a separate council for Unani research reinforced a strict separation between Unani and Ayurveda which contributed to the systematization of Unani, while at the same time maintaining an ambiguous relation to biomedicine characterized by a rhetorical distance and practical closeness.

The practice and training of Unani medicine as well as the production of Unani pharmaceuticals is regulated by the Indian state. The AYUSH Ministry is the umbrella institution which allocates funds to all the recognized non-biomedical forms of medicine in the country. Several states have their own AYUSH directorate, and it is up to them to make proposals which were subjected to approval of the AYUSH headquarters in New Delhi. On the other hand, the AYUSH Ministry is the organism in charge for the approval of Unani colleges, which is done under the evaluation carried on by the CCIM (Central Council for Indian Medicine). The CCIM, on its part, is not only in charge of evaluating the capacities and infrastructure of the colleges and college hospitals every year, but it is also the organism in charge of the central registration of practitioners, establishing the training curriculum for the Bachelor in Unani Medicine and Surgery (BUMS).

All these institutions maintain websites offering practical information and resources about Unani. For those outside India, the internet may be the first source of information about Unani medicine. The CCIM website makes the BUMS syllabus and government notices related to the colleges available to the public. The CCRUM website offers information on Unani medicine, its principles, history, and present status, while the AYUSH website gives a short historical introduction about the different systems of medicine, including Unani. The representations of Unani in these government online portals was in line with the official recognition of Unani as a system of medicine. In them, the historical outline of its development is given in a simplified linear way, commonly consisting of the Greek origin of Unani medicine, its further development by Arab and Persian physicians like Razi and Ibn Sina, its introduction to India by trading Arabs, a 'golden age' thanks to Mughal patronage, a decline due to lack of support by colonial authorities, its survival through the efforts of the well-known Sharifi and Azizi families, and official recognition after independence.

This representation of the history of Unani is contested. Several works have demonstrated that the past of Unani medicine is not as simple as this seven-point linearity suggests (Attewell 2007; Mukharji 2007; Speziale 2010a). However, from the perspective of Unani physicians, BUMS students, as well as government officials working in institutions related to Unani, this is the history of Unani. The definition of Unani medicine as a system of medicine with distinct principles and a continuous linear history is the product of influence of nineteenth-century orientalists (Hardiman 2009: 272). Unani is enacted as a system of medicine in official publications and websites based on a simplified historical outline and descriptions of uniform principles underlying its practice. A publication by the AYUSH department entitled *Unani System of Medicine. The Science of Health and Healing* describes Unani as follows:

> The Unani System of Medicine is a medical system that deals with the management of health and diseases. It provides preventive, promotive, curative and rehabilitative healthcare with holistic approach. The fundamental framework of this system is based on deep philosophical insights and scientific principles, including the Empedoclean theory of four Elements, i.e. Air, Water, Fire and Earth; four proximate Qualities (*Kayfiyāt*) i.e. Hot, Cold, Wet and Dry described by Pythagoras, and the Hippocratic theory of four humours (*Akhlāṭ*) – Blood (*Dam*), Phlegm (*Balgham*), Yellow Bile (*Ṣafrā'*) and Black Bile (*Sawdā*). Admixture of different Elements and their Qualities in specific ratio in particular entity, whether living or non-living, denominates the Temperament (*Mizāj*). [...] Any disturbance in the equilibrium of humours causes disease, and therefore treatment aims at restoring the equilibrium by giving factors (including drugs) of opposite temperament (Department of AYUSH 2013b: 1, capitals in original).

Official documents such as pamphlets, publications, and websites offer similar descriptions of Unani medicine, introducing the reader to the so-called basic principles, i.e. elements, four proximate qualities, humours, temperaments and the concept of health as the balance between the four humours. It is, however, no secret that the principles used to define Unani are not always applied in practice. In India, this problem affected especially government institutions (Attewell 2007; Langford 2002; Speziale 2010a). In spite of a common ground reality pointing out to new institutionalized forms of Unani medical knowledge and practice which integrate biomedical ideas and practices, official representations insist in portraying Unani medicine as a distinct system of medicine. These portrays emphasize a profound difference between Unani and biomedicine through a distinct underlying Unani epistemology and history that grant legitimacy to Unani as a medical tradition and as science, and, consequently, as a coherent system of medicine.

Enactments of Unani in official publications and websites mirror the regulations and policies that define it as a secular system of medicine in postcolonial India by stressing its Greek origin and neglecting its connection to Islam (Speziale 2005). The pursuit for recognition by international scientific standards goes hand in hand with the aims of the postcolonial secular Indian State to give space to all religious communities in the country. When thematizing the Colonial Period, official representations portrayed Hakim Ajmal Khan—one of the most important figures in the modern history of Unani—as a national hero who not only defended the cause of Muslims, but of all Indians. In the modern revival of Unani or Islamic medicine during the late Colonial Period, the emphasis was secular and not religious, as Islamic symbols were used in a communal and not in a religious sense (Metcalf 1985). In postcolonial India, the state continues to enact Unani largely as scientific and detached not only from religion, but also from communal associations. However, this separation is no longer guaranteed, neither does it necessarily apply to hakims who practice privately, as discussed in Chapter 6.

The Prescription of Drugs

Practitioners commonly distinguish the system used not on the basis of the principles employed to interpret health and disease, but rather on the medications that are prescribed. This is especially the case in government settings, where the medications are provided free of cost. They have to be medications belonging to the system in question because only these are allocated and available for the respective OPDs. Because the government settings enforce a strict separation of dispensaries, patients in a hospital could not expect to get free biomedicines from a Unani consultant physician, even if such a dispensary was available, as for example in the Dr. R.M.L. Hospital. In other settings where there are neither biomedical consultations nor dispensaries, like in some Unani college hospitals, biomedicines are still prescribed but are not handed out at the dispensary. Whenever a practitioner deemed the prescription of allopathic medications necessary, he would write the prescription in a separate piece of paper and instruct the patient to purchase the medication from a private pharmacy.

A consultation in the OPD of a Unani college hospital illustrates the distinctions made between Unani and biomedicine on the basis of drugs. A woman approached the female Unani doctor attending a general OPD. The patient had high sugar levels in blood according to the examination report she brought along. The Unani practitioner asked her if she has been taking medications for that. The patient said that she had been taking *angrezī golyāṉ* ('biomedical pills') before, but she was no longer taking them. The practitioner explained that it was important that she continued taking them, and wrote a prescription. The patient asked her if the medicines that she was prescribing right now would help her, and the physician said: 'Allopathic pills are necessary to keep the [blood] sugar [level] under control, the [blood] sugar will not get better from only taking indigenous pills.' Then she wrote an order for a new blood test in order to measure the current blood sugar levels.

In this brief yet representative consultation in an institutionalized setting, the Unani practitioner clearly differentiated between *angrezī* ('allopathic')[12] and *desī* ('indigenous') pills, to which Unani count as part of. Dialogues like these are common, this brief example reveals not only the differences made between Unani and biomedicine based on the medications, but also how modern diagnostic methods are used for the assessment of the patient's health, thus being integrated into Unani practice. Although the Unani practitioner also integrated biomedical pills in the treatment, it was through them, the pills themselves, that a differentiation between allopathic and indigenous medicine was made explicit. Because neither the diagnosis was established using traditional Unani methods such as pulse reading, nor the treatment prescribed was Unani medication, it may seem difficult to classify this consultation as a Unani one. And yet, because it took place in a Unani OPD and was conducted by a Unani practitioner, within the legal frame of Unani medical practice, it was officially recognized as such.

The patient was diagnosed with 'sugar', which is a common term used for diabetes. Diabetes (both mellitus and insipidus) is commonly equated with *ẕayābeṭus*, which in Unani corresponds to a debilitating condition 'caused by increase in the innate heat of kidneys' (CCRUM 2012: 237). The etymology of the word diabetes points out towards its Greek origin, which

12 Here I used the term allopathic medicine to refer to biomedicine, since it is the English term preferred in India. I use both terms interchangeably throughout this book.

Unani and biomedicine share. It may be possible to agree that there is no major conceptual gap regarding the symptoms of the condition as understood by a Unani physician and by a biomedical doctor, and that the differences may be found in terms of the root cause of the disease. In other words, the disease would be considered the same if assessed by a Unani or a biomedical practitioner, but the treatment prescribed would be, in theory, different, because the root causes would be understood differently. Practically, however, Unani practitioners may resort to both biomedical and Unani remedies, as the example above demonstrates.

When practitioners stated that they practice 'pure Unani', as was often the case in institutionalized settings where the dispensary arrangements and regulations made cross-prescription within the institution difficult if not impossible, they meant that the treatments given in the OPDs were Unani drugs only. This idea of 'pure Unani' practice embodied in the prescribed drugs underlies the assumption that treatments reflect the epistemic framework of disease causation. Even when physicians use modern diagnostic methods, their practice is considered Unani as long as the therapies are prescribed according to the Unani concept of the root cause of disease.[13] The prescription of Unani drugs, thus, is important in enacting Unani as a distinct system of medicine.

The prescription of biomedical pharmaceuticals by Unani practitioners is a contested practice, criticized by biomedical doctors and hakims alike. The former see Unani and other so-called AYUSH practitioners as unqualified to prescribe allopathic medicines, while the latter condemned these practices arguing that those who indulge in them were acting in a way that 'harms the system', i.e. damages the reputation and status of Unani medicine. While AYUSH practitioners who prescribe biomedical drugs are blamed as quacks by many hakims and biomedical doctors alike, there is actually no clear regulation regarding the permission for Unani physicians to prescribe biomedical pharmaceuticals applying to the whole country. In India, each state regulates this matter on its own. The Drugs and Cosmetics Act from 1940 regulates the standards of drug import, manufacture, distribution and sale of drugs, but there is no central law explicitly regulating their prescription. Drug prescription is implicitly acknowledged under the general term of 'practice', which is regulated by the Indian Medicine Central Council Act from 1970. Because it is not explicitly mentioned as part of the medical practice of any specific medical system, the prescription of biomedical drugs is allowed in some states. Others have banned the practice after individuals

13 This concept is explained in Chapter 3.

and associations defending the interests of biomedical doctors were able to push their agendas.

The ambiguities in the regulations led to an inquiry by the Rajya Sabha (the Indian upper house of parliament) about the legal status of AYUSH practitioners prescribing allopathic drugs. In 2007, the Minister of Health and Family Welfare of the time clarified that after the examination of a case presented to the supreme court by a non-biomedical practitioner against the State of Punjab, Section Two of the Indian Medicine Central Council Act granted practitioners of Indian Medicine and Homeopathy the right to prescribe biomedical drugs as long as there were no state regulations explicitly prohibiting it. Following the unprecedented judgment of this case, the Minister of Health, at that time the authority competent for AYUSH, sustained that AYUSH 'practitioners can prescribe allopathic medicines under Rule 2 (ee) (iii) only in those States where they are authorized to do so by a general or special order made by the concerned State Government in that regard' (Press Information Bureau 2007). This act allowed AYUSH graduates to prescribe biomedicine explicitly on the grounds that college trained practitioners have received basic training in allopathic medicine in order to discern the necessity to prescribe allopathic drugs under specific circumstances. This measure can be interpreted as a strategy to legalize the great number of AYUSH graduates employed in government facilities to practice biomedicine. Although these measures were portrayed as 'emergency' treatment, it was well known that it constituted a systematic approach by the government of India to tackle the shortage of trained MBBS doctors, especially in rural areas. The National Rural Health Mission, a government initiative launched in 2005 with the aim to provide health care coverage in rural areas, provides a good example of this practice. More recently, the highly contested National Medical Commission Bill Act 2017—a new legislation seeking to replace the Indian Medical Commission Act of 1956—initially allowed the introduction of a bridge course in pharmacology for AYUSH graduates in order to allow them to prescribe biomedical drugs. This bridge course was later dropped from the bill draft after massive protests called in early 2018 by the Indian Medical Association, the professional association of biomedical doctors in the country.

The case of medications is extremely interesting because it reveals the fissures of the system and the ambiguities of Unani medical practice in spite of clear efforts of demarcation and differentiation from other forms of medicine by the Government of India. In their study on Western pharmaceuticals in Africa, van der Geest and Whyte argued that the 'charm' of medicines arises from their 'concreteness as substances' which makes it possible to objectify knowledge (van der Geest and Whyte 1989: 345ff.). While these authors discussed how this objectification created the notion that medical substances contained medical knowledge in themselves, hence making it accessible to anyone (1989: 348), in the case of Unani medicine this objectification is used to establish the boundaries among medical systems, as the distinct medical knowledge of Ayurveda, biomedicine and Unani, for example, is enacted through the medicines themselves. The objectification of medical systems in general and of Unani in particular is problematic, however, because Unani therapies are not only pharmaceutical in nature and also because Unani as a form of medicine cannot be reduced to its therapies only, even though ideas of disease causation are reflected in the choice of therapies and advice. Following van der Geest and Whyte, I would argue that the materiality of medicines constitutes a powerful enactment of Unani as a system of medicine. This enactment has been influential to the extent that the two major medical anthropological works dedicated to Unani medicine focused on Unani pharmaceutical products (Bode 2008; Bright 1998).[14]

The National Formulary of Unani Medicine and the Unani Pharmacopoeia of India

The boundaries between Unani and other forms of medicines are also delineated through The National Formulary of Unani Medicine (NFUM) and The Unani Pharmacopoeia of India (UPI), the two publications setting the standards for Unani drugs in the country. The NFUM, which was published by the Ministry of Health and Family Welfare for the first time in 1981, was set up by the Unani Pharmacopoeia Committee of that time. The first Unani Pharmacopoeia Committee was constituted in 1964 and it has been reconstituted ever since (CCRUM 2007b: xviiiff.). The committee was formed by 'Hakims, Chemists, Botanists and Pharmacologists' whose function was to compile the formulary upon consultation with 'various organizations, institutions, pharmacies and hakims in different parts of the country' (CCRUM 2006 [1981]: v). The formulary consists of 'compound preparations that are frequently used in Unani practice in the country' (ibid.). It offers a description of the methods of preparation and storage, and establishes the

14 It should be noted that at the time when these studies were conducted, medical anthropologists had been increasingly concerned with the study of pharmaceuticals. See for example Leslie (1989), Nichter and Vukovic (1994), and van der Geest and Whyte (1988).

formula used for classical products according to the 'authoritative sources' as required in the Drugs and Cosmetics Act.

The NFUM sets the standards for the measures to be used in the formulations as well as detailed descriptions of the preparation procedures. For measures like weight, the Indian units commonly used in Unani literature were converted into metric ones. To simplify the measurements, the weights were approximated. The NFUM sustains that 'the equivalence are [sic.] for the convenience of the prescriber and are sufficiently accurate for pharmaceutical and other purposes' (CCRUM 2006 [1981]: xxix). The Weights and Measures Act of 1956 officially implemented the metric system in postcolonial India. Although the metric system had not been fully adopted in daily life throughout India (Chakrabarti 2007), the hakims whose practice I observed—even *k͟handānī* ones—used the metric system when writing prescriptions. The adoption of the metric system 'for pharmaceutical purposes' (CCRUM 2006 [1981]: xxix) suggests that its introduction was part of the agenda of modernization of Unani seeking its acceptance as a system of medicine at the global level. The formulations listed in the first volume did not follow 'scientific standards' (i.e. they do not use pharmacological or phytochemical parameters) because of the lack of availability of such information when the volume was published. Thus, the committee recommended to make the standardizations of drugs a priority programme by the government (CCRUM 2006 [1981]: vi). The process of standardization of drugs following pharmacological parameters was undertaken later on with the joint efforts of the CCRUM and other research institutions in the country, resulting in the second part of the UPI.

The UPI, whose completion was an ongoing process, fixed the standards for single (Part I) and compound drugs (Part II) according to pharmacological and phytochemical parameters. It can be seen as the continuation of the NUFI, where the drugs selected had been only standardized in terms of the version of the formula used, but not regarding the standards of each ingredient. As an instrument for the standardization of Unani drugs, the goal of the UPI was to ensure that all mass-produced classical medications were of the same quality and that their products were manufactured following its specifications, as required under the functions of the Unani Pharmacopoeia Committee (CCRUM 2007b: xxvii). The foreword of one of its volumes emphasized the developments carried forward by the Unani Pharmacopoeia Committee over the years, including the introduction of chemical standards quick to operate and 'reproducible in any laboratory', explicitly acknowledging the WHO's concern regarding 'the need for effective maintenance and quality of these herbal products including those used by Unani Medicine' (CCRUM 2010: v). The methods used for standardization, thus, were selected to conform to international standards of scientific research which favour reproducibility. Hakims manufacturing drugs for their own patients were, however, exempted from following the standards set in the NFUM and the UPI, as stipulated under section 33EEB (c) of the Drugs and Cosmetics Act (Government of India 1940).

The decisions pertaining to the formulae included in the NFUM (some of which have been later standardized in part II of the UPI) are highly contested among hakims and manufacturers of Unani medicines. The NFUM claimed repeatedly in its introductions that it 'represents the consensus and opinion of experts in Unani medicine' (CCRUM 2006 [1981]: v). From a list of 588 formulations that were considered, 440 were finally selected 'on the basis of popularity, frequency of use by Unani physicians, their large-scale manufacture and sale by the Pharmaceutical firms' (ibid.). The formulae selected as standard were chosen from among sixteen Unani books considered as authoritative. Formulae obtained from the *Bayāẓ-i Kabīr* ('Kabir's Notebook')[15] by Hakim Kabiruddin and the *Qarābādīn-i Aʿẓam* (which could be translated both as 'Azam's Pharmacopoeia' or 'The Great Pharmacopoeia') by Hakim Muhammad Azam Khan (Ḵẖān 2004) were among the most frequently selected. The second part of the NFUM presented an even more narrow selection of texts—only eight. Moreover, all formulations for *ḥubūb* ('round pills') and *aqrāṣ* ('tablets') in the second part of the NFUM were selected from one single book, namely the *Qarābādīn-i Aʿẓam o Akmal* mentioned above.

It is remarkable that ingredients present in classical formulae were eliminated or substituted in the standardized forms. For example, the original formula for *Javārish-i zarrʿūnī ʿanbarī* (a stomachic) was changed through the omission of musk (CCRUM 2007a: 94f.). The original formula from the second volume of the *Bayāẓ-i Kabīr*, included two *māshah* (approx. 1.94 grams) of 'genuine or unadulterated musk' (Kabīruddīn 2008: 27). Musk is an animal product obtained from a secretive gland of the musk deer and a very expensive ingredient whose sell or offer for sale is prohibited in India under the Wildlife Protection Act, 1972.[16] The official formulae of Unani

15 In the context of Unani medicine, the Urdu term *bayāẓ* refers to a notebook kept by hakims containing prescriptions and other notes on medical theory or practice. I met several hakims—most of them considered *ḵẖāndānī* hakims—who kept their own *bayāẓ*. The prescriptions of several hakims have been published under similar titles, for example *Bayāẓ-e Ajmal*, by Ḥakīm Ajmal Ḵẖān (2010), or the above mentioned *Bayāẓ-i Kabīr* by Ḥakīm Kabīruddīn (2008).

16 This is stated in Chapter 5, 40 (2) of The Indian Wildlife Protection Act (1972).

medicines, thus, have been adjusted to the legal framework prohibiting certain animal products.

Formerly, the musk deer was killed in order to extract the gland which secretes the substance. Nowadays, techniques have been developed for the extraction of the substance without killing the animal, which is bred in farms. The Central Council for Research in Ayurvedic Sciences (CCRAS) runs a musk deer farm in Mehroori (Bageshwar, Uttarakhand), where musk is extracted without killing the deer. An informant who visited the farm expressed concern about it, saying that the musk extracted was supposed to be used for the production of research medicines by the production unit of the CCRAS. Since medicines containing musk are banned in India, research using the ingredient poses questions regarding the consistency of policies. Because musk is so expensive, even if proved efficacious through the CCRAS research, the drugs containing it would probably not be available free of cost in government facilities—as it was the case with medicines handed out in government run dispensaries—, and pharmaceutical companies would not be allowed to produce and sell them unless the law is changed. Therefore, this interlocutor argued, it made little sense to maintain such a farm and conduct research on musk. He suspected that the musk produced in the farm ended up in the black market. It is possible, however, that the research conducted by the CCRAS was oriented towards the breeding of deer and methods of extraction of musk instead of the pharmaceutical uses of musk itself.[17]

Substitution in order to comply with the law, however, was not the only motivation behind the removal of certain ingredients in the standard formulae of the NFUM. The formula for *Maʿjūn-i alkulá,* (an electuary) was also modified through the omission of a different ingredient: grey ambergris. Like musk, ambergris is also an animal product. Because whales were killed for their collection in the nineteenth and twentieth centuries, some countries like the US banned it. Grey or white ambergris is considered of higher quality than black ambergris, for this reason the price of the former is much higher. Its removal from the original compound suggests that the committee in charge of the NFUM not only changed original fomulae based on the incompatibility of ingredients with the law, but also for cost reasons. *ʿAnbar ashhab* ('grey ambergris') (Kabīruddīn 2008: 177) was not

17 A media article with an interview with the research officer in charge of the project points out towards this direction (Kasniyal 2009). A bulletin by the CCRAS stated that 'breeding Deer Musk in captivity' was among the objectives of the research institute, but it offered no details about the purpose of musk deer breeding in captivity, suggesting that it might be an end on its own (CCRAS 2013: 20).

substituted by black ambergris but it was completely removed from the list of ingredients instead.

This kind of omissions or substitutions are controversial among hakims. A researcher working for a prestigious Unani institution complained about Part V of the NFUM, whose formulations were all taken from a single book: the *Qarābādīn-i Majīdī* (Āl Īnḍyā Yūnānī Ṭibbī Kānfrans 1984 [1951]). This *qarābādīn* ('pharmacopeia') was originally published by the Hamdard Davakhanah in 1951. According to him the book was intended to address the *ʿām ādmī* ('common man'). Thus, he and other informants claimed, the pharmacopoeia was characterized by the substitution of expensive ingredients through affordable ones. We may, indeed, find such substitutions in the book, for example the recipe for *ḥabb-i misk surk͟h* ('red musk tablet') does not contain musk in its list of ingredients even though it is mentioned in its name (Āl Īnḍyā Yūnānī Ṭibbī Kānfrans 1984 [1951]: 97). It is possible that the ingredient was removed from the recipe for the 1984 edition in order to comply with the country's wildlife protection law. The presence of ambergris in some of the formulae may speak for this possibility. However, I could not access any edition of the book older than the Wildlife Protection Act, hence I was not able to check if the removal of musk took place before or after its ban.

I discussed with the manager of a Unani pharmaceutical company if the substitution of musk affected the efficacy of Unani drugs. He said that the medicines still worked, but their effects were not as optimal as when musk was used. Similarly, a hakim claimed that the substitutions affected the quality of the treatments negatively, having a detrimental impact on the reputation of Unani as a whole. Others blamed a particular pharmaceutical company for its influence on the selection of standard formulae and the substitution of expensive ingredients, which they claimed was based on profit-oriented interests. Some hakims expressed concerns about the approval of modified formulae as a standard. They considered it being against patients and practitioners who trusted and relied on certain well-known classical formulations which, thanks to the approval of the NFUM, may be produced now using cheaper substitutes, thus lowering their quality. This, they complained, was exploited by Unani pharmaceutical companies. Some interlocutors regarded with great suspicion the fact that just a few months after the publication of Volume V of the NFUM in July 2008, the then chairman of the Unani Pharmacopoeia Committee, Dr. G.N. Qazi, was appointed Vice-Chancellor of Jamia Hamdard, the university linked with Hamdard Laboratories, the biggest producer of Unani medicines in the country. A few sustained that Dr. Qazi was only appointed by Hamdard because the committee approved the *Qarābādīn-i Majīdī*, thus allowing the company to legally produce remedies which some considered as substandard. Opponents also argued that this pharmacopoeia made it possible to 'fool the patients'. They lamented that this could have negative consequences for the whole Unani system in the long term, because patients would not obtain the desired results from the low-quality medicines any longer, and consequently they would not trust Unani medicine anymore. Although persons having their own manufacturing units of branded Unani drugs have been part of or even chaired the committee as well—Hakim Abdulhamid from Hamdard, Hakim Fayaz Alam Islahi from Islahi Dawakhana (later Islahi Drug House), and Hakim Khalifatullah from Niamath's are some examples—, the involvement of Jamia Hamdard's Vice-Chancellor was also controversial because, unlike the hakims mentioned above, he has no training background in Unani. Instead, he is a trained biochemist and microbiologist. However, that was not the first time that the Committee was chaired by a non-Unani person, something that reflects the interests of the government to standardize Unani medicine following international scientific standards. The issue of substitutes, however, seemed to be the greatest cause of concern among critical informants, even though it seemed clear that they were not exclusively found in the formulae adopted from *Qarābādīn-i Majīdī*, but they appeared to be a characteristic of the whole NFUM instead.

The decision-making process related to the NFUI has been questioned by higher authorities as well, although not formally. In conversation, Hakim Khalifatullah, then CCIM president Unani and former chairman of the committees constituted in 1994 and 1998, expressed doubt if the committee had taken the correct decisions regarding the approval of specific formulae as a standard. He argued that the committee set an inquiry among practicing hakims regarding which formulae were mostly used by them, and no studies were conducted regarding their efficacy. Thus, the selection criteria were based on the popularity of formulae and not on beneficial qualities backed by research. It appears plausible that, because of the substitution of expensive ingredients, the use of modified formulae was indeed widespread among the practitioners consulted by the committee. Being the popularity of formulae an important criterion for inclusion in the NFUI, this decision may not appear much surprising. Yet some competitors of Hamdard as well as hakims not involved in the Unani pharmaceutical industry alike complained that Hamdard had 'tricked the committee'. Hamdard Laboratories sold mostly through its strong brand, which is well-known all over India. Patients buying over the counter as well as Unani practitioners who prescribe Hamdard drugs make it the strongest Unani pharmaceutical company in India, as it produces 70 percent of the Unani products in the country (Bode 2008: 54). In other words, Hamdard is the greatest representative of Unani in the realm of drugs.

Some interlocutors feared that the production of classical drugs using cheap substitutions would risk the reputation of Unani medicine as a whole, because the Unani medications that most people used, that is branded drugs produced following the official standards, were considered to be of an inferior quality and, as such, not able to offer the best results. A researcher complained about the substitution of expensive ingredients in branded products, arguing that there was a Unani formula which contained four grams of saffron for each ten grams. According to him, a package sold in the market contained 60 grams of medicine, that would make 24 grams of saffron per package. The market value of saffron, he argued, was Rs. 200/- per gram, hence just the cost of saffron for the whole package of medicine should be as high as Rs. 4800/-. According to this person, the 60 grams package produced by a specific Unani brand cost Rs. 70/- but its label stated that it contained four grams of saffron for each ten grams of medicine. 'So, is there saffron in the medicine? Of course not! And the patients are being fooled, also the practitioners are being fooled' he argued. Although I was not in a position to prove this claim, similar complaints against Unani pharmaceutical companies and the substitution of expensive ingredients were widespread, revealing tensions and disagreement among members of the Unani fraternity (the informal professional group of Unani practitioners, see below).[18]

While many hakims relied on branded Unani drugs, especially those manufactured by Hamdard, it was difficult to assess to which extent critics were right regarding the loss of reputation of Unani. However, it became apparent that the commercialization of Unani created looping effects that established the officially accepted, and hence legally binding, formulae ascribed to the Unani system of medicine. An examination of the NFUM reveals how interest groups—be them private pharmaceutical companies, wildlife protection groups or the WHO—shaped official representations of Unani medicine which in turn enacted versions of it. The standardized formulae of the NFUM worked as a unifying force which, although not absolute, was bounding for pharmaceutical companies and individuals who produced and marketed classical Unani medicines on a large scale

18 The substitution of expensive or unpalatable ingredients from classical formulations is known to be practiced in the Ayurvedic pharmaceutical industry, too (Ganguly 2014: 117).

outside the context of the clinic. This phenomenon resonates with Pordié & Gaudillière's work on what they call the 'reformulation regime' of Ayurvedic pharmaceuticals (Pordié and Gaudillière 2014a, 2014b). This reformulation is not simply a change of formulae, but it is better understood as a myriad of dynamics involving 'industrialization, pharmaceuticalization, and globalization' (Pordié and Gaudillière 2014a: 7). The corpus of officially sanctioned classical Unani drugs, thus, is not just the product of a 'given' tradition, but it is continuously on the making. The codification of medical formulae and the standardization of drugs are part of the efforts to present Unani as a unified system of medicine, to resolve variations of formulae, and to select what is considered worth of being part of the Unani corpus. This process, by which one particular reality of Unani is enacted and given authority over others, exemplifies Mol's concept of coordination, whereby one enactment 'wins' over other ones in a particular locality (2002: 53ff.). Following Mol, coordination is required in order to achieve coherence when faced with contradicting facts, and it is done by establishing a hierarchy (2002: 63). By standardizing drugs and codifying Unani's formulary, influential actors in the Unani scene exercise their power to prioritize their version of Unani medicine above others through official recognition. The Government of India, in turn, complies with international pressure to impose standards helping regulate Unani practices. The results, however, are contested. This is especially the case when practitioners are considered more authoritative than any government institution.

Unani Practitioners

Doctors or Hakims?

The figure of Unani practitioners, particularly *k̲h̲andānī* ('familial') hakims, may be among the strongest images of Unani as a unified whole, because old hakims are still popularly seen as the embodiment of authentic Unani knowledge and, hence, as bearers of the medical tradition. The individual clinical practices of different Unani physicians were so diverse and heterogeneous that they make problematic to call Unani a system of medicine. And yet, as bearers of Unani medical knowledge, Unani practitioners played an important role in the systematization of Unani medicine.

The practices of Unani physicians vary, and so do their denominations. In common usage, some practitioners use the denomination hakim interchangeably with (Unani) doctor, while others make a strict distinction between the two. Unani practitioners have been addressed differently across time and space. Hakim is the most common denomination found today, but older sources refer to practitioners as *ṭabīb* (pl. *aṭibbā'*), the Arabic term for physician. While *ṭabīb* is now rarely used in India outside Unani circles,[19] female Unani practitioners are addressed, interestingly, both as *ṭabībah* and as *ḥakīmah*, whereby the first denomination seems to currently prevail.

With the increase of college graduate Unani practitioners, the term 'Unani doctor' has become common for both male and female practitioners. Some insisted that there was no difference between calling a practitioner a Unani doctor or a hakim. During fieldwork I collected almost a hundred business cards from differently trained Unani practitioners. Most of the college graduates used the title 'Dr.' in front of their names. While in Germany the use of the doctor title is prohibited by law to those who do not hold the required academic qualification, in India its usage is common among BUMS graduates, even by those without a postgraduate degree. The Medical Registration Acts passed in all provinces between 1912 and 1919 allowed the use of the title 'Doctor' for qualified practitioners of Western medicine only (Berger 2013: 67f.; Jeffery 1988: 53). This regulation was challenged by practitioners of indigenous medicine, leading to its withdrawal after independence. Among those with institutionalized training, only a few preceded their names with 'Hakim' or its abbreviation 'Hkm.' in their business cards; only one of them wrote 'Dr. & Hakim' in front of his name. Those holding high posts in colleges used 'Prof.,' and some added their degrees in parenthesis after the name, i.e. '(BUMS, MD)'.

Although most Unani practitioners take pride in being called 'doctor sahib', this is not always the case. An old hakim from Hyderabad who was a well-known practitioner in his area and held no Unani degree angrily scolded patients who addressed him as a 'doctor sahib' telling them, to their annoyance, that they should address him as 'hakim sahib' because he was no doctor. The term *ḥakīm* derives from the Arabic root *ḥikma*, meaning wisdom. Hakim refers not only to a medical practitioner, but to a wise person, meaning both sage and physician (Speziale 2010a: 307). There is no clarity regarding a strict differentiation between the terms hakim and *ṭabīb*. In India, the term hakim is not used exclusively for practitioners of Unani

19 Attewell mentioned a preference to use *ṭabīb* over *ḥakīm* by elite physicians in 20th Century India (2007: 1). However, it is not clear when the usage of the term hakim became more common. I would suggest that it was due to its use as title in bibliographic publications and also in signatures and auto-denomination, in contrast to *ṭabīb*, which is not interchangeable with hakim in front of names.

medicine. Street vendors of medications against male sexual disorders are also addressed as hakims, even though their medicines and treatments are not necessarily recognized among Unani professionals. However, this kind of practitioners may never be addressed as *ṭabīb*. In my search for non-registered hakims in Delhi, I ended up meeting two self-named hakims who claimed to practice *'jaṛī būṭyon̠ kī paṭī'* ('herbal medicine'). After a long conversation it was clear that they did not practice Unani medicine: neither did they make claims of belonging to the tradition, nor was the epistemic framework of Unani medicine present in their understanding of disease causation and treatment. They saw themselves as practitioners of herbal medicine and not of Unani, and they naturally called themselves hakims.

In the context of medial representations of Unani practitioners, newspaper articles commonly referred to practitioners trained in the so-called Indian Systems of Medicine or those forms of medicine falling under the purview of the AYUSH Ministry as 'ISM practitioners' or 'AYUSH doctors'. These denominations are clearly influenced by the state policies that named the institutions in this way. The term AYUSH, which is an acronym for Ayurveda, Yoga, Unani, Siddha and Homepathy, is also a common Hindu name (*Ayush*, meaning 'having a long life'). The name AYUSH has been already internalized by Unani practitioners as the term for non-biomedical forms of medicine. On one occasion, a family brought a child to a hakim for examination. After finding out that the boy's name was Ayush, the hakim told his parents to change his name because AYUSH stands for Ayurveda, Yoga, Unani, Siddha and Homeopathy. The Hindu family, however, did not seem to understand what was wrong with the name.

The personal context of practice as well as the own aspirations play a crucial role in the self-denomination of practitioners. Once I was invited to the home of a Unani graduate pursuing an MD in Unani pharmacology (*'Ilm al-adviyah*). She introduced me to her older sister. When she told me that her sister was also a BUMS graduate, I said to her 'Oh, so you are a *ṭabībah*!' but she frowned and refuted: 'No, I am a doctor! I practice allopathy.' I asked her how that is possible. She said that in the government hospital where she worked, they hired BUMS doctors to practice allopathy. The way in which she told me this—with wide open, shining eyes—transmitted a feeling of pride. Later on, she told me that she always wanted to become a doctor. Those BUMS graduates who practice allopathy feel more comfortable with being called 'doctor' than 'hakim'. In contrast, some BUMS graduates who actually practiced Unani feel proud to be addressed as hakims, as they argued that anyone can graduate from a Unani college, but not everyone can master Unani medical knowledge to become a real hakim. An old hakim suggested that not all BUMS graduates deserve to be called hakims: 'all graduates are doctors but not all graduates are hakims'. While the denominations hakim or *ṭabīb* do not necessarily apply to all BUMS graduates, not all hakims are practitioners of Unani medicine, as mentioned above.

The variety and overlap of denominations of practitioners is important because it shows that without an established framework—there is currently no regulation pertaining how to address a practitioner of Unani medicine—, practitioners can stress their role as practitioners of indigenous medicine or accentuate their institutionalized training. More than the denomination, however, what matters most for establishing and maintaining medical authority is the recognition of the practitioner among patients and among the community of Unani professionals—the Unani fraternity.

The Old *Ḵẖandānī* Hakim as Embodiment of Unani Knowledge

The figure of the hakim is a fascinating one. During the Colonial Period, court hakims were respected, influential figures. A hakim was not necessarily a practicing physician, but primarily a person having vast knowledge on literature, well versed in Arabic and Persian who embodied etiquette and refinement, following the understanding of 'a healthy body as a cultured body', whereby individual well-being was crucial for health (Alavi 2008: 860). In the imagination of scholars, government employees, and patients, the figure of the hakim is often associated with a learned man with deep knowledge about the world and the human body.

An ideal hakim should not only be knowledgeable on medicine, he should have a noble personality as well: serving without expecting personal reward, using reason and logic to arrive at conclusions, applying his vast knowledge on diseases, their causes, and how to treat them in everyday practice. Although there are female Unani physicians, biographical books of eminent physicians list often exclusively male practitioners (Ḥabīburraḥmān 2000 [1988]; Iṣlāḥī 1987) and to date there are, to my knowledge, no female authors of well-known Unani medical books. Hence, a good hakim was thought to be a man, an old man for instance, because Unani medical expertise requires a lifetime of scholarship as well as own experimentation and experience in order to be mastered. The intricacies of accurate pulse reading and uroscopy were revealed over time, thus being reserved for those with many years of clinical exposure. This also applied to the knowledge of *mufradāt*, or single drugs, and also to the *murakkabāt* or compound drugs, as they were all matters that required deep knowledge in order to identify, assess and apply the substances correctly for the treatment of disease.

Hakims are, without doubt, considered the most authoritative persons in Unani medicine. A young practitioner told me that patients expected the hakim to be an old man wearing a long white kurta or a sherwani coat (the men's buttoned kurta associated with the reformist movement in Aligarh, worn by Hakim Ajmal Khan in famous portraits) with a cap on his head and, most probably, having a long white beard. In short, a common South Asian style for male Muslims. A hakim's wardrobe was often important. Although nowadays most Unani students are not only young but also female—this became apparent during my visits to different Unani colleges and was confirmed through conversations with students and college staff—, the image of the old hakim as an old man prevails. This was considered problematic by some young practitioners who, wearing jeans and shirts, at times felt that they were not taken seriously by their patients, who were expecting to find an old 'hakim sahib' and would prefer to be examined by their fathers instead. A few young practitioners told me that they dressed up before attending patients in order to gain their respect during the consultations.

The image of the hakim as an old, experienced practitioner was not only based on physical, exterior characteristics, but also on narratives attributing almost miraculous skills to them, including stories of 'those days' when hakims would diagnose correctly through pulse only and could cure even cancer. Hakims do not only embody Unani knowledge in their person, but also the idea of a 'golden age' of Unani before its decline during the British period. The decline of hakims is connected to a decline of Unani medicine. In an interview, an old family hakim who also held a high post in a government institution referred to this, saying that the situation of Unani is very difficult nowadays. He mentioned that the people teaching Unani these days were not knowledgeable about it. They do not know how to read the pulse and relied on modern diagnostic techniques instead. He said that the modern diagnostic techniques were being taught in the BUMS course because it was necessary for the students to know how to assess an ultrasound or a pathological examination report, but Unani practitioners were not supposed to rely on them to establish diagnosis. Now, he said, there was no physician in India like the ones before, no *nabbāẓ*, i.e. no person fully knowledgeable about pulse diagnosis. Is Unani endangered because of that? He said 'no, it is not endangered, it is decaying. Unani in its practice and teaching is decaying.' In this context, the cult of eminent hakims constitutes an important source of legitimation and identity for young Unani practitioners.

The Cult of Eminent Hakims

Unani practitioners often mention eminent personalities linked to the history and development of Unani medicine as their source of inspiration, model roles, and heroes. Urdu publications on the history of Unani tend to focus on the lives of eminent physicians, and biographies thereof are also an important genre in the Unani literature.[20] The focus on eminent personalities is characteristic of the historiography of Unani by those involved in the spheres of Unani medicine (Speziale 2010a). This kind of books include short descriptions of the hakims' lives, stressing their commitment to society and to the advancement of Unani medicine through *k̲h̲idmat* ('service') as well as their medical and scholarly achievements. A list of publications by the hakims and anecdotes that stress the hakims' skills in diagnostics and therapies are also common in these books. The title *Aṭibbā' ke ḥairat angez kārnāme* ('Physicians' Amazing Achievements', (Fārūqī 1995) is an interesting example. A compilation of anecdotes of Unani physicians, the book includes sayings about several ancient Greek scholars, not only Hippocrates and Galen, but also Aesculapius, Aristotle, and Plato. In this way, ancient Greek thinkers were consciously integrated into the Unani tradition by the author.

Although these kinds of books are not compulsory for BUMS students, their reading is encouraged in order to increase students' interest in and motivation for Unani. Abdunnasir Faruqi was a lecturer at the *Jāmi'ah Ṭibbiyah Deoband* (a Unani college), in the preface to his book he stated his aim to show students exemplary stories of excellent Unani physicians (Fārūqī 1995: 9). BUMS students learn the biographies of prominent hakims under the subject *Tārīk̲h̲-i ṭibb o ak̲h̲lāqyāt* ('History of Medicine and Medical Ethics'). During a visit to his clinic in Mumbai, Hakim Muhammad Islahi, grandson of Hakim Muhammad Mukhtar Islahi, handed me the biographies compiled by his grandfather, along with other texts on *mu'ālijāt* ('clinical medicine') and *murakkabāt* and *mufradāt* ('compound and uncompound drugs') to take home and read in order to enhance my knowledge about Unani.

20 Publications about the history of Unani focusing on biographies of eminent physicians include Rahbar Faruqi's *Islāmī Ṭibb* ('Islamic Medicine') (1999 [1937]), Azmi's *History of Unani Medicine in India* (2004), and Hakim Sayyid Muhammad Hasan Nigrami's *Tārīk̲h̲-i ṭibb* (*Ibtidā tā 'ahad ḥāẓar*) ('History of Medicine from the Beginnings to Present Times') (2009). Contemporary biography compilations may be dedicated to a particular lineage of *k̲h̲andānī* hakims, like for example Syed Us̱mani's *Taẕkirah K̲h̲āndān-i 'Us̱mānī* ('Biography of the Usmani Family') (1987) and Hakim Syed Zillurahman's *Taẕkirah K̲h̲āndān-i 'Azīzī* ('Biography of the Azizi Family') (2009).

Unani practitioners commonly narrated the stories of the great achievements of old hakims presented in these books to patients and to me. With noticeable nostalgia, a Unani practitioner who was in charge of one of the most important Unani college hospitals in India told me about an old hakim who had already died and who was very famous. This hakim, he explained, would have the patients sitting in a room and he would come to each patient instead of letting each patient approach him (as it is commonly done in consultations). He had a *nusk̲h̲ah navīsī* ('prescription-writer') who followed him while he walked and dictated the prescriptions. The hakim accurately diagnosed diseases only by taking the pulse of the patients. He would not keep a record of the patients and what medicines he had given to them before. Instead, he checked the pulse every time the patients came and assessed in this way the progress of the treatment. I asked if this hakim had children, the hospital director said with regret that this hakim's children followed another path (i.e. a different profession) and that all his medical knowledge got lost when he passed away. The director then told me about another hakim from Lucknow who was also very famous and whose *nusk̲h̲ahjāt* ('recipes') got lost forever after his death because he did not have any children. Not only the skills of the old hakims were stressed, but also the loss of Unani knowledge was a central topic in this narrative, a loss associated with the death of the hakims and the lack of offspring ready to inherit medical knowledge. Whether the hakims would reaffirm their status through a connection with the fabulous physician of their narratives or not, these narratives seem to evoke glory and splendour, and the deeds of eminent hakims are recalled with a certain form of pride and strong identification. In these accounts, the grandeur and skills of the old hakims is stressed above their person, sometimes their names are not even mentioned. In oral accounts, the deeds often prevailed above the hakim's person, as if it did not matter who was the one performing them. The cult for eminent hakims, thus, is not always personalized.

Eminent physicians are also venerated through quotes and images along the corridors of government institutions and Unani colleges. I became familiar with the images of a bearded man with a turban (Ibn Sina) and that of a bearded man with a dark, buttoned suit and a broad topi (Hakim Ajmal Khan), as well as with the portrays, real or imagined, of many other physicians whose names resonated again and again during conversations, or who were referred to as important authorities in different publications related to Unani medicine. I have chosen the two men mentioned above to explain what I call the cult of eminent hakims that characterizes the Unani scene in India.

Known as Avicenna in the West, Ibn Sina was a Persian philosopher and physician born in a village near Bukhara who lived from around AD 980 to AD 1037 (Gutas 2011 [1987]). His masterpiece *Al-Qānūn fī al-ṭ ibb* ('The Canon of Medicine') is considered 'the most authoritative and comprehensive codification of the Graeco-Arab system of medicine' (Hameed 1993: xiv). Ibn Sina was not only a physician, he also wrote on logic, theology, physics and other natural sciences (Ullmann 1997 [1978]: 45). *The Canon of Medicine* is so thorough that it was used as a standard text in medical in training in European and middle-Eastern contexts until the seventeenth century and it was among the medical books most frequently printed in the fifteenth and sixteenth centuries (Ullmann 1997 [1978]: 46; Weisser 2011 [1987]). Unani physicians in contemporary India see in Ibn Sina a Muslim wise and a scientist whose knowledge surpassed that of Europeans. As such, the figure of Ibn Sina is a powerful symbol that stands for the scientificity, historical importance and the superiority of Unani medicine and Muslim culture. In the preface to the English translation of the Canon published by Jamia Hamdard, Hakim Abdulhamid recognized not only Ibn Sina's scientific achievements, but also the relevance of his religious works (Hameed 1993: xiii).

Ibn Sina is commonly celebrated in Unani circles as one of the most important Muslim scholars of all times. The omnipresence of his person as a figure giving a sense of continuity to Unani medicine is evident in the Indian context, giving name to institutions such as the Ibn Sina Academy of Medieval Medicine and Sciences in Aligarh—a research and educational institution which hosts a library and a museum—, an Ibn Sina Tibbiya College in Uttar Pradesh, as well as many Ibn Sina Unani clinics and dispensaries across the country. The Ibn Sina Academy of Medieval Medicine and Sciences grants an Ibn Sina Award to distinguished Unani scholars and practitioners. Representations of Ibn Sina embody the figure of a Muslim scholar whose scientific achievements had a great influence that reached even Europe and lasted for centuries.

Many centuries after Ibn Sina's lifetime, in 1868, Hakim Hafiz Muhammad Ajmal Khan was born in Delhi (Ẓillurraḥmān 1995: 243). Belonging to a family of physicians, Hakim Ajmal Khan was a hakim with a high social status who was not only respected among Muslims, but who also enjoyed friendships with some British officials (Metcalf 1985). Hakim Ajmal Khan was perhaps the most influential hakim in contemporary India, being commonly referred to as an inspiring figure by practitioners. He is 'remembered as a "nationalist" and a "modernist"' (Metcalf 1985: 2) and 'became the most famous defender of Muslim traditional medicine in Colonial India' (Speziale 2011). Apart from his service during the struggle for independence, which was seen as a service provided to all Indians—whether Muslims or not—, his contribution to the development of Unani medicine was mainly through the modernization of teaching, as the Karol Bagh Tibbiya College exemplified, as well as through his impetus for the scientific (i.e. pharmacological and chemical) research of Unani formulations (see Chapter 5). He was also the founder of the All Indian Unani Tibbi Conference, created to oppose the new Medical Registration Act of 1910 passed by the British government which was seen as detrimental for practitioners of Indigenous medicine (Berger 2013: 70; Liebeskind 2002: 61).

Apart from his service to the nation and to Unani, Hakim Ajmal Khan was portrayed as an excellent Unani physician. There are several anecdotes accounting for his mastery in pulse reading, his accurate diagnostic abilities, and his almost miraculous cures (Fārūqī 1995). Also, hakims told me stories about his excellent medical abilities. For example, Hakim Muhammad Islahi once told me a story about how Hakim Ajmal Khan managed to cure a patient using a curious method to administer mercury avoiding the poisoning of the patient. Hakim Ajmal Khan would mix the mercury in the food given to a chicken. After a few days following this feeding procedure, the chicken was slaughtered and a broth was cooked, which was given to the patient to eat. The patient soon recovered successfully. Hakim Muhammad Islahi saw himself as part of the lineage of Hakim Ajmal Khan because his grandfather Hakim Muhammad Mukhtar Islahi was a student of Hakim Ajmal Khan. Hakim Muhammad Islahi saw Hakim Ajmal Khan as a great inspiration and was very proud of the master-pupil connection of his family with him, which he invoked with pride to legitimate his own practice.[21]

Hakim Ajmal Khan was named *Massīḥʿ al-mulk* ('The Messiah of the Country')[22] because of his excellent abilities in the art of Unani, meaning bedside care and knowledge of diseases and their cures, as well as for his role in the independence struggle. Hakim Ajmal Khan embodies the ideal hakim because his person and legacy combine extraordinary healing skills, commitment to society through free consultations and treatment for the poor in his *davāk̲h̲ānah,* his commitment to the nationalist cause, as well as his efforts to modernize Unani in order to make it competitive in times of enormous changes. He did not only have a noble origin and a family background with records of service in court. It was through the efforts of

21 Practitioners of Tibetan Medicine also saw 'institutional education as a way of maintaining lineage-based legitimacy' (Craig 2012: 96).

22 The usage of the term *massīḥʿ* in Muslim contexts is related to descriptions of Christ as a person with extraordinary healing powers. I thank Susanne Kurz for helping me clarify this point.

Hakim Ajmal Khan that Unani became modernized following the model of Western medicine (see Chapter 5). While a few informants criticized him arguing that his support towards Ayurveda led consequently to the neglect of Unani in the postcolonial state, it was still commonly agreed that without his efforts, Unani would probably have never been recognized as an official form of medicine in postcolonial India at all, and that hardly any person would have seriously considered the possibility to validate Unani medicine using scientific standards as done nowadays. The sum of these characteristics makes him the most important hakim of modern times; his cult among Unani circles in contemporary India is the greatest. There are many publications dedicated to the life and works of Hakim Ajmal Khan (some of them published in Pakistan),[23] his relevant role in the modern history of Unani found a special place in official representations of Unani medicine, where he is portrayed as 'the pioneer of modern research in Unani System of Medicine' (Department of AYUSH 2013b: 8).

Ibn Sina and Hakim Ajmal Khan are considered exemplary personalities that embodied the ideal hakim: a wise Muslim scholar with noble intentions whose life was dedicated to the service of humanity. Their biographies and the cult of their persons provide testimonies that the Unani system of medicine is not only enacted through medical knowledge, but also by the practitioners who embody this knowledge, wisdom, and values. These prominent hakims are seen in Unani circles as reminders for new generations of the venerable tradition of knowledge, scholarship, and service. The so-called Unani system of medicine is represented and understood as strongly attached to these virtues, which are embodied in the personalities of eminent hakims. Their cult operates as a reminder of the greatness of Unani, the legacy of hakims being passed through generations of familiar or master-pupil lineages and, since the late nineteenth century, also through educational institutions. These loopings were manifested, for example, through the commemoration of the World Unani Day, which is celebrated every year on 11 February on occasion of Hakim Ajmal Khan's birthday, and through other activities organized by members of the Unani Fraternity in remembrance of these great hakims.

The Unani Fraternity

Scholars of Unani medicine, including old and well-established practitioners and persons holding relevant government positions in the field of

23 See for example *Ḥayāt-i Ajmal* (Ḵẖān 2002), *Ajmal-i Aʿẓam* (Ḥussain 2003), and *Ḥakīm Ajmal Ḵẖān* (Ẓillurraḥmān 2004).

Unani, exchange professional views and gossip inside what they call the 'Unani fraternity'. This fraternity can be defined as a group of professionals engaged in Unani medical practice, research, and marketing, as well as government officials working in Unani-related institutions, all of whom pursue the common goal of further developing Unani medicine in order to attain recognition outside their own Unani professional milieu. The Unani fraternity is no official association, but rather an informal, loose group of people who are well connected and who maintain more or less cordial relationships with each other. Members of the Unani fraternity include hakims or scientists holding posts in Unani-related government offices and institutions, respected and/or popular Unani practitioners, owners of pharmaceutical companies and scholars of Unani medicine. They gather at conferences, grant themselves awards, and write prefaces for the publications of other members. Social capital in the form of a vast social and professional network is an intrinsic quality of this fraternity, whose goal is arguably to represent, advance, and promote Unani medicine.

In the same way that the fraternity members keep their connections warm, those outside of it are not considered bearers of Unani. During fieldwork, it was very difficult for me to obtain access to the informal sector, mostly because my informants were members of the fraternity and disapproved of those outside of it. Thus, it became evident that only the members of the fraternity were considered by other members as 'worthy' representatives of Unani, and, hence, worth being included in the present study. In this way, through the inner dynamics of the fraternity, its members are actively involved in the drawing of boundaries of what is considered to be Unani and what is not. Although for some the fraternity is a loose group that included the whole professional community of Unani practitioners, officials, teachers, research scholars and manufacturers of Unani products, others mean by it a selected group of eminent persons involved in the spheres of power of Unani as well as those around them. BUMS graduates are not automatically considered members of the fraternity; those who actively network with members eventually become part of it, as do persons holding postings in government settings or important Unani colleges.

During the Colonial Period, *k̲handānī* hakims looked down upon non-*k̲handānī* hakims (Quaiser 2012b: 122). However, this did not always happen in the Unani fraternity. The democratization of Unani through its institutionalization (Liebeskind 2002; Speziale 2010a) made training accessible to a wider portion of the population. In independent India, most Unani practitioners did neither belong to an old physician lineage nor to the elite of the country, as it was the case until the late Colonial Period.

Access to government jobs for Unani graduates, which became possible in the 1970s through the recruitment of staff for the newly founded CCRUM as well as other government institutions related to Unani, enabled a significant number of Unani college graduates to pursue a career in government service and to eventually secure influential positions. Others made their careers in educational institutions like Unani colleges, obtaining posts as professors or rectors. Thus, access and mobility to and within the Unani fraternity did no longer depend on a familial background. An influential position in any Unani government or educational institution can be even more important for the recognition among peers and for inclusion in the fraternity, depending on the case. Through fraternity networks, members can secure jobs thanks to their connections with decision makers or with those influencing them.

Practitioners who neither have a strong, that is eminent, family background nor hold positions in influential institutions can build their access to and position in the fraternity using other strategies. For example, a Unani practitioner who neither held a Unani degree nor had a family background had self-promoted himself as a 'great hakim' over the years. He had built several imposing clinics in his small town and, through a timely use of mass-media, had become very well-known and popular in his locality and beyond. His children and their spouses pursued Unani degrees and worked in his several clinics, thus establishing an own family tradition. This family kept warm ties with important figures of the fraternity, thus cementing its status as recognized members themselves. Eventually, they secured government support for the construction of Unani facilities on their property.

The creation of foundations and other organizations such as research institutions and charities offering medical services for free is also common among members of the fraternity. *Ḵẖidmat*, thus, remains an important feature for recognition of hakims among peers. It could also be said that the fraternity's vast network contributes to overcome tensions over different conceptions regarding the development of Unani medicine, notoriously the conflicts between the Azizis and Sharifis that are often referred to in the historiography of Unani during the late Colonial Period (Alavi 2007; Liebeskind 2002). For example, the principal of the *Takmil uṯ-Ṯibb* College in Lucknow—the educational institution established by the Azizis—at the time of my visit, Hakim Sikandar Hayat Siddiqi—, had obtained his BUMS degree from the Ayurvedic and Unani Tibbiya College in Karol Bagh (established by the Sharifis) and his MD from Aligarh. While the BUMS training is the same everywhere, as every college has to follow the curriculum established by the CCIM, tensions echoing the ideas of the two schools remained. However, these are not as antagonistic as they were during the late Colonial Period, since the dominant view among the fraternity embraces the development of Unani through the integration of modern scientific advances.

Although nowadays most practitioners hold a BUMS or equivalent degree, and nearly all of those working in government service certainly do, the democratization of Unani (Liebeskind 2002; Speziale 2010a) changed the ways in which hakims legitimize their status as members of the fraternity. While the fraternity may be understood as an informal professional group, through its events and actions it grants recognition to some of its members as authoritative and influential. Prize events are very common, they are organized privately by companies such as Rex Remedies, which award the 'All India Hakim Azmad Khan Award' (Rex Remedies 2014), or by private practitioners like Dr. Ahmad Ashraf and his wife (also a Unani practitioner) in Hyderabad, who, through their 'Hakim Ashraf Memorial Society' stage an award function in memoriam of Dr. Ashraf's father, late Hakim & Dr. Ahmad Ashraf Farhat. Government institutions also organize functions where distinguished guests and fraternity members receive recognition for their work and service to the Unani cause. Among those who have received prizes we find mostly persons holding high posts in government Unani institutions and practicing hakims.

The awarding of these recognitions not only brings together members of the fraternity in staged events that are at least attended by the important personalities who receive the awards, but it also gives the organizers a strong legitimation as members of the fraternity. Pictures of them together with eminent Unani figures are then displayed in websites or social media. One hakim, for example, kept several photography albums of the staged award ceremonies. Many pictures were displayed in one of his clinics in the centre of Hyderabad. When I visited his clinic for the first time, I was hoping to see how he treated patients. Instead of showing me the consultations, he showed me all the pictures displayed in the waiting room which pictured mostly his father, himself, and other hakims holding high ranking posts in government institutions during different events. He would tell me 'this is my father with hakim so and so' or 'hakim so and so is a friend of us.' There was also a collection of press-cuttings mentioning his clinic in one wall, another wall displayed several awards. The hakim invited me to his office, where the staff had brought several big photo albums, like those used for wedding photographs in India. Most of the photographs displayed a memorial meeting in honour of his father (also a hakim), with several prominent hakims as distinguished guests.

Other events such as conferences are also staged by government and private Unani institutions. During fieldwork, a conference on Unani taking place in the United Arab Emirates was a common topic of conversation, as I witnessed different members of the fraternity talking about it. While some were critical about the event, most seemed proud about such a conference being held in the Gulf, seeing it as proof for the spread of interest on Unani medicine around the world. Although I heard rumours that some of the prizes were given to those who paid the best price for them, there is no doubt that—whether paid for or not—the awards granted by and to members of the Unani fraternity are powerful enactments of professional recognition. I saw awards displayed in the waiting rooms and offices of many Unani practitioners and manufacturers of Unani products, they are displayed for legitimating purposes in a professional environment where degrees are not the most important sources of professional recognition.

Textual Sources of Authority

Unani Medicine is often portrayed as a textual tradition. Undoubtedly, there is a corpus of medical texts considered as authoritative. This corpus is considered an integral part of Unani by those who practiced it, offering a material distinction between the knowledge tradition of Unani and other forms of medicine. Medical texts attributed to the Graeco-Islamic medical tradition do not only outline the knowledge upon which Unani is arguably based upon, but they also convey a sense of tradition and continuity, a line of delivered knowledge that has been passed from physician to physician over the centuries. The works of Graeco-Islamic scholars attesting to the grandeur of Unani medicine and the intellect characterizing early authors at times when Western medicine was anything but scientific are commonly evoked by hakims to ascribe cultural superiority to Unani medicine and Islamic sciences. They are also considered proof of Unani's cosmopolitan character and scientificity, as scholarly authors kept continuously integrating new medical knowledge acquired in different geographical settings.

The Unani system is said to have originated in ancient Egypt and Babylon, where medicinal plants and surgery were reportedly used as forms of treatment and uroscopy used as diagnostic method (Department of AYUSH 2013b: 2). Unani's beginnings as a textual tradition are most commonly located in the works attributed to Hippocrates. He was not only considered crucial for the further development of Unani medicine, but his importance for medicine and science in general is emphasized in official documents (ibid.). Another government publication mentions Hippocrates as the one 'who freed Medicine from the realm of superstition and magic, and gave it the status of Science' (Central Council for Research in Unani Medicine 2009: 3). Hippocrates is considered to be the person who established the basis of the humoral theory of Unani medicine. Also, the *Muʿāhidah-i Buqrāṭ yah* ('Hippocratic Oath') remains important in Unani medicine and it is part of the BUMS curriculum (Qadīr 2011 [2001]: 286ff.). Hippocrates' name also resonates among practitioners of Unani because of recipes attributed to him such as *Ambrosyā* ('ambrosia') for stomach and kidney ailments, and *Maʿjūn-i Buqrāṭ* ('Hippocrates' Electuary') against sexual weakness (Iṣlāḥī 1987: 19). The latter was often prescribed by some of the hakims whose practice I observed.

Galen's works are also considered fundamental. From the perspective of historians of medicine, his works shaped Unani medicine, as it was he who established the humoral theory as accepted in Unani today, the four grades in medicines, as well as other elements which are still present in the understanding of contemporary Unani (Ullmann 1997 [1978]: 10). Apprentices and students of Unani may not read the works by Galen, but his teachings still reach them. The following saying attributed to him was kept in the *bayāẓ* of a *k̲h̲andānī* hakim in Lucknow:

> A person asked Galen about the four humours and requested him to kindly describe them. Galen answered:
> 1) Blood is a purchased slave, but sometimes the slave may also beat the master.
> 2) Yellow bile is a fresh and moist garden; the watch dog of the human body may also bite his master.
> 3) Phlegm is a king and leader; if a door is closed to him, he opens another gate to get out.
> 4) Black bile is a big solid [*kaṭan*?] soil; when it shakes all what is on it starts moving.[24]

The source of this anecdote remains obscure, it probably has a South Asian origin.[25] This saying was handwritten in Hakim Atiq Ahmad's *bayāẓ,* an old daily planner used as a notebook which apart from this anecdote contained different fragments of Unani medical knowledge, some of which were written in rhyme, as well as his *qaul* (vow), which specified the knowledge he had acquired in training and that he was capable of in terms of medical practice.

24 I thank Mudassir Iqbal for his kind help with the shaky Urdu handwriting.

25 I am in debt with Hans Hinrich Biesterfeldt for his kind help tracing the origins of this anecdote. Neither him nor several of his colleagues knowledgeable about Galen's work could link this anecdote to any Greek or Arabic source.

Interestingly, although Plato and Aristotle find a place in books dedicated to hakim's biographies (Iṣlāḥī 1987), Dioscorides[26] rarely appears in contemporary representations of Unani, even though his contribution has been acknowledged in some official representations (Department of AYUSH 2013b: 3). In contrast, Hippocrates and Galen figure widely in both official and non-official accounts of the history of Unani medicine. They are portrayed as the scholars who laid the basis of the Unani system of medicine. The focus on ancient Greek scholars such as Hippocrates as the precursors of Unani medicine can be read as an attempt to establish Unani as science through the location of its common origins with Western science. The influence of Greek authors, especially Hippocrates and Galen, on Unani medicine in India rests not directly on the texts attributed to them, but rather on works influenced by those, including translations and commentaries thereof—notably Ibn Sina's *Qānūn*. Such medical works proliferated during the Mughal period in Persian language, as Iranian scholars were employed in the Mughal administration 'and gave a fundamental impulse to the translation and commentary of Avicenna's *Qānun* in India' (Speziale 2011); it was also then (sixteenth century) that the first known works on Avicennian medicine were composed in Sanskrit (ibid.).

There seems to be a clear consensus among Unani practitioners and students about the most influential personality in the Unani textual tradition. Ibn Sina's *Al-Qānūn fī aṭ-ṭibb* ('The Canon of Medicine') is arguably the most influential and important textual source. When I asked for relevant Unani books, practitioners and students of Unani medicine alike would answer almost invariably '*Ibn Sīnā kā Qānūn*!' ('Ibn Sina's Canon!'). Although most have actually never read the book, it is considered one of the most important textual sources since it defined medicine in a way that is still considered of paramount meaning for Unani medicine today.

Apart from the Canon of Medicine, which itself and its abridgments 'were especially the objects of some important Indian commentaries' (ibid.), works from the Abbasid period (750-1258AD) are mentioned as integral parts of the Unani textual tradition. In his annotated bibliography *Ṭibbī Ṣaḥā'if* ('Medical Books'), Hakim Ashhar Qadir—a lecturer at the Faculty of Medicine, Jamia Hamdard—described Al-Tabari's *Firdaus al-Ḥikmat* ('Paradise of Wisdom') as one of the most influential medical books of all times, situating it among the principal and most complete sources of medical knowledge (Qadīr 2004a: 19). The book is further known for giving an overview of Indian

26 For the relevance of Dioscorides' works and posterior translations and adaptations see Chipman (2018 [2014]) and Chipman (2018 [2012]).

medicine (i.e. what we know as Ayurveda today) (Ullmann 1997 [1978]). Apart from Al-Tabari, Razi and Sahil Massihi are also mentioned in official representations of Unani as 'some great physicians of that [Abbasid] period' (Department of AYUSH 2013b: 4). The *Ẕakẖīrah Ḵẖvārzimshāhī* ('Treasure of the King of Khvarzim'), composed in Persian by Jurjani also deserves special mention, as it has been described as one of the most popular medical works of Unani's textual tradition. The *Ẕakẖīrah,* as it is known by Unani scholars, is a medical encyclopaedia that was influential throughout the Persian-speaking world (Liebeskind 1996: 60; Storey 1971: 207).

Government publications establish the eight century as the time when Unani was introduced in India (Department of AYUSH 2013b: 5),[27] whereas the period between the thirteenth and seventeenth centuries is described as its 'heyday' (Central Council for Research in Unani Medicine 2009: 3f.). The role of the Delhi sultans, the Tughlaq dynasty and the Mughal emperors as patrons of Unani physicians is highlighted, as well as the scientificity of the works by the 'scholars and physicians of Unani Medicine' of that time (ibid.). The major developments of this period are said to be the application of the principles established by the Arabs and Persians as well as the discovery and integration of new drugs already known to Ayurveda (Department of AYUSH 2013b: 6). Official representations emphasized the works of Indian authors such as Arzani, Gilani, and Yusuf Harvi during this time (ibid.). Arzani, who lived in Aurangzeb's times, was the most prominent among them. His works were known at least by name to many Unani physicians. The *Mīzān aṭ-Ṭibb* ('Standard of Medicine') and the *Ṭibb-i Akbarī* ('Akbar's Medicine') were considered his most important works and several hakims, particularly old ones, mentioned them as important readings. While the rich exchange between Unani and Ayurvedic scholars during the Mughal Era contributed greatly to the development of Unani medicine, the cross-fertilization between both traditions is neglected in official representations, which stress the Graeco-Arabic tradition and underplay the Perso-Indian heritage, contributing to foster separate identities as distinct systems of medicine (Speziale 2018, 234f.).

The identification of the textual tradition with a lineage of prominent physicians is crucial, particularly in times where master-pupil training has become the exception, regardless if the textual knowledge of the classic books is applied or not in practice. Notwithstanding the fact that Unani was

27 This date coincides with the time where '[p]roper dissemination of Islam in India' begun (Azmi 2004: 2). However, only from the twelfth century do we have evidence of Muslim physicians settled in India (Speziale 2010a).

not called 'Unani' at the times when these classical works were composed (Speziale 2005, 2010a), the textual tradition constitutes a framework for identification which enabled Unani practitioners to be part of a chain of knowledge transmission starting from the ancient Greeks up to our days. Thus, while many students and practitioners would mention classical authors as important contributors to Unani, only a few would mention particular books—with the exception of Ibn Sīnā's *Qānūn*—, and even fewer would know details about their content.

Classical authors and their works are part of the BUMS training under the subject History of Medicine and Ethics, whereby the textbooks addressed briefly the textual sources, and the original sources are not read. The reading of the classical Arabic and Persian texts or their translations does not constitute a requirement for the BUMS course. Hardly any Unani practitioner had actually read the original Arabic or Persian textual sources, let alone the Greek ones. This was because of a lack of language skills, since knowledge of Arabic was usually limited to Quran reading and Unani students of the last two or even three generations rarely knew Persian (Speziale 2018, 234). Whoever is interested in reading these works can access Urdu translations, notably those published by the CCRUM. This lack of familiarity with medical knowledge of the classical texts is regretted by some learned hakims such as Hakim Zillurrahman. Having himself dedicated his life to the study of these sources, using his skills in Arabic and Persian, he claimed that having access to the original texts granted access to the real knowledge. This is because certain terms could not be accurately translated, thus losing meaning in translations. Similar claims were articulated when the topic of translating Unani medicine into English was addressed. The loss of knowledge through translation was acknowledged with distress by those capable of reading the original sources, who claimed that Unani and its knowledge would be lost if translated to English. Some members of the Unani fraternity expressed their wish of making Arabic and Persian compulsory for the study of Unani, while others claimed that it was only through English translations that Unani could survive and attain recognition as a scientific system of medicine at the international level. Urdu remains the most important language for Unani. It is not surprising, thus, that Urdu modern classics have become the most read sources of Unani medical knowledge in contemporary India.

Some modern works are also considered classics among several college-trained Unani practitioners. Indeed, many of these texts are adaptations of old classics. Hakim Muhammad Azam Khan is considered among the most famous hakims of the nineteenth century. Born in Rampur, he had a *maṭabb* in Indore. He wrote in Persian, among his works the adaptation of the *Aksīr-i*

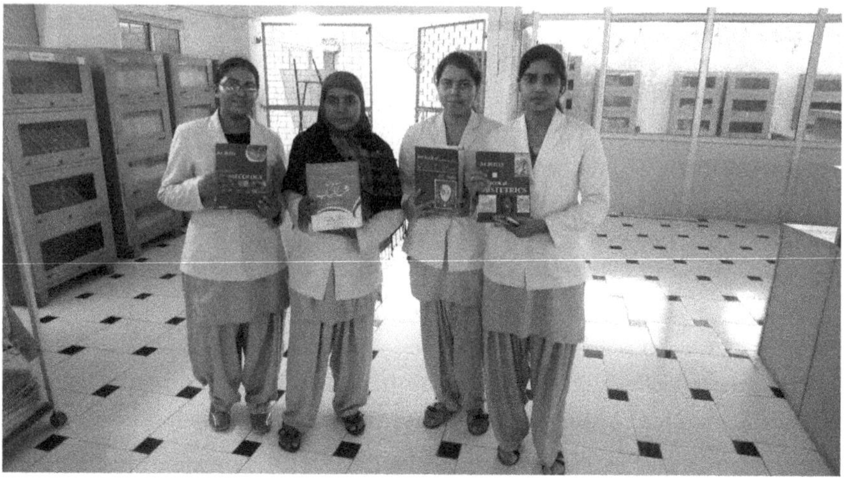

1. BUMS students at their college library holding Hakim Kabiruddin's adaptation of the *Sharhaḥ-i Asbāb* and biomedical textbooks on Gynaecology and Obstetrics (2012).

Aʿẓam was considered one of the most important, comprising four volumes on *muʿālijāt* ('medicine'). He wrote several other books on medicine, but the *Qarābādīn-i Aʿẓam* is considered among members of the Unani fraternity '[...] his best, most complete and standard literary work' (Ṣiddīqī in K̲h̲ān 2004). The book is a compilation of prescriptions by prominent hakims as well as his own. Notwithstanding the importance of Hakim Azam Khan, the most salient author of the modern period was Hakim Muhammad Kabiruddin. His authority in contemporary Unani medicine ranges from nosologies to formuale adopted in the National Unani Pharmacopoeia of India. He has been described as 'the most influential writer and translator of *yūnānī* medical texts into Urdu' (Speziale 2011). Hakim Kabiruddin was born in 1894 and trained in the Ayurveda and Unani Tibbiya College in Karol Bagh. He was a student of Hakim Ajmal Khan and followed his steps in the revitalization of Unani medicine. After graduation he was appointed as a lecturer in the college, where he taught before establishing his own Unani college, the Jam'iah Tibbiya, with colleagues (Liebeskind 2002: 62). Years later he moved to Hyderabad, where he taught at the Nizamia College (ibid.). Hakim Kabiruddin published in Urdu, which at that time was established as the common language of the Unani milieu. He wrote in a simple and accessible style which, paired with his favourable stance towards Western medicine, placed him among the standard authors read by BUMS students nowadays. Hakim M.M. Islahi brought the relevance of Hakim Kabiruddin's works to the point:

> The truth is that his fundamental miraculous power or splendid deed in medicine come to light in his books, where in contrast to English terminology, he established easy and appropriate [Unani] medical terminology. To introduce new medical terminology from the customary terminology of a foreign language into another language is not an easy task. It is for this reason that he and his companions, who made the passing through difficulties very easy for future ones, receive praise and deserve compliments (Iṣlāḥī 1987: 221).

This resonates with the opinion of many informants who agreed that it was thanks to Hakim Kabiruddin that Unani medical texts became accessible to those without training in Arabic or Persian. He did not only translate Unani classical works, his versions also introduced biomedical terminology. This modern approach to the composition of Unani medical books was favoured by the Indian authorities, who included many of his works in the BUMS curriculum. According to some students, some of Hakim Kabiruddin's books are compulsory, hence he was perhaps the most widely read Unani author among BUMS students in India. Although the *Qānūn* was almost always mentioned as important, modern authors such as Hakim Kabiruddin were preferred because of their accessible style. And yet, representations of Unani tend to focus on the complete legacy of its textual tradition, with an emphasis placed on the Graeco-Arab tradition.

There is no doubt that the modern works have much to owe to classical authors of the Greek, Arabic and Persian traditions. Many paragraphs in recent books do, indeed, mirror classical Greek sources. However, it is important to remember that the classical sources are not static entities (Speziale 2014a). Elements from Indian medicine have been integrated into the Graeco-Islamic tradition since the Abbasid period, and in South Asia several medical scholars from the Graeco-Islamic tradition dedicated themselves to the translation, evaluation, and integration of local medical knowledge (Speziale 2018). Just as physicians during the Mughal period integrated materia medica from the knowledge of the vaidyas, modern sources adopted a substantial amount of biomedical knowledge, too. As long as Unani continues to be represented as a medical system, students and practitioners keep holding to this rich textual tradition as the basis of what they consider a unified Unani system of medicine, in spite of the obvious influence of biomedical knowledge, especially in institutionalized training.

Systematization and Looping Effects

The Systematization of (Unani) Medicine: Historical Overview

Before independence, and before the British introduced Western modern medicine, no writing on Graeco-Islamic medicine bothered much about how to name medicine. It was simply named *ṭibb* ('medicine') (Kurz 2014: 40; Speziale 2005: 18). The adjective Unani (Arab. *yūnānī*, lit. 'Greek') was rarely used to refer to the form of medicine discussed here, it seems to have appeared first during the eighteenth century (Speziale 2005). During the Mughal period, *ṭibb* was understood as a global medicine by authors writing in the Graeco-Islamic tradition, as they considered their principles the only logically acceptable framework in a similar fashion as biomedicine understands itself (Kurz 2014). That self-confidence, which has long been eroded through the developments during the Colonial and Postcolonial Periods, made the question of differentiation of Graeco-Islamic medicine from other forms of medicine rather unnecessary at that time (Speziale 2018: 197). Although authors distinguished between *hindī*[28] and *ṭibb*, this distinction was attributed to the authors and physicians themselves, as they would be referred to as 'the physicians/scholars from India' or plainly as 'Indian' in order to be separated from *ṭibb*, which was not addressed specifying the region of origin of its authors (Kurz 2014: 30). Although the differences between these forms of medicine were clear without being separated into systems—they were mainly established on the lineage of the physicians, who followed a certain knowledge tradition transmitted through it—it seems that there was no interest or necessity for a strict demarcation of the medical traditions as systems based on the epistemological basis, because the fundamentals of *ṭibb* were taken for granted as the only possible correct ones, and not just one possible way among many (ibid.). Hence, medicine was just medicine (*ṭibb*),[29] its own understanding as global medicine did not require any effort of differentiation (Kurz 2014). It was only when the dominance of the Graeco-Islamic paradigm was confronted to Western medicine that a need for differentiation emerged. The difference between Unani and Western medicine helped delineate a Unani system of medicine.

28 The adjective *hindī* in Perso-Arabic sources means 'Indian' and addresses anyone or anything coming from *Hindustan*, or the land across the Indus. Here, Indian medicine refers to what we know as Ayurveda today.

29 Medicine has also been referred to as *ḥikmat* (wisdom, of the same Arabic root of the word hakim). This is still the case in Pakistan, for example.

Competition over medical authority during the Colonial Period was broadly characterized by hakims aiming to attain equal recognition and rights as medical practitioners, and the struggle of doctors of Western medicine to retain their authoritative and superior status (Berger 2013). Much of the systematization of Unani medicine was owed to professional hostilities between hakims and biomedical doctors. The Medical Registration Act from 1910, for example, threatened practitioners of Unani and Ayurveda and prompted Hakim Ajmal Khan to establish the All India Ayurvedic and Unani Tibbi Conference in the same year (Liebeskind 2002: 61). The Medical Registration Act of 1910, whose stated object was the 'protection of the public and the medical profession from irregularly qualified practitioners', contributed significantly to the delineation of boundaries among systems of medicine, regulating professional activities (Sivaramakrishnan 2006: 90ff.). The legislation was contested by hakims and vaidyas alike, who criticized that the regulation treated them as unqualified, making no distinction to quacks (ibid.). The identification of legitimate practitioners, thus, became a concern for elite hakims who wanted to be considered the sole bearers of authoritative medical knowledge (ibid.; Alavi 2007; Attewell 2007). The importance of the Medical Registration Act and the Medical Degrees Act rested on their influence on ideas and forms of private practice, being even more influential than other efforts for professionalization such as the establishment of hospitals (Sivaramakrishnan 2006: 96). The peak of this antagonism took place in 1940 with efforts by biomedical doctors to reserve the title of 'modern scientific medicine' for what was previously allopathic or Western medicine only (Liebeskind 2002: 59).

Although the majority of Indians kept accessing the services of indigenous practitioners of medicine (Arnold 1993: 3), Western medicine was gaining popularity among Western-educated middle classes (Arnold 1993: 12). The role of Orientalist scholars (Alavi 2007; Liebeskind 2002: 70) as well as the imposed superiority of Western modern medicine contributed to the systematization of Unani medical knowledge in a way that emulated Western modern medicine, culminating in the institutionalization of training and practice. The idea behind was the need to scientize Unani medicine following modern institutional standards in order to place it at the same level as Western modern medicine. The need to do so rested on the idea that Western medicine and the regulations favouring its practitioners threatened practitioners of Unani.

At that time, debates on the modernization of Unani medicine were taking place. The most salient was the divide between the modernist Sharifi family from Delhi, to which Hakim Ajmal Khan belonged to, and the Azizis from

Lucknow, who followed a more conservative stance. Although having different positions on how Unani medicine was supposed to be carried forward, both families reacted to the perceived threat to which Unani medicine was subjected to. The families also shared the idea that the establishment of Unani colleges emulating the British medical school's model was the only way to compete face-to-face with Western medicine. Through the introduction of *ṭibbiyah* ('medical') colleges, minimum requirements of teaching and learning had to be established. Although minimum requirements were already existent in the apprenticeship system that dominated before institutionalization, for example through the granting of certificates based on the mastering of a range of knowledge and practices (ibid.), the requisites for obtaining them had not been standardized. The introduction of colleges marked a process where the knowledge content of each system of medicine had to be clearly defined. Although training in colleges was not standardized for the whole country until the CCIM was created, the distinction between systems of medicine was already imposed through them.

A further development in need of consideration was the increased tension of hakims vis-à-vis vaidyas which started to develop during the Colonial Period and acquired communal tones with the pass of time. The proceedings of the former All India Ayurvedic and Tibbi Conference, the association of hakims and vaidyas funded in 1910 by Hakim Ajmal Khan with the aim to defend the interests of Unani and Ayurvedic practitioners against the Medical Registration Act, were a testimony for it. The Tibbi and Ayurvedic Conference, which was established in cooperation between hakims and vaidyas unified in the struggle against the non-recognition by the British government, was instrumental in making traditional Indian medicine a symbol of the nationalist freedom struggle (Metcalf 1985). Increased communalism in society at that time poured through the conference, and the differences became such that the vaidyas' attendance diminished by 1920 (Attewell 2007: 184). Competition between hakims and vaidyas, thus, became greater, contributing to a greater emphasis in the distinction between Unani and Ayurveda as separate systems of medicine instead of building on their similarities as Indian medicine. The divide between vaidyas and hakims and their respective medical practice was cemented during the Postcolonial Period. Official representations of Unani stressed its being a system which, although it had integrated Indian medical knowledge, was distinct from it (CCRUM 2009: 4).

To summarize, the denomination Unani arose during the Colonial Period (Speziale 2005) as a way to present itself as a distinct form of medicine. The new self-identification of Unani as a system emerged in part as a response to the pressure acted upon Unani physicians by the discriminatory regulations introduced by the British (Berger 2013; Speziale 2005) in combination with the role of Western historiography in establishing categories of representation (Ebrahimnejad 2009a: 4). The idea of Unani as a distinct system of medicine was solidified through communal tensions that arose in the late Colonial Period and lead to divisions among practitioners of Unani and Ayurveda. Also, the introduction of Unani medical colleges, where knowledge had to be systematized for teaching purposes, contributed to the making of Unani as a system of medicine. The 'Unani System of Medicine' was consolidated through post-independence policies on indigenous forms of medicines that took them for granted as systems, reinforcing boundaries among different forms of medicine through regulations such as those related to training and practice as well as the systematization of drugs as in the Unani Pharmacopoeia of India and the National Formulary of Unani Medicine. These boundaries, however, are not static, as exemplified by the practice of allopathic medicine by BUMS graduates integrated in the health care system of the country.

Enactments and Loopings

In spite of the critique in social science literature, why does the definition of Unani medicine as a system of medicine remain ubiquitous in everyday use? Already in 2005, Pool & Geissler argued that even when anthropologists no longer state that there are different systems of medicine, people still perceive and refer to forms of healing as such (2005: 39-45, cit. in Krause et al. 2012: 18). Hence, while historians and anthropologists have been avoiding the term systems of medicine when referring to forms of medicine of any kind (biomedicine included), the hakims and government officials I met during fieldwork used the term interchangeably with Unani or *ṭibb*. What social scientists no longer considered as a homogeneous unit was still defined as such by those engaging with it on an everyday basis.

Variations in medical practice have been regarded as problematic because medicine is supposed to be based on solid, scientific grounds (Andersen and Mooney 1990: 1). But as philosophers, historians of science, and scholars adhering to the tradition of science and technology studies agree, science and epistemology cannot be separated from society, culture and history (Daston and Galison 2010 [2007]; Hacking 2002; Latour and Woolgar 1986 [1979]). Because of its history and the confrontation with modern science and biomedicine since the Colonial Period, Unani was systematized in order to retain its recognition as a formal form of medical practice, as opposed to folk medicine or quackery. Hence, Unani was enacted, through representations in official institutions, publications, narratives and through its professionals, as a fixed system in order for its variations to remain legitimate and accepted. Any fragmentation in its representations could be turned against Unani's recognition as a valid form of learned medicine. The systematization of medicine in the representations of Unani appeared as a recourse to avoid Unani being considered unscientific. The construction of a medical tradition is based on a tangible textual corpus and advanced by lineages of eminent physicians, the configuration of institutions dedicated to training and the advancement of scientific knowledge of Unani medicine, the professional groups of Unani practitioners as well as the strict differentiations of medicines and medical practices as belonging to what was called the Unani system of medicine.

The Unani system of medicine came to existence through the historical processes described above. Hacking argued that there is a connection between what comes to existence, the historical dynamics of naming, and the subsequent use of a name manifested in 'dynamic nominalism' (Hacking 2002: 26). A system of medicine such as Unani is the product of this process and its looping effects, brought about by the unifying efforts discussed in this chapter. Those involved in the practice or research of Unani did not question whether Unani was a system of medicine or not because this was invariably assumed to be the case. However, that assumption was not free of ambiguities. Government officials applying the concept of system in their daily speech revealed a broader and more inclusive understanding of Unani that could not be confined within the official enactments of Unani as a system. The same applied to the clinical practices of hakims who integrated concepts which were apparently different from the fundamentals of Unani considered as the basis of their medical understanding. It was the non-questioning of Unani's cohesiveness, this taken for granted-ness as a system of medicine what made it possible for Unani to remain malleable. The fixation on Unani as a homogeneous and continuous system of medicine was precisely what allowed it to be so inclusive and diverse in practice.

Unani is Unani in many ways, its multiplicity varies according to circumstances and context, depending on what is enacted and for what purpose. The enactment of Unani as a system of medicine allows it to vary in practice without compromising its status as an officially recognized form of medicine with claims of scientificity and efficacy in the global medical market. The unifying forces discussed above are not always evoked at once and by all, the enactments are distributed. Incoherence is coordinated through the imposition of hierarchies (Mol 2002: 53ff.), for example through the establishment of official standards like the NFUM. Attending to what version of Unani is enacted in a particular time and place reveals the politics involved in the process, allowing us to examine whose authority counts in which context. It also reveals the limits of authority and the fluid nature of enactments of Unani. As the next chapter discusses, efforts to standardize the Unani profession and its medicines remain contested. These contestations are possible thanks to Unani being enacted as a system of medicine, leaving room for multiplicity in spite of enactments focusing on homogeneous cohesiveness.

2. Authority, Originality, and the Limits of Standardization

One of the most important consequences of the institutionalization of Unani medicine was the systematization of Unani knowledge and the establishment of regulations for the recognition of its professionals at different levels. These new forms of knowledge transmission and authority have not eroded older ways completely. As a consequence, various and sometimes conflicting forms of medical authority, legitimation, and practice coexist in contemporary Unani medicine. This chapter discusses the problem of state legitimation versus professional recognition by peers and patients, scrutinizing forms of knowledge creation and transmission as well as the limitations of state regulation. Apart from analysing the influence of these processes on the enactments of Unani and the looping effects emerging from them that shape what Unani is today, I discuss multiplicity as inherently characteristic of Unani medicine, arguing that it persists in spite of efforts of standardization.

Creation and Transmission of Medical Knowledge

Becoming a Hakim

Before the spreading of formal teaching institutions, Unani medical education was commonly imparted through an *ustād-shāgird* ('master-pupil') apprenticeship system that remained greatly unchanged (Liebeskind 1996: 39). Practitioners trained mostly in informal settings like homes (Metcalf 1985: 4; Kutumbiah 1962, cit. in Jefffery 1988: 46). Also, training in institutionalized settings was most probably imparted in madrasas, such as during Akbar's reign (1556-1605) (Speziale 2012b: 160), and there are indications that this was the case in Punjab in the late nineteenth century, too (Attewell 2005: 389). Basic medical training in madrasas did not only target hakims-to-be, but also religious and other scholars (ibid.). Although the textbooks, mostly in Arabic and Persian, constituted an important part of medical training (Attewell 2005: 390), practice itself had a dominant role, both as clinical training or bed-side instruction (Jaggi 1977: 26; Liebeskind 1996: 40). Students learned how to examine patients and how to diagnose and treat through practice (ibid.). Also, the preparation of drugs was a constitutive part of their learning and an important aspect of the family practice (ibid.; Speziale

2010b: 177f.). Part of this medical knowledge was not in the books. In order to become a Unani practitioner, apprenticeship with a practicing hakim remained necessary, and physician-families offered more sustainable forms of knowledge transmission than hospitals (Speziale 2012b: 161).

Family settings remained among the most important medical institutions of the Muslim milieu, especially during the Colonial Period (ibid.). Training through apprenticeship within one's own family was easier when there was already a family physician running a *maṭabb* with a *davāḵẖānah* attached to it. Many family hakims today have a *maṭabb* attached to their homes, often on the ground floor while the family resides on the upper floor. Many practitioners still profit from a family lineage. If hakims could not trace their medical legacy from their family tree, they could resort to experience and experimentation, as these remained important sources of legitimation.

Unlike Tibetan medicine, in Unani lineages were considered to be vehicles for the transmission of exclusive knowledge, but not of healing powers (Besch 2006: 62ff.). Because they are not necessarily blood-bounded, knowledge-lineages in Unani were not exclusively family-based and could also be established in a master-pupil relationship that did not involve familial relations at all. Some BUMS graduates and others lacking a family background interested in becoming hakims sought apprenticeship from renowned, non-related Unani physicians. Even some celebrated Unani practitioners learned from non-related renowned hakims (Attewell 2005: 391; Ḥabīburraḥmān 2000 [1988]: 166). The knowledge obtained from training with other physicians was of added value to that from their own family, as each lineage shared some exclusive knowledge, especially regarding *nusḵẖahjāt* ('recipes' or 'prescriptions'). Hakims with a family background, and sometimes also older hakims who trained with a non-related established hakim, were to this day commonly referred to in Urdu-speaking contexts as *ḵẖāndānī* ('familial') hakims. This denomination was reserved mostly for hereditary practitioners (Attewell 2005: 391), but it was also used for hakims without a family background who were known and reputed as experienced, in contrast to most institutionally trained BUMS graduates without additional training.

Being families and lineages so important for the transmission of Unani medical knowledge, it is not surprising that the first institutions for formal Unani medical training in the Subcontinent were created by members of such families. This is the case of the *Takmil uṭ-Ṭibb* in Lucknow and the Ayurveda and Unani Tibbi College in Delhi introduced in Chapter 1.[30] The

30 As mentioned above, formal educational institutions including medical training existed previously, but they were not primarily aimed at instructing Unani practitioners.

institutionalization of Unani training by elite families was also pursued in order to regain the authority that had been jeopardized through the spread of the printing press and the vernacularization of Unani medical texts and knowledge (Alavi 2007; Attewell 2005: 393).

The introduction of Unani medical colleges gradually supplanted the master-pupil system as the main form of transmission of medical knowledge, especially after a college degree became a requirement to register as a practitioner. However, even after the establishment of Unani medical colleges, family training retained a higher prestige than institutionalized education (Speziale 2010b: 76), and some BUMS graduates sought apprenticeship from established hakims to complement the knowledge acquired in institutionalized settings. Some of the shortcomings of this form of training were already becoming evident by the beginning of the twentieth century, as revealed in a letter from a student of the *Takmil uṭ-Ṭibb* College. He complained about teaching practitioners keeping their family recipes concealed and also about omissions in the treatment of certain parts of the body, as in the case of anatomy class (Attewell 2005: 400ff.; 2007: 129ff.). The letter does not only suggest that the paradigms of medical authority were contested (ibid.), but it is also fascinating because the issues it addressed remain relevant after more than a hundred years.

Institutionalized Training and its Shortcomings

The institutionalization of training contributed greatly to the democratization of Unani knowledge (Liebeskind 2002; Speziale 2010a) even though institutionalization in North India was originally conceived by elite families in order to regain their authority lost through new forms of knowledge circulation and the commercialization of traditional medicines (Attewell 2005: 393). Institutionalization has also been blamed for having led to irrevocable changes in Unani medicine itself due to its inherent inadequacy to foster the transmission of exclusive knowledge, to convey expertise on skills based on long exposure and experience, as well as through the introduction of new subjects in the curriculum aiming at modernizing Unani. The instruction of traditional medicine in South Asia was deeply influenced by Western medicine, leading to a new 'configuration' in which biomedicine, in the case of Ayurvedic education, gradually supplanted Sanskrit concepts and categories (Pordié 2014a: 336). The same applies for the institutionalized training in Unani colleges.

In 2015, the training in Unani medicine was imparted by 42 officially recognized private and state-run Unani medical colleges (CCIM 2015d).

The Central Council of Indian Medicine (CCIM) was the regulating body establishing the syllabus and conducting inspections in order to ensure that the colleges' infrastructure and staff met the minimum standards. However, the AYUSH department (now AYUSH Ministry) had the final say in granting the permissions to the colleges to admit new students in the undergraduate and graduate courses each year. The establishment of the CCIM followed the post-independence efforts by the Indian state to promote and regulate the practice of indigenous medical systems. Set in 1971, the CCIM's role was to implement standards of training and practice, including the maintenance of a central register of qualified practitioners (CCIM 2015a). Its inception marked the beginning of the end of the official recognition of *k͟hāndānī* hakims who did not possess a degree in Unani medicine as well as the introduction of the BUMS course as the standard of Unani training and practice. Before the CCIM was founded, there was no unified curriculum for Unani training (Attewell 2005: 395).

Institutionalized training turned the traditional *ustād-shāgird* form of knowledge transmission onto its head. This signified not only a change in terms of knowledge transmission, but also of knowledge itself. Some hakims emphasized that Unani medicine was both a science (*'ilm*) and an art (*fann*), and institutionalized training privileged the science part, neglecting the art. The tension between theoretical and practical instruction is at the heart of institutionalized training of traditional medicine in India (Pordié and Blaikie 2014; Sieler 2013). While transmission of practical knowledge is covered in the BUMS curriculum, it cannot be compared to years of apprenticeship with a practicing hakim, as the practical training established by the BUMS curriculum requires only twelve months of clinical exposure. Moreover, 50 per cent of the 'compulsory rotatory internship' that students have to complete has to be done in biomedical institutions. A notification for the regulation of the BUMS degree specified that the one year internship shall be divided between six months clinical training in a Unani hospital and six months in a primary health care centre or a rural, district, or civil hospital, or any government hospital of modern medicine, and that only when there is no provision of a hospital or dispensary of modern medicine the full year can be completed in a Unani college hospital (CCIM 2013: 13). This regulation is revealing not only in terms of why BUMS graduates are not sufficiently competent in the art of Unani, but also because it masks an important agenda: that of training practitioners in Indian medicine to work in the health care services in rural areas, where there is an acknowledged shortage of MBBS graduates (Priya 2013: 25).

In their analysis of Tibetan medical education in India, Pordié & Blaikie used the term 'taskscapes'[31] to characterize different learning contexts with different aims as to what a physician should know, hence influencing the content of what is taught and learned (Pordié and Blaikie 2014: 341). While each mode of training is associated with a different social and professional status, Pordié & Blaikie argued that they cannot be strictly separated from each other because practitioners interact through overlapping placements and social roles (2014: 359). In this way, their status as legitimate practitioners is context-dependent and contingent based on transformations of the social environment (ibid.). In accordance with this idea, while the state recognizes BUMS graduates as qualified medical practitioners and employed them—albeit for a smaller salary than their MBBS colleagues—in public health care facilities like for example those of the National Rural Health Mission (NRHM), *k͟hāndānī* hakims claim that BUMS graduates know little about Unani medicine and condemn institutionalized training for failing to provide adequate knowledge of Unani as a medical art. In parallel, MBBS doctors struggle against measures that allow AYUSH graduates to prescribe allopathic medicines, claiming that they are not qualified to do so in order to protect their own professional interests. The professional recognition of BUMS graduates, thus, is not guaranteed through their degree in all taskscapes. While a BUMS graduate working in a biomedical public facility can be entitled to officially do so, he is not recognized as a member of the Unani fraternity, not just because he may lack knowledge of, say, pulse diagnosis, but because he was perhaps not interested in contributing to fostering the advancement and support towards Unani. In other words, he would be considered a Unani practitioner statistically speaking, as he was registered by the CCIM as such, but he would not be considered a hakim by the fraternity.

The influence of institutionalized training on Unani practices became apparent in the case of diagnostic methods. For example, the practice of pulse taking has been affected by the new forms of training and practice (Attewell 2005: 410). Pulse taking remains greatly absent as the sole or main form of diagnostic practice among the college-trained generations. Among those who still use it, many confessed that they did so in order to fulfil the patients' expectations and to establish rapport with them. Although taking the pulse is still a standard in nearly all the consultations with a Unani practitioner, de facto it often fulfils a more performative role instead of a

31 The term 'taskscapes' was coined by Pordié & Blaikie (2014) in analogy to Appadurai's five dimensions or scapes in his framework for the study of modernization and globalization (1996).

diagnostic one. I discussed this with a young practitioner at his clinic, who told me that no BUMS graduate learned how to read the pulse. I asked him if he learned that from the hakims he sought training from after graduation, and he replied that, honestly, he could not read the pulse, saying that the skill required long experience to master, which he lacked. He took the pulse in the consultations 'for the patient's satisfaction'. Similarly, several other young practitioners with a BUMS background explained that they took the pulse because 'it is what a hakim is supposed to do' or 'it is what patients expect'. Other not so young hakims explained that their knowledge of pulse diagnosis was not sufficient to be used as the sole method of diagnosis, as it only gave them a rough idea of the patients' condition and their temperament which required confirmation through other diagnostic methods, hence the need for pathological and other forms of examinations.

Many teachers in Unani colleges do not have a family background and were exclusively trained in Unani colleges. Their teaching is characterized by a mixture of Unani and biomedicine. In Unani college hospitals, the pulse of the patients is usually not recorded according to the Unani style as described, for example, by Ibn Sina: considering the ten features of the pulse, including the pulse's length, breadth, and thickness; its emptiness or fullness, and its rhythm (1993: 289ff.). Rather, they measure the pulse in biomedical fashion. Pulse reading following the traditional method is considered to be a difficult skill in the Indo-Muslim milieu (Speziale 2010b: 190), while pulse taking following the biomedical style is easy to master: one only needs to count the beats per minute. Pulse diagnosis, although still present, has changed in purpose and scope. Old diagnostic methods no longer serve only their original purpose, not because they have become useless but because learning them is difficult in the institutionalized context. The long years of practice and clinical experience required are not granted during the five and a half years of BUMS training. This is accentuated by the fact that many students pass a significant part of their compulsory internships in biomedical facilities, as required by the BUMS curricular regulations.

Students and practitioners agreed that the use of old diagnostic methods, such as pulse or urine diagnosis, were no longer central because modern diagnostic techniques were easier to handle, were widely available, and were even more accurate than the traditional methods, with which they did not feel confident enough. Taking the pulse continues to be a token of Unani medical practice, though, but its main purpose had changed, as it is seldom used mainly as a diagnostic method. However, not all patients were aware of this shift: older patients continued to stretch their arms automatically toward the hakims at the beginning of the consultations, whereas most younger patients did so only after the physicians asked them to, commonly during an ongoing anamnesis in the case of first-time patients. It seems as if the younger generation of patients is largely unaware of its diagnostic purpose, while the elderly continue to have faith in it. I could observe this generational gap among hakims, too. A BUMS graduate who came from a family of Unani physicians and who was working in one of the several RRIUMs (Regional Research Institute of Unani Medicine) talked about the traditional practice of his father, a *k̲h̲āndānī* hakim, and the one of his brothers, a BUMS graduate like him:

> BUMS graduate: It's like this, I do not practice. Our father, and the rest, who are brothers, sisters, and uncles, they do practice. You should understand my practice as distinct from theirs. My father, he takes the pulse, pulse, [and] there is the urine, right? Urine. He looks at the urine and says what it is, what the patient… which disease, what is it. My father's elder brother, he also saw the pulse, he saw the pulse and told you what disease you had. Now, my father does not use a stethoscope and all that, he just looks at the urine, the morning urine, right? He grabs the [bottle with] urine, looks at it and says what is in it, and says what disease is there, he tells you immediately, and he also takes the pulse. So, like that, he looks at that and without any tests and all that. Scans and all that, my father does not use.
> KS: He does not?
> BUMS graduate: No. Pulse, and the first urine in the morning… the first that comes out. He looks at that and he tells.
> KS: And your brother? Does he also use that?
> BUMS graduate: [Laughed] He, there are the modern methods, he uses them…

This dialogue exemplifies the differences between new and old generations. Although some hakims still trained younger ones in traditional diagnosis, the majority of the new generation felt more comfortable using modern diagnostic techniques than old methods due to the emphasis given to them in college training. Because college training emphasizes the science part of Unani, pulse reading as an art is neglected. Based on the claims made by BUMS graduates, uroscopy has completely banished from practical training in Unani colleges. As a consequence, BUMS graduates are not skilled in these traditional forms of diagnosis. This is not so much a consequence from the growing use of modern diagnostic methods alone, as I discuss in Chapter 4, but rather the product of institutionalized training. College training curtailed the individual and experience-based training of master-pupil lineages. The officially recognized form of knowledge transmission—focused on the production of medical professionals able to tackle different taskscapes from primary health care delivery to the coverage of the demand for traditional medicine—consequently, has modified medical knowledge itself (Sieler 2013), leading to a displacement of practices (Attewell 2005).

Family Lineages and Secret Knowledge

A family background or lineage remains an important source of legitimation for hakims, especially for those without a degree. The practice of Unani in India was largely a family matter, some practitioners could trace their lineage for centuries. Young *k̲h̲āndānī* hakims did not only have access through their families to a pool of medical knowledge which could be considered both reliable and powerful thanks to its secrecy (Attewell 2007: 37), they also benefited from the forefathers' reputation and experience. Patients considered lineages a source of authority and trust and hakims with a family background benefited from using the names of their forefathers if these were hakims. During informal conversations in the waiting room of a clinic, several patients pointed out that the family background was decisive when they opted for a certain hakim. A young BUMS graduate whose father runs a Unani clinic told me that in Unani, patients look at the name of the hakim, whereas in allopathy people look at the name of the hospital. The reputation of a family name is attributed to all practising members of that family.

The importance of a family background rests in the assumption that medical reputation is based on an original form of practice considered to be the product of a hakim's *tajribah* ('experience' and 'experimentation') and exclusive knowledge transmitted through generations. Patients expect hakims with a family background to have inherited the knowledge of their forefathers. Some young Unani graduates interested in actually practicing Unani seek to spend some time with one or several well-established hakims in order to gain some extra training and deepen their clinical knowledge. Conversely, it is common for hakims' children to pursue a BUMS degree in order to comply with the regulations for taking up their relatives' clinics and to make use of their family names, which attracted patients to their establishments. However, a renowned name does not stand on its own. If the family *nusk̲h̲ahjāt* can effectively treat certain diseases, the hakims and their descendants can build their reputation upon them. As their family trademark and basis for their reputation, this knowledge is commonly kept inside the family and is rarely shared with outsiders. Moreover, as I was told by a young Unani physician, it is considered discourteous to ask a hakim for his family *nusk͟h͟ahjāt,* being something to share—if at all—only with a selected and intimate group.

It is not a secret that medical practitioners have for centuries zealously kept their knowledge concealed in order to preserve their reputation and to offer exclusive treatments. Recent scholarly work has dealt with secrecy as an important aspect of medicine and science in different cultural and historical contexts (Leong and Rankin 2011; Sieler 2015). In the case of Graeco-Islamic medicine, a practitioner's reputation was and continues to be closely connected to the number of prescriptions collected or inherited by him. A BUMS graduate who had a directing charge in one of the branches of the CCRUM told me about the importance of collecting rare recipes. He said that when he was in college, back in the 1970s, everyone would keep their own Unani books, especially old ones, hidden or under lock and key. The reason was 'to avoid others putting eyes on them', i.e. to conceal rare recipes that were potentially exclusive and effective. He explained that if no one else had these recipes, they could help a hakim to build a great reputation and, with it, a livelihood. Sharing the recipes printed in those books would mean sharing a potential trademark of competitiveness among other graduates. This knowledge was especially coveted among BUMS students who lacked a family background and who depended on other sources of prescriptions or their own innovation in order to build an own reputation.

Secret knowledge has historically defined heritages of intimacy in medical contexts, meaning the circle of people with whom knowledge is shared (Weiss 2009: 155; Welch 2008: 135). Apprenticeship was sought also outside familial boundaries, but that was no guarantee for the obtainment of exclusive knowledge. Young hakims who had trained with non-relatives after completing their BUMS course reported that not all hakims were open regarding their practices, as some of them reportedly used tricks to conceal their knowledge such as asking the trainee to step out of the *maṭabb* during certain consultations.

A young hakim named Munis who had no formal training in Unani but belonged to a long family tradition talked about his own experience regarding concealed knowledge. According to Munis, the big problem in Unani medicine was the politics and the jealousy among physicians. He complained that hakims preferred to take their recipes along to their graves instead of sharing their knowledge with the newer generations—a complaint that resonated with critiques from other hakims. Munis told the story of an old villager who had a powerful cure for snake bites. The healer was an old, very rude man without education, Munis did not like him at all. The man had learned to produce the antidote through his father and did not charge for his services. Munis asked the man to teach him, but the man refused, upon which Munis cursed him, saying: 'You will die without passing your knowledge, many people will die because of your greedy fixation on not sharing your secret, you shall be cursed'. Time passed, and one day the healer called Munis saying: 'Do you still want to learn? Come to my village!' Munis asked his father (a respected *k̲h̲āndānī* hakim) to arrange his consultation schedule because he would take leave to visit the healer. He left immediately. The old man told Munis the secret, under the condition that he shall never take money for his healing services, and Munis accepted this condition. Munis explained that, in part, he lied to the healer because he earns money through the consultations in his clinic. However, he would not charge money when using the old man's antidote. A week after sharing the secret, the healer died. Munis said that unlike that man, many hakims died before they shared their knowledge. 'Why is that?', I asked. He shrugged, hesitating: 'Pride, jealousy?' He did not know; he only knew that people were not ready to share their knowledge. He instead claimed to be open to share his knowledge and so was his father. Munis' family was well-known in the Unani fraternity; his ancestors were court physicians hundreds of years ago. He had both a family lineage and family recipes, but he was still eager to gain more medical knowledge and obtain a successful recipe from a folk healer. Munis run a fancy clinic employing other Unani physicians in a big Indian city. He had no formal training in Unani.

Young hakims do not only profit from inherited recipes, but from inherited names. A young Unani practitioner told me that his clinic was only well consulted because his father's name was mentioned on the board. His father, a self-made hakim whose qualifications consisted of several courses in naturopathy, acupuncture and herbal medicine as well as an apprenticeship with a renowned hakim, held a reputation stemming from the medical preparations he had formulated based on what he claimed were his own research and experimentation. Through active self-promotion, he had attained great popularity in his region and beyond. Patients expected this hakim's sons and relatives, some of whom were also Unani practitioners, to share the hakim's knowledge. One of his sons, Dr. Arif, admitted that he never really learned how to read the pulse, neither during his BUMS training nor during short internships with other practitioners.[32] As he

32 I infer that his father was also unskilled in pulse reading, otherwise he could have taught his own son.

further explained, pulse reading required a skill that needs many years of training and experience. And yet, even though he could not diagnose from the pulse, he still touched the wrists of his patients. He said that he does it because this is what is expected from a hakim and also because it helped him to establish patients' trust which, according to him, was a crucial aspect of the healing process.

Like Munis, Dr. Arif complained that some hakims were reluctant to share their knowledge. He told me that after finishing his BUMS, his father suggested that he sees other hakims, to sit with them and learn from their practice. Dr. Arif went to see the son of his father's *ustād*, but that would be of no use. This practitioner would, like others also did, send him out of the consultation when a patient was coming, only to call him back when the patient was gone. There was no sharing of knowledge and Dr. Arif was very disappointed. He communicated this disappointment to his father, who advised him to clearly express to the hakim in question what he was expecting from the apprenticeship. Dr. Arif did so, but it was of no use: the hakim remained reluctant to disclose his knowledge. Dr. Arif said that he later spent time as an apprentice with another prominent hakim from whom he learned a lot. There are very few good old hakims left, Dr. Arif regretted, and this one was sadly an exception. He spent two days with that hakim. He obtained most of his knowledge from another prominent hakim who would show him everything—except the *nusk̲h̲ahjāt*— and with whom he spent ten days.[33] Dr. Arif's father advised him to ask the hakim whatever he wants to know, except the *nusk̲h̲ahjāt*, because it was a taboo to ask for them. He added that the tragedy was that old hakims were not sharing their *nusk̲h̲ahjāt* and were taking them along to their graves.

It may appear paradoxical that these young practitioners expect healers to share their knowledge whereas it is known that keeping knowledge concealed is necessary for obtaining and retaining a professional reputation. But there is a difference between sharing practical skills, like for example about pulse reading, and sharing knowledge about *mujarrab nusk̲h̲ahjāt* ('tested recipes'). A physician who shared his knowledge and experience in terms of diagnosis was considered to be a good hakim, without having to share the actual recipes used for treatment. Hakim Sadiq in Hyderabad, for example, was training one of his own sons, Dr. Sabir, as well as Dr. Farzanah, Sakinah, and the pharmacists and physiotherapists that also worked in his clinic. Dr. Farzanah was very confident in terms of establishing diagnoses

33 I was surprised by the short apprenticeships, since Dr. Arif himself emphasized the necessity of many years of experience in order to master certain skills, see below.

and prescribing treatment, but when it came to the treatments, she almost always sought Hakim Sadiq or his son for confirmation. Moreover, while she knew the names of the medicines prescribed, she did not know how to prepare them all. As Hakim Sadiq told me at the beginning of my fieldwork in his *maṭabb*: I could write down the names of the medicines he prescribed, but that would be a waste of time since I would find those medicines only there. They were modified formulae of well-known medicines, all produced in the dispensary at his home. Dr. Farzanah had been working with Hakim Sadiq for one and a half years at the time of my fieldwork and she still learned from him and his son. She would bring an old daily planner which she used as a notebook to the *maṭabb*. There, she copied prescriptions given by Hakim Sadiq and his son Sabir in special cases. Sakinah also copied these in her own notebook, sometimes she copied Dr. Farzanah's copies. Hakim Sadiq and his son discussed the cases with their apprentices. On one occasion, Hakim Sadiq asked Dr. Farzanah to learn from a case presented in an old *qarābādīn* (pharmacopoeia). He gave her the book with the section in question marked and left. Dr. Farzanah read the case study from the book to us (Sakinah and I), aloud and slowly. She wrote the title of the book in her notebook and then parts of the text. Later on, when Hakim Sadiq came back, he asked her if she made use of the prescription given in the book, Dr. Farzanah shook her head in negation. Hakim Sadiq said nothing and left the room. She seemed to interpret his silence as disapproval, and eagerly opened the book again and copied the complete prescription in her notebook. After a few minutes, when no patients were coming, she got up, took the book and went to see him in his private chamber, where he usually rested after mid-morning.

The discussion of cases among Hakim Sadiq, his son, and the two apprentices took place very often. Hakim Sadiq and Dr. Sabir often called the two women when special cases came, telling them how to establish a diagnosis and how the patients should be treated. The prescriptions were also communicated, but not the recipes of the compound drugs. In some of the rare moments when no patients were coming, Dr. Farzanah would go to the room in the back side of the house to chat with the women preparing the medicines, asking them for the herbs and other ingredients they used in the manufacturing. Their knowledge, she told me, was not comparable with her college training, and she estimated that it would take her another few years to learn about the preparation of the medicines, too.

The distribution of diagnostic and therapeutic training became apparent on another occasion too, when I asked Hakim Sadiq what he 'sees' when seeing the pulse. As he started telling me, a *davāsāz* ('compounder') who was standing behind him made gestures signalizing to me to take notes of what Hakim Sadiq said. When Hakim Sadiq was gone, he came to me and asked, showing great curiosity, what the hakim had told me, being very careful about not to be seen talking to me, something that did not seem to bother him on other occasions when we exchanged words. The lineage of knowledge transmission outside the family was exclusive, and this *davāsāz*, perhaps because of the nature of his role at this clinic, seemed to be aware that he did not belong to the circle of intimacy with whom Hakim Sadiq shared his diagnostic knowledge. He may have known about the medicines and what they were prescribed for, but he was not supposed to learn about diagnosis, in the same way that Dr. Farzanah knew much about diagnosis and treatment, but less about the preparation of the medicines dispensed at the *Shifa Mahal*. Division of labour, thus, was a way to ensure the monopoly of original medical knowledge even in a setting where medical knowledge was shared and exchanged. In this way, Hakim Sadiq secured his position as the most knowledgeable physician in the *maṭ̣abb*, mastering diagnosis as well as different forms of treatments ranging from manual techniques to the preparation of medicines. He personally trained his staff on these skills and knowledge, but this training was distributed among the different staff working for him: physiotherapists learned techniques like massage or how to apply compresses, the *davāsāz* knew all about packaging the dosages of the prescribed drugs, drug producers were in charge of cleaning raw materials and preparing Hakim Sadiq's recipes, while the trainees were learning how to diagnose and what to prescribe. Only his son, Hakim Sabir, was acquiring knowledge in all the areas of expertise in order to one day assume the role of his father.

Degrees and (Un-)Official Practice

The Regulation of Practice

The first regulations pertaining to the registration of medical practitioners were introduced during the Colonial Period. The British government dropped first plans to introduce a registration system for practitioners of Indian Medicine in the 1880s due to expected hostility from vaidyas and hakims (Jefferey 1982: 1836). Later, Medical Registration Acts were passed around 1913 based on the discussions about 'quackery' that emerged around the 1880s (Mukharji 2011: 7). These targeted only practitioners of Western medicine and marginalized indigenous practitioners (Berger 2013: 67). Registration patterns reinforced the subordinate position of practitioners of indigenous medicine vis-à-vis doctors of Western medicine (Jeffery 1988: 56). Over the years, successful acts of different presidencies granted legitimation to Unani professionals to different degrees, but still their role continued to be subordinated to that of Western practitioners. It was not until the 1920s that practitioners of indigenous medicine began to be considered to become part of the healthcare system, and that the standardization of training and practice became part of the provincial health administration plans (Berger 2013: 74). However, it was only shortly before independence that the Indian state attempted to regulate indigenous medicine (Lambert 2012: 1033).

In order to regulate the practice of traditional medicine, the State Governments established so-called Boards of Indian Medicine in the 1940s and 1950s which distinguished between 'A registrations' (those with a college degree on a particular form of medicine) and 'B registrations' for those who did not possess a formal qualification but learned in the traditional manner (ibid.). 'B registrations' required passing an examination and five years of practical experience, and were licensed until 1976 (ibid.). Since 1979, whoever wanted to practice Unani medicine in India was compelled to register in the Central Register of Indian Medicine. In order to be eligible for such registration, a Unani practitioner should hold a diploma or certificate in Unani, commonly the BUMS degree or an equivalent.[34] Because B-registrations were no longer licensed, *k̲h̲āndānī* hakims without a degree in Unani were no longer officially entitled to practice: the Supreme Court decided in 2010 against Ayurvedic physicians who continued to practice in spite of not being registered because they had no degree (Lambert 2012: 1034). However, it is known that unregistered practitioners still practice, some of them quite openly, indeed.

BUMS graduates are not automatically allowed to practice after obtaining their degree, a registration with the CCIM in their respective state is necessary. The CCIM prescribes a code of conduct for registered practitioners, who receive a registration number and a certificate of registration. Many Unani practitioners display this certificate in the walls of their clinics. In the case of hakims without a Unani degree, the registration of the *maṭabb* runs often in the name of a relative (commonly a son or younger brother) holding a BUMS degree and registered as a practitioner. Although not conforming

34 Other degrees include former equivalents to the BUMS that were granted by different colleges before training was completely standardized, such as the DUMS (Diploma in Unani Medicine and Surgery) or the GCUM (Graduate of College of Unani Medicine), as stipulated in The Indian Medicine Council Act, 1970.

to the regulations, this kind of practice is tolerated. Most practitioners in question have no major problems with the authorities because they enjoy respect in their communities, among patients, and occasionally even among the staff of Unani colleges nearby. The authorities still allow—or at least do not oppose—the practice of old and well-established hakims with long years of experience. Even though they are not officially registered, they are considered to represent the last vestiges of the former training system. As such, they are recognized as legitimate Unani practitioners, as opposed to quacks. A few unregistered but reputed hakims even have a consultant status in government institutions and are approached by government officials seeking for cooperation. Old hakims without a degree are still commonly called 'B-practitioners' in Unani circles. These hakims are emblematic of the shortcomings of institutionalization and efforts of practice regulation because they are recognized as legitimate Unani practitioners due to their experience and knowledge, albeit this recognition is only unofficial and as such at the margins of legality. Thus, the government has failed to establish itself as the sole authority in terms of Unani professional recognition, since knowledge and experience continue to be recognized by many as more important sources of medical authority than a Unani degree, leading to concurring legitimating systems.

Qualified and Registered Practitioners

Old hakims without institutional training are seen as bearers of Unani knowledge, a status that BUMS graduates without additional practical training can hardly claim for themselves. From this emerges the subtle, yet clear, distinction employed in Unani circles between the terms 'qualified' and 'unqualified' to refer to hakims. Here, qualification does not mean institutional qualification acquired through college training and official registration. Rather, it means the capacity in terms of knowledge and skills based on experience and experimentation and sanctioned by the Unani fraternity, regardless if acquired through self-learning or through a family tradition, through an apprenticeship or through a formal degree course. Formerly, some hakims trained in a lineage system received a permit (*ijāzah*) from their masters through which prominent physicians attested the skills and knowledge of their pupils (Attewell 2005: 3f.). 'Qualified hakim' means, in the jargon of the Unani fraternity, a physician who mastered the art and science of Unani medicine through lineage training or own experience, as well as a physician who is officially entitled to practice. In contrast, an 'unqualified practitioner' can be described as a quack or at least as a less knowledgeable physician. Because of their malleability, the adjectives 'qualified' and 'unqualified' are purportedly employed by hakims to establish their own legitimation and authority vis-à-vis other practitioners.

The need for registration forced many *ḵẖāndānī* hakims to pursue degrees in Unani. Hakim Faruqi, an old hakim from Lucknow, claimed he had over 80 pupils during his long life as a practitioner, a life that started very early because he learned from his father while he was still a young boy. I asked him if the pupils had a BUMS degree, and he said of course, otherwise they would not be allowed to practice. 'But then why do they seek apprenticeship?', I asked. Hakim Faruqi told me that the degree is a must, but it does not equal an understanding of the practice. He explained that he also had to go to college because a degree was required, but college for him was like learning the ABC, so basic and simple, he claimed that it was no contribution to his knowledge. He criticized the 'new system' (i.e. the requirement of college education for Unani practice) that started some 50 years ago, complaining about the six months of the practical year that had to be passed at an allopathic hospital as a requirement for the Unani degree. People get degrees as easily as that, he claimed, but they have not been exposed intensively to practice. 'Suppose you don't know how to swim and you want to learn. For that you read a book on swimming. You know the book by heart and then you jump into the water. What will happen? Yes, you will drown!' While those physicians practicing without being officially registered are not necessarily considered to be quacks, holding a BUMS degree is not a guarantee for recognition as a Unani physician among the fraternity. The failure for the BUMS degree to produce recognized hakims rested not only on the lack of sufficient exposure to Unani clinical training, but also on the motivations behind Unani college education and the health care system in India in general.

BUMS as Second Choice

A crucial aspect for the understanding of the contemporary state of Unani education and practices is knowledge about the BUMS student's background and aspirations. For practitioners and students with a Unani family background, official Unani training is the natural way to ensure that they would continue with the family lineage (and business), as they require the qualification to register as practitioners. However, the majority of Unani students and a significant number of practitioners and even some teachers

I talked to were primarily interested in pursuing studies on biomedicine before enrolling in a Unani college. Because they did not receive admission to the MBBS course, they opted for Unani medicine instead. I hardly met any Unani practitioner without a family background whose interest was to study Unani in the first place.

A senior government official in a Unani institution told me in conversation that he was previously not very interested in Unani, as he did not come from a family of physicians. He decided to study Unani because he saw a good opportunity to obtain a government job through it. According to him, those times were different, nowadays Unani graduates hardly get government jobs, although many continued opting for the study of Unani medicine having a government job in mind. Back then, he explained, many took up government jobs. He joined the RRIUM he now directed from its very beginnings, in the early 1980s. A researcher working for another RRIUM explained that his uncle was professor for Botany at university and it was him who saw a future in Unani medicine as a profession for his nephew, so he went to study Unani out of state. When he returned to his hometown he got three job offers for government service, from these offers he decided to work for the RRIUM. While the prospect of getting a government job with a BUMS degree was no longer a safe bet at the time of research as it was 30 years ago when the CCRIUM was a new institution looking for staff, students who did not know much about Unani still pursued college training in Unani. One of these young students told me, a bit ashamed, that she did not have any contact or experience with Unani medicine before enrolling into the Unani college she was attending, all she wanted was a career in the 'health sciences'.

The interest in pursuing a career in the health sector is seemingly the greatest motivation among students in Unani colleges. They passed courses in Physics, Chemistry and Biology at school, since these were eligibility requirements for MBBS and BUMS courses. It is not surprizing, thus, that subjects concerning the basic concepts of Unani medicine are perceived by students like the one above as particularly difficult because, coming from a science background, the fundamental principles of Unani do not seem to match what she was taught in high school. This problem was also acknowledged by a senior lecturer who commented that students with a science background had problems with taking Unani's basic principles seriously if the teachers were not able to adapt knowledge to modern concepts.[35] Another student explained that the terminology used in the

35 While dominant, this view was not shared by all the students I spoke to.

Unani books in Urdu was very complicated, so she and her fellow students had to spend a substantial amount of time looking up for the meaning of the medical terms, mostly of Arabic and Persian origin, that they were not acquainted with. If all was in English, she wished, it would be easier to study. She considered the subjects taught using biomedical texts to be easier to learn than those using Urdu ones, and claimed that those were preferred by many other students, too.

Language is an important issue. Training in Unani is mostly in Urdu, a language that has come to be identified as a symbol of Muslim identity in (North-) India. Most students of Unani medicine in India are, indeed, Muslims (see Chapter 6), and students coming from more affluent families are less likely to study Unani because they would not have visited an Urdu medium school if their parents were able to afford English medium education. Added to that, those who can afford better school education and have a better socio-economic position often prefer to study biomedicine. This is the case of the children and grandchildren of several well-positioned *k̲h̲āndānī* hakims. Students who are not very good in Urdu, let alone Arabic or Persian—the languages that constitute the basis of Unani medical terminology, just as Greek and Latin in biomedicine—have problems understanding the texts. While some teachers are very enthusiastic about making Unani training accessible in English, a step which would enable to expand Unani practice beyond the South Asian Muslim milieu, the majority remains cautious, arguing that translations are full of pitfalls and that it is difficult to find equivalents in English. They fear that translations into English could jeopardize a proper understanding of Unani medical concepts.

Some Unani practitioners who were critical about the BUMS degree remarked that many, if not the majority, of the students were mostly interested in biomedical subjects and knew beforehand that they would not practice Unani once they graduate (Latif 2008: 11). This motivation seems to be reflected in the practice of biomedicine in private or public facilities by AYUSH graduates, which has been said to be characteristic of them (Bode and Hariramamurthi 2013; Jeffery 1988: 186).

Practicing 'Allopathy' with a Unani Degree

The practice of biomedicine by BUMS graduates encapsulates the ambiguities of institutionalized Unani education: whereas college training grants a recognized degree, qualifying holders to practice Unani medicine officially, most BUMS graduates without a family background or additional traineeships with hakims do not feel confident enough to practice Unani medicine in terms of diagnosis and treatment. At the same time, they are not allowed to prescribe allopathic medicines in many states, although they are expected to do so when employed in government biomedical facilities in rural (and even urban) areas with shortage of MBBS doctors (Naraindas 2014b: 121; Pordié and Blaikie 2014: 354). The result of institutionalized training is a mixed form of practice which, in the case of Ayurveda, was described by Bode & Hariramamurthi as an 'hybrid form of medicine marked by biomedical diagnosis, biomedical drugs, and industrial Indian medicines' (2013: 10). This practice has been described as a creolization of therapeutic languages, whereby the language of biomedicine dominates (Naraindas 2014b: 123ff.) Bode & Hariramamurthi estimated that only 10,000 of the over 500 thousand registered ISM practitioners actually practiced mainly Indian medicine in terms of diagnosis and treatment (2013: 2).

In spite of a general consensus about the massive amount of biomedical knowledge integrated into the BUMS curriculum, some members of the fraternity downplayed its influence on Unani medical practices. A prominent hakim who used to direct a department at a renown Unani college claimed that biomedicine had only a minor role in Unani college training. He explained that anatomy and physiology were the same in every medical system, and only surgery could be seen as purely allopathic. Still, he argued, surgery had a minor part in training. He explained that the students were not exposed to allopathic pharmacology, so how could they practice allopathy? I asked him what about the practical year that most students completed in biomedical facilities? He claimed that it poses no problems because students had to learn how to use modern diagnostic techniques, and those were not exclusive of allopathy but were the product of inventions made by scientists and technicians, hence their use did not compromise Unani medicine or its fundamental principles (see Chapter 4). According to him, X-rays, stethoscopes, blood tests and other modern diagnostic methods were really useful for Unani practitioners. 'As long as the treatment remains Unani, there is nothing to be afraid of.' He claimed that BUMS graduates did not prescribe allopathic treatments, saying that it was something he was completely against, claiming to rise his voice loud against those who do so.

When I started fieldwork in May 2012, my initial contacts were all members of the Unani fraternity. My original plan was to include the informal sector into this study, and I searched for Unani practitioners at random places, walking through Muslim areas in different Indian cities, asking people in the street and in pharmacies for a hakim or a Unani *davāḵẖānah*. I also approached practitioners in private clinics who announced their BUMS degree on the board, but soon I learned that unless the board explicitly mentioned Unani, those BUMS physicians did not practice Unani but biomedicine or even Ayurveda instead. One of those practitioners was a man in his mid-thirties with polished English, he had a small clinic close to a slum in Mumbai. When I introduced myself telling him that I was conducting research on Unani medicine, he immediately said that I had come to the wrong place, because he practiced allopathic medicine. I still wanted to talk to him, and he agreed. He answered many of my questions before I could even pose them. He explained:

> Dr. Yunis: Out of ten doctors in this area, eight are BUMS doctors who practice allopathy. Only two are MBBS doctors. The statistics show that there are not enough MBBS doctors to cover the population. If BUMS doctors would not be taking this job, what would happen to the people? Where would they go?
> KS: Were you trained to become a doctor or a hakim?
> Dr. Yunis: [Laughed] The aim of the BUMS course is to produce doctors, not hakims. Most of the people who studied MBBS prefer to go for specialization areas which are not clinical. They would not sit in a general practice seeing patients here. I charge little to my patients, they would not pay more, it is not attractive for the [MBBS] doctors and they do their MDs in other areas. BUMS doctors have to practice allopathy, the patients need malaria treatment which is allopathic and not Unani treatment for most of the cases. If I was to set a Unani clinic, then it had to be something big, because patients look at that. A big clinic with a big board for herbal medicines, that would work. But not a small clinic like this. And money is what thrives human beings. It is as simple as that. Everyone needs money nowadays to survive, everyone opts for an option which offers the best possibilities. Here, 90 percent of the patients are illiterate. It is a poor area, and a few MBBS doctors would work as general practitioners here.

Not only did this practitioner explain that BUMS graduates like him practiced biomedicine because they have been trained to do so, but he also justified this practice as a form of social service. While he claimed that working as general practitioners in slum areas was not profitable for most MBBS doctors and hence they preferred to specialize in non-clinical areas of expertise, BUMS doctors filled the gap and provided primary health care as needed by the patients. Hence, practicing allopathy for this practitioner was not only the logical consequence of his insecurity in Unani medical knowledge, but also a moral duty. BUMS graduates practicing biomedicine often articulated, apologetically, the need for income as a reason for their practice but, more importantly, they stressed that their practice was a service towards patients neglected by MBBS physicians as a way to justify their practice. While practitioners like Dr. Yunis, who work in low-income urban areas, claim legitimacy of their practice based on a structural problem of health care delivery, they are blamed indirectly both by the Unani fraternity for not promoting Unani medicine, and by MBBS professional groups for being quacks, using the argument of practicing a system of medicine they are not entitled to.

Unani practitioners prescribing allopathic drugs are often the target of verbal attacks in social media like Facebook, where they are criticized by peers for not advancing Unani or for putting their personal and economic interests before the advancement and promotion of Unani as a system of medicine. Some practitioners have understanding for their colleagues—this is especially the case of practitioners having a family background—, arguing that these colleagues might prescribe allopathic medicines simply because they do not feel confident practicing Unani (i.e. the college degree does not grant sufficient knowledge on Unani medications in order to apply it in practice). However, it is still widely argued that BUMS graduates prescribing allopathic drugs are actually practicing allopathy. This practice is condemned by many as a form of treachery against the Unani system of medicine.

The situation of these practitioners remains ambiguous because of a lack of clear regulations pertaining to the prescription of medicines. The ban imposed towards AYUSH practitioners regarding the prescription of biomedical pharmaceuticals in certain states triggered protests and strikes at the time of my first fieldwork in 2012, some of which even lead to violent confrontations between the protesting practitioners and security forces, as reported in Lucknow.[36] AYUSH practitioners demanded the right to prescribe allopathic drugs in emergency cases as well as during employment in the NRHM. Although the argument of these demands was the patients' interest, who in rural areas might not have access to public biomedical facilities, informants agreed that the protests were primarily aimed at decriminalizing cross-prescription practices in urban areas. As protests by AYUSH practitioners continued, they were driven by a rather different agenda, namely the rise of salaries.

The employment of Unani graduates in government-run biomedical facilities represents a double-standard in the treatment of Unani practitioners: on the one hand, their training in biomedicine is conveniently used to

36 For newspaper reports on the strikes in Karnataka see for example IBN Live (n.n. 2012c) and *The Times of India* (n.n. 2012c). For reports on the violent protest in Lucknow see for example India TV News (n.n. 2012a) and *The Times of India* (n.n. 2012b).

overcome a shortage of MBBS practitioners in the public sector, while on the other the private practice of allopathy by BUMS doctors continues to be largely condemned, at least on paper. The state's approach is a pragmatic one. However, while different state governments have lifted the bans for AYUSH practitioners to prescribe allopathic medicines and even to perform minor surgeries, MBBS professional groups have issued harsh criticism. The Indian Medical Association (IMA), which is the biggest professional group of MBBS doctors in the country, strongly opposed the lifting of the ban in Maharashtra and has since then continuously fought the appointment of AYUSH graduates to fulfil biomedical tasks (Shelar 2015). More recently, the IMA pressed against the recent draft of the new National Medical Commission Bill that would allow AYUSH graduates to practice allopathy after passing a bridge course (Dutta 2018). The IMA's president claimed that this course would 'open up the floodgates to allow backdoor entry to crosspathy thereby promoting quackery legally' (ibid.).

The BUMS degree is looked down by MBBS practitioners, leading to an 'inferiority complex' as described by some high-ranked hakims. BUMS graduates in government service are paid less than MBBS graduates, and their status in the hospitals is also lower. A BUMS graduate that was formerly employed in a government biomedical facility narrated that she felt discriminated against by her MBBS colleagues, who looked down upon her for having 'only' a BUMS degree. However, BUMS graduates and students claimed that the study of the BUMS course was even more difficult than the MBBS course because they had to learn both Unani and biomedicine. But while they were certainly exposed to both forms of medicine during training, it was recurrently reported that graduates were not fully accountant with any of them. A BUMS graduate who sought an apprenticeship with an established hakim explained that the BUMS degree was not sufficient for practicing Unani. Moreover, according to him the BUMS degree was 75 per cent allopathy and only 25 per cent Unani. How was he supposed to practice Unani if he did not learn it properly? The BUMS is only a degree, he said.

While BUMS graduates do not usually master Unani in terms of traditional diagnostic methods and treatment (including the preparation of medicines) unless they seek apprenticeship with an established hakim, neither do they master all the subjects needed to be a qualified biomedical practitioner. The anatomy and physiology classes attended by the BUMS students may be the same as those attended by their MBBS counterparts—in fact, teachers of these subjects in Unani colleges held often MBBS and not BUMS degrees—, but biomedical pharmacology, for example, is not part of the BUMS curriculum.

The prescription of biomedical drugs by BUMS graduates is not only a symptom of the equivocal status emanating from institutionalized training and its modes of knowledge transmission and content, but also the product of ambiguous health and profession policies. The integration of Unani professionals in the health care sector grants Unani graduates a status superior than that of folk practitioners, but lower than that of biomedical doctors (Bode and Hariramamurthi 2013; Priya 2013). Even though they have a degree that they can hang on the walls of their clinics, BUMS graduates do not enjoy the same recognition that old and respected *k̲h̲āndānī* hakims do. As Lambert put it: 'formal qualifications do not necessarily equate to the acquisition of genuine therapeutic expertise or ensure the provision of high quality care' while at the same time 'a lack of formal accreditation does not necessarily signify the complete absence of therapeutic expertise' (2012: 1035). The Unani fraternity, the patients, and even the government of India are aware of this situation. In this way, recognition of Unani medical professionals varies depending on the context, accounting for the multiplicity of the Unani profession, too. The professional recognition of hakims is distributed between the state, the Unani fraternity, and patients, who define it according to the different taskscapes (Pordié and Blaikie 2014).

Defying Standards

Individualized Treatments and Clinical Falsification

Attention to the individual constitution of the patient through tailored therapies has been addressed as characteristic of humoral forms of medicine (Bode 2008: 166), and also official representations stress the individualized and holistic approach of Unani. Hakims often contrast Unani with biomedicine, emphasizing the former's focus on the individual patient and its environment and not just on isolated organs or affected body parts. Therapies, according to members of the fraternity, have to be adjusted to the temperament of the patients. In practice, however, this is not always done. While observing the clinical practice in a Unani college in Delhi, it became apparent that patients in that facility were treated symptomatically only, using standard formulations for the same ailments in different patients. BUMS students and teaching physicians in that clinic seemed to be under great pressure to treat quickly given the number of patients waiting for a consultation.

When asked about the role of *mizāj* ('temperament') in Unani practice, a teacher and consulting physician in this college apologetically explained that *mizāj* is a very important concept in Unani, but she did not have the time to assess the temperament of the patients in the OPD. Establishing a patient's temperament takes time, and she could not afford to waste time since many patients were queuing waiting to be seen by a doctor. If she took enough time to do that, she would not be able to attend to all the patients. How could she send patients home when they had been waiting the whole day to be seen by a doctor? Later on, she told me that 'the temperament of the patient has no clinical importance, it is irrelevant.' This teacher had successfully pursued post-graduate Unani education in a prestigious Unani institution in another city and had been teaching for two years. While this direct dismissal of the clinical relevance of the temperaments was not representative for all Unani practitioners, it neither constituted an isolated case, especially in institutionalized settings.

Institutionalized training introduced biomedical categorizations and technologies. Their influence is prominent in the clinical practices of many Unani college hospitals and dispensaries where physicians work under time pressure, rely primarily on modern methods to establish diagnosis, and treat diseases using the limited number of ready-made drugs available at their dispensaries. Moreover, medicines are known to be on short supply in many government facilities, forcing practitioners to constrain their therapeutic options. Once I witnessed a consulting physician dictating a prescription: the drug that the physician wanted to prescribe was not on stock at the hospital's dispensary, nor was its substitution. He changed the medicine five times until he found one which was available.[37]

Not all college hospitals have standardized their treatments, an important exception being the Nizamia Hospital in Hyderabad. There, *davāsāz* compound medicines in a 'traditional' dispensary attached to the college, where also decoctions are prepared individually for the patients staying at the IPD.[38] Generally speaking, however, it can be said that the clinical practices in institutional settings have been largely standardized, hence individually tailored therapies constitute the exception rather the rule in these facilities. Maarten Bode was very critical about the role of the government and the

37 The authorities were aware of this problem. The then AYUSH department issued 'Essential Drugs Lists' (EDL) for Ayurveda, Homeopathy, Siddha and Unani in 2000 and reviewed these in March 2013 in order to 'ensure that the essential medicines are regularly available in the health facilities and the people does not have to suffer from paying medicines' costs from their pockets' Department of AYUSH (2013a). The Essential Drugs List for Unani, which contains 288 drugs, is online available at the CCIM website.

38 Following the claims of patients, this college hospital was also affected by a shortage of medicines. See also an article in The Hindu (Iftekhar 2012).

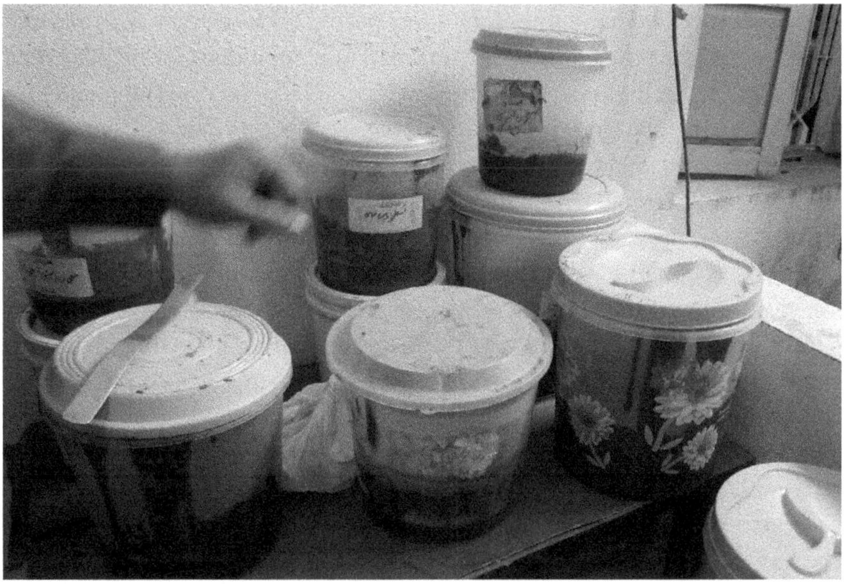

2. Home-made medicines at the compounding table of a hakim in Hyderabad (2012).

pharmaceutical industry regarding the de-individualization of Ayurvedic and Unani therapeutic practices in India. For him, de-individualization is the consequence of efforts to develop Indian medicine to keep it at par with modern medicine, identifying the reliance on ready-made drugs as one of the main threats against the individual approach to disease in Ayurveda and Unani (2008). Others have similarly argued that the pharmaceuticalization of Ayurveda, through its focus on active ingredients and description of action based on biomedical categories, lead to changes regarding 'the internal structure and epistemology of this knowledge system' (Banerjee 2008: 201). Therapeutic practices have also been affected, as diseases were approached through biomedical categories and treatments, treating diseases and not patients (Gaudillière 2014b: 175; Naraindas 2006, 2014c: 27f.).

Despite the fact that the temperament of patients is seldom explicitly acknowledged in clinical consultations, the observation of private clinical practices revealed that Unani treatments given by some hakims are still, indeed, often individualized, even when hakims treated with branded drugs. Hakim Ahmad and Hakim Sadiq in particular followed a prescription procedure based on a trial-and-error approach. Here, the hakims tried to identify the cause of a patient's problem not only through diagnostic methods, but also through the testing of therapies and the assessment of a patient's reaction to it. When the actual cause of the disease had not been identified yet, the hakims prescribed medicines for a short period of time in order to observe how the patient reacted to them. Hakim Sadiq, for example, always asked his patients to tell him how many days should he prescribe the medicines for, because he charged the medicines per day. In this way, patients could buy the medications according to what they could pay at the moment. For example, once he had a patient suffering from diabetes, hypertension and kidney problems. After the consultation, which included pulse and urine diagnosis, the hakim asked the patient to get different laboratory tests. He asked the patient to bring the results the next time, arguing that he should find out the cause of the disease. 'If you do them today you will get them in three days', he said. The patient asked the hakim to give a prescription for a whole week. Hakim Sadiq looked at the patient and said: 'Fine, you should rest a bit and don't walk much. I'd better give you medicines for three days and today only, so that I can give you the medicines according to the tests results.'

If no improvement (*farq*, lit. 'difference') was achieved with the treatment, the hakim would change the prescription and try with other medicines, addressing the individual reaction to the drugs as well as targeting another possible cause of the condition. This treatment approach resembles that of Ayurvedic practitioners in Sri Lanka analysed by Obeyesekere, who referred to it as 'clinical falsification' meaning that 'if a prescription does not work, it is abandoned' (Obeyesekere 1992: 172). In the case of Unani, clinical falsification assumes that different patients present different reactions to the same drugs. This assumption stands in clear contrast to a standardized approach where the same prescriptions are utilized for the same diseases. Hakims focus on the temperament of the disease as they also attend to the individual responses of the patients to the administered drugs. These responses are said to be influenced not only by the patients' humoral constitution, but also by the environment, dietary habits, lifestyle patterns, and other aspects constituting the six-essential factors in Unani medicine, a concept whose relevance is discussed in the following chapter.

Some patients seemed skeptical about the constant change of prescriptions and asked hakims why this was needed, to which hakims responded that it is 'the Unani way of treatment' or 'we will see if the medicines work'. A few patients did not return to the clinics after their prescriptions were changed for a second or third time. Perhaps the changes were interpreted as a sign of inconsistency and hesitation from the physicians' part, as biomedical practitioners who changed prescriptions several times may generate the impression of a lack of medical competence. In the case of Unani medicine, however, the individualized approach as well as clinical falsification often required making changes of this sort. As argued by Obeyesekere for the case of Ayurveda, clinical falsification is clearly congruent with the idea of targeting the root cause of diseases (1992). In this way, variations in treatment, thus, were not just accepted in Unani medicine, but were moreover required if the root cause of the disease was to be targeted.

Pulse Diagnosis and the Limits of Standardization

One of the most significant moments during a consultation with a Unani physician was the moment of pulse taking. Often, patients and physicians stopped talking during it. For a few seconds, silence reigned inside the *maṭabbs* and the time seemed to stand still once the hakim placed two or three fingers over one of the wrists of his patient. During this instant, the patients tended to search for the eyes of the hakim with an avid expression, as if trying to decipher from them any clue about their problems. In this special interaction, only the patient seemed to matter. While the patients' excitement was hard to oversee, the expression of the hakims was difficult to unravel: some hakims frowned, some held an inexpressive face while others fixed their gaze on some invisible point on the wall or closed their eyes. Most hakims seemed to be gone for an instant, sometimes as short as a wink. Not a few hakims asked the patients for the other wrist, and the procedure was repeated once again on the other arm. Some hakims asked questions while feeling the pulse, sometimes it was the patients themselves who revealed details about their complaints while the physician was feeling the pulse. It was usually a moment of intimacy—even when done in public—that seemed to seal the roles of the hakim and the patient, the latter submitted to the hakim's authority, waiting for relevant information concerning the own health.

Although the patterns described above are not always present in all consultations—I also saw hakims attending phone calls or reading text messages on their mobile phones while feeling a patient's pulse—, in most consultations it is an important moment where hakim and patient seem to get closer. On a few occasions I even felt like a silent intruder in a very intimate moment. The haptic connection between patient and healer is for some hakims an important recourse to establish a bonding of trust and intimacy (Sieler 2015: 147). In institutionalized settings, however, more often than not pulse examination is conducted in a rush and, admittedly, for the patients' satisfaction only. Also, a few very popular family-hakims felt their patients' pulse for no longer than a few seconds, sometimes even after they had written the prescription. In this context, asking about the role of taking the pulse in contemporary Unani practice is justifiable, because pulse reading can be seen not only as a method to establish rapport with patients and arrive at diagnoses, but also as a token of differentiation from biomedicine and a symbol of Unani medical authority and skill.

The first time I met Hakim Azim, I asked him how he diagnosed. He told me that the pulse was very important in his practice. Through it, he could identify what a patient had, and that experience was crucial for pulse diagnosis, and lack of it was the reason why so less Unani practitioners were skilled in pulse diagnosis nowadays. Not even a year later, after I had spent some weeks observing his clinical practice, Hakim Azim told me once again that the pulse was very important in Unani medicine, but this time he added that he could forgo it for diagnosis. He always conducted pulse examinations for the patients' satisfaction, because patients expected a hakim to feel the pulse, even though they often came with examination reports and already knew their diagnoses. To give me an example, he reminded me of a patient who, without uttering a word, automatically stretched her arm towards him once she sat inside his tiny *maṭabb*. I remembered that situation very well: the patient expected Hakim Azim to provide a diagnosis from the pulse only. However, he had to ask questions, too, as he could not rely on pulse alone as a diagnostic method. Pulse examination was an important part of his clinical practice, but it was more about creating a bond with the patients in a ritualized moment of silence than about establishing a diagnosis. Hakim Azim not only had to satisfy patients' expectations of a hakim as someone who feels the pulse, he also had to establish rapport with them. Since an important part of his practice was related to the satisfaction of patients and re-assuring that they would soon be fine, he used pulse not mainly as a diagnostic method, but as part of the therapeutic process. As Langford pointed out, 'Pulse reading sparks the faith that fires the healing process' (1999: 40). For diagnostic purposes, Hakim Azim would rely more on observation and questioning as well as on the examination reports brought by his patients, and not on the pulse.

Dr. Hussain routinely checked the pulse of his patients, too. With no need to presume to be knowledgeable about pulse diagnosis, since he openly claimed to practice allopathy, he told me that through the pulse he could get an idea of the patient's temperature, of hypertension and hypotension. He also said that quite often there was no need for an examination of the blood pressure with the sphygmomanometer after feeling the pulse, but he still did it for the patients' satisfaction. Once, Dr. Hussain was examining a patient and, while feeling the pulse, asked him if he had fever, the patient said yes. Dr. Hussain turned to me: 'You, see? I could feel that through the pulse, it is very easy. Anaemia we can find, it is manifested in a feeble pulse. Hypertension we can feel, cardiac arrhythmia we can feel'.

For a long time, pulse diagnosis had a very special place as a form of authoritative medical knowledge. This skill was often the reason for a hakim's fame (Attewell 2005: 390). *Nabbāẓī*, or the mastering of pulse diagnosis, was considered a source of professional recognition and respect among patients and colleagues alike. Biographical accounts of elite hakims included anecdotes on accurate diagnosis based only on pulse taking or an account of the physician gaining knowledge about the patient's profession or habits solely through feeling the pulse. These anecdotes exalted the hakims' skills and knowledge through accounts of their expertise in pulse reading. Today, many Unani practitioners and government officials regret that there were no longer experts in pulse reading. The rector of one of the most prestigious Unani medical colleges in India told me about a famous hakim known for his pulse diagnostic skills; when he died, his knowledge died with him. He regretted that old diagnostic methods such as pulse were getting lost forever because the new generations were not learning these practices in college. Even his own generation (he was above 50 years old) was not able to teach that knowledge properly anymore. He claimed that unlike the regimental therapies, which were being revived, pulse diagnosis could not be revived, because it required training based on experience which could not be transferred through books: 'when the practitioners who had that knowledge are no more, how can it be revived?'

The combination of diagnostic methods was sometimes interpreted as the decay of pulse diagnosis. However, it is difficult—if not impossible—to know if hakims in the past really diagnosed only through the pulse as the narratives of *nabbāẓ* suggest. The idea of great hakims diagnosing solely from the touch of their patient's wrists seems to be more a myth than reality, as even Ibn Sina advocated the combination of different diagnostic methods in order to ensure reliability. However, today less and less Unani practitioners are acquainted with pulse diagnosis. According to Guy Attewell, pulse and urine diagnostic methods became marginalized during the twentieth century due to the establishment of institutional training, the decay of training apprenticeships, and through the integration of modern diagnostic methods (2007: 134). I agree with Attewell in that institutionalized training and practice contributed enormously to the loss of knowledge on pulse diagnosis. However, I have reservations regarding the integration of modern diagnostic methods as a cause for it. Hakims knowledgeable on pulse diagnosis knew how to complement it with new diagnostic procedures, avoiding substitution. On the other hand, younger practitioners like Hakim Azim, who did not seem well versed in this skill, argued that this knowledge was not clinically relevant because questioning and observation were more useful to diagnose. For these reasons, the blame for the decline of pulse as a diagnostic method cannot be placed only on the use of modern diagnostic methods.

In spite of its decay as a diagnostic tool, feeling the pulse remains an important symbol of Unani medical practice. Pulse reading is used by many hakims to create a solemn moment of silence where the patient occupies a central space and is cared about. Moreover, pulse continues to play a crucial role in the representations of Unani medicine. The practice of feeling the pulse, thus, can be said to have experienced a shift of purpose: from a diagnostic tool to a symbol of Unani medicine. Pulse examination escapes observation, it privileges other senses instead. For more than two thousand years, pulse reading was investigated with far more interest than other diagnostic methods such as observation and questioning (Kuriyama 2002 [1999]: 19f.). Unlike other forms of diagnosis except for palpation, pulse is intrinsically related to the sense of touch, and hence with feeling. Many efforts have been made to render this subjective knowledge objective, the most common being attempts of visualization. These ranged from linear representations of the different kinds of pulse in analogy to animals—as done by Galen (Müller 2012)—to transcriptions of the pulse as musical notes in the sixteenth and eighteenth centuries, for example (ibid., Kuriyama 2002 [1999]: 81). At the time of fieldwork, a research project at the Ajmal Khan Tibbiya College in Aligarh Muslim University was developing a device to allow the visualization of different patterns of the pulse. This effort is interesting because it would not only tell us about the selection of parameters to be visualized (i.e. which ones are considered to be useful in diagnosis), but also because it was a development motivated by the perceived need to rendered the physicians' experience objective, hence 'proving' the existence of the different parameters through visualization, which until now could only be identified subjectively through the physician's feeling.

Apart from offering a visual proof of the different parameters used in Unani pulse diagnosis, this device may compensate for the lack of Unani practitioners sufficiently skilled in conducting pulse diagnoses in the traditional way, and Unani students in the future may not need to bother to train the skills if a device can help them to perform this task. Opinions about the usefulness of such a device were divergent. An old *k̲h̲andānī* hakim and government official expressed concern that such a tool would make Unani practitioners 'lazy'. Practitioners would rely on the machine only, he feared, which is problematic not only because machines are vulnerable, but also because a good hakim is supposed to make a diagnosis based on his knowledge and interpretation, assessing the temperament of the patient from the moment he sets a foot in the *maṭabb*, observing gestures, voice, and behaviour. A machine, he argued vehemently, cannot do that:

> Machines give us a wrong clue and they cannot be trusted alone, the human capacity of reasoning is the basic, *manṭiq* [logic] and *falsafah* [philosophy], this is why these subjects are important in Unani! But the new generations are lazy. Unani is not only a science, it is also an art. This is something that everyone should remember.

If and how this device will be used by Unani practitioners remains to be seen. Although the role of pulse reading as a diagnostic method seems, in the case of most practitioners, subordinate to its symbolic imaginary as a token of Unani practice and a recourse to establish trust in patients through touch and through the atmosphere of intimacy that often characterizes the moment of pulse taking, it continues to be practiced by almost every hakim. Whenever I asked about diagnostic methods, the pulse was commonly mentioned first as the most important one. Hakims usually feel the pulse at the beginning of almost any consultation, before or during questioning or when patients narrate their complaints. Through its convenience—feeling the pulse only requires a patient and a practitioner, and unlike urine diagnoses no hygienic issues are involved—and its embodiment of a physician's knowledge and skill, pulse reading has been retained in Unani practice and is considered characteristic of Unani medicine. Whether as a diagnostic method or as a performative tool, whether felt by the physician or visualized with a device: *nabẓ* remains, for the time being, an integral part of Unani medical practice.

Exclusive Knowledge and the Pursuit of Originality

Hakims consider innovation in terms of treatment an important virtue. Only experienced and skilled hakims possess the ability to integrate their own experimentations and to go beyond the teachings of the books during the diagnosis and treatment of patients. When a practitioner told his patient that the medicines he was giving were formulated by himself, he did so as to establish the difference from other practitioners, as only good practitioners are considered to have the knowledge to formulate good remedies. The results of these experiments, if proven effective, are very valuable. They are used as a trademark for the hakim in question and his family, becoming exclusive knowledge. Such is the case of hakims who have a specialized practice in which they mainly treat patients suffering from specific diseases for which they have a tested (*mujarrab*), own recipe. One hakim in Hyderabad, for example, treated only heart patients. His family *nuskhah* ('recipe') had been formulated by his father, the first hakim in the family, and it was the only medicine given out at that *maṭabb*: a special heart tonic that, judging from the number of patients queuing outside the clinic early in the morning, seemed to enjoy a great popularity among different sections of the city's population (Schmidt Stiedenroth 2019a). This hakim's son, who had a BUMS degree, also practiced in the clinic they run attached to their residence in a middle-class neighbourhood in Hyderabad.

In India, the production and marketing of medicines is regulated by the Drugs and Cosmetics Act, 1940. An amendment made in 2010 established that a good manufacturing practices (GMP) certificate should be issued to producers of Unani medicine in order to obtain a manufacturing license. However, practitioners like Hakim Sadiq, who manufacture their own medications in their dispensaries, do not require to adhere to GMP standards or any other regulations stipulated in the act (The Drugs and Cosmetics Act 1940, 33EEC (c)). In this way, the law not only recognizes, but also allows the use of exclusive knowledge as well as experience and experimentation when it comes to the preparation of drugs by hakims in their private practice. Standards, thus, are not universally applied to Unani medicines, and hakims legally retain autonomy regarding the preparation of medicines as long as they do not use banned ingredients such as musk.

During my search for practitioners in the Phydoonie area of Mumbai, I met a man in his early forties who had a shop selling Unani medicines where he also offered free consultations. I asked him questions about clinical practice, but he kept avoiding answering those. As it turned out, he did not see many patients, as he was mostly busy with his own manufacturing company and his activism within the Unani fraternity (which included being the editor of a small Unani magazine). He seemed apologetic while explaining why he hardly saw any patients. I asked him about his company, and he showed me some printed advertisements and packaged medicines, he gave me a free sample of a syrup for menstrual pain. He said that these were his own recipes, 'the product of my own experimentation and trial with patients'. This was his own wording, in English. By experimentation and trial, this practitioner did not mean modern scientific research, but rather an aspect ubiquitous in Unani medical practice: the testing of different treatments and the observation of its effects on patients. I later spoke to his elder brother, who also practiced Unani. Unlike his younger brother, he neither spoke

English nor did he pursue formal Unani education. He told me that he teased his younger brother by telling him that a degree means nothing. I asked him why he said so? He opened his eyes widely and said that experience is very important: 'What is a degree without experience?' The man told me later about his own recipes, and explained that many hakims keep their knowledge secret, but he was willing to share his knowledge because it was something that god has given to him. As proof of that, he wrote down a recipe for me. The first letters of each ingredient formed the name of the formula. He told me that in this way, sharing knowledge was easier, as we both would remember the ingredients just by remembering the name of the compound. Interestingly, this recipe included neither instructions nor measurements, it was merely a list of ingredients.

In a similar way, Hakim Sadiq claimed to have created his own formulations. Although some of them had common names, he assured me that they were variations of the classical formulations, and that I would not find the same medicines anywhere else. His son Sabir also told me this one time as I was copying one of his prescriptions: there was no point for me in copying the names of the medicines because those medicines were only available there. Exclusiveness was very important for Hakim Sadiq's monetary income, because he did not charge for the consultations and only earned through the therapies. He had one powder for weight loss which was packaged in a plastic container with a coloured printed label that included a picture of him and his name. The rest of the medicines were individually packed for each patient by the *davāsāz* in inconspicuous containers: electuaries and stomachics in plastic tins, syrups in glass bottles, and powders and tablets in newspaper slips. Hakim Sadiq and his colleagues wrote prescriptions containing lists of ingredients and instructed the patients on how to prepare the decoctions at home. Patients were sent to buy the ingredients at a medicinal herb shop just around the corner.

For the practitioners I spent time with, adding uniqueness to their own practices was central for attaining reputation. It constitutes a way to create a signature treatment for those who do not have a family background and, thus, have not inherited *nuskhahjāt* ('recipes'). The creation of own efficacious prescriptions or formulae through experimentation and innovation allows practitioners without a familial background to establish a reputation on their own. Establishing an own lineage is possible, provided that there is unique and efficacious knowledge to be transmitted. This was the case of many of the family-hakims I met: even those trained in Unani colleges had the option of using their own experimentation and experience in order to produce unique knowledge and, through it, to establish an own lineage, as the example of the Unani heart clinic mentioned above or the case of Hakim Sadiq, whose knowledge was the product of his own self-study, demonstrate. These hakims profited from the democratization of Unani medicine, which allowed even for those without a renowned family background to attain a reputation as skilled hakims. I met several practitioners who claimed to be *k̲h̲āndānī* hakims and whose family lineage could be traced only a few generations back. For a few hakims the lineage consisted only of the self-taught father, as the case of Hakim Sabir or Hakim Azim. The idea of lineage suggests that it is a continuous chain of knowledge transmission, but except for elite families whose genealogies can be traced for centuries back, as claimed for example by Hakim Khalifatullah from Chennai and Hakim Zillurrahman from Bhopal, not all *k̲h̲āndānī* hakims nowadays can trace their lineages for many generations. In fact, only few hakims could trace their background for several generations. As the families of elite hakims enjoyed a better socio-economic position which allowed them to send their children to English medium schools, the better-off newer generations could opt for more prestigious degrees such as MBBS or studies abroad. With the decline of Unani medicine as elite medicine during the Colonial Period, the profession ceased to be attractive for the offspring of elite practitioners. Apart from that, some *k̲h̲āndānī* hakims did simply not have (male) children to pass on their knowledge, and their lineage died with them.

When a practitioner does not prepare medications on his own, uniqueness can be sought using other strategies. For example, Dr. Hussain, who practiced mainly biomedicine in Mumbai, told me that through his long experience and experimentation he had increased the recommended dosage of a certain antibiotic. This became clear while he explained to me how he was treating a patient whom he had diagnosed with cystitis. The patient was afraid of having a kidney failure, but Dr. Hussain assured him that he had nothing of the sort and that he would get well soon. The physician explained to me that he was treating the symptoms with Unani, Ayurvedic, and allopathic medicines. While he was preparing an injection for this patient, he turned to me with the filled syringe in his hand and explained that the usual dosage for that antibiotic was two cubic centimetres, but he used three cubic centimetres instead. He had augmented the dosage based on his experience through the years, and this is what made it a unique treatment. 'It is my uniqueness, my policy' he proudly said, explaining that no other doctor would do that, and that made him stand apart from other practitioners. 'It is not written in the books', he remarked. He further explained that he used the three cubic centimetres of that antibiotic for gonorrhoea, STDs in general and urine infections as he injected the medicine into one of the patient's buttocks.

The practice of Dr. Hussain is interesting because it reveals how biomedical drugs—in this case antibiotics—were prescribed following a prescription logic characteristic of Unani: one pursuing innovation through modification. While the over-usage of antibiotics in India is a subject on its own and it is embedded in a complex web of practices, including self-medication and wide availability through government support to the pharmaceutical industry, among others (Saradamma et al. 2000), Dr. Hussain's motivation to use a larger dosage than the recommended one was rooted in his interest to create a unique treatment in order to satisfy patients and enhance his reputation. Experimentation, thus, is not exclusive of practitioners involved in the manufacturing of medicines, nor of traditional hakims. Originality of practice is also open for those who rely on branded medicines, standard formulations or even allopathic drugs, as the practice of Dr. Hussain suggests.

Standardized Drugs

Standardization is considered one of the keys for the recognition of Unani medicine among the scientific community, it is seen as the basis to ensure the safety and quality of Unani drugs by the government authorities.[39] The standardization of Unani drugs is deemed a high-priority area because the safety and the reputation of Unani is considered to depend upon it. Standardization work is conducted in different institutions like for example the *'Ilm al-adviyah* ('Pharmacology') Department of the Ajmal Khan Tibbia College in Aligarh Muslim University. Its head, Dr. Abdullatif, explained that they check for contamination of the drugs included in the UPI and that they created standards for those medicines in the NFUM which had not been previously standardized. For this, they used the standards and parameters for herbal medicines laid down by the WHO.

The quality of raw materials has arguably deteriorated with the growing demand of herbal medicines, pointing out that the supply of medicinal plants for the production of medicines 'remains unwieldy within the unorganized sector' (Banerjee 2008: 203). In order to curb this development, the standardization of medicines takes place at three levels: raw materials, manufacturing processes, and final product (Banerjee 2004: 90). The standardization of raw materials is crucial because the efficacy of herbal medicines is ascribed to a variety of factors, including the place of growth of the plants (climate and soil condition, for example), the times for collection or harvest, as well

39 For a detailed description of the standardization process as conducted by the CCRUM, see Bright (1998: 172ff.).

as transportation and storage (Banerjee 2008: 203). Also, complaints of adulteration and substitution are not seldom. I once witnessed the arrival of the wrong herbs to the *Shifa Mahal* in Hyderabad. Hakim Sadiq ordered many of the raw materials he used for the production of the medicines in his *davāḵẖānah* from Khari Baoli, the medicinal herbs bazaar in Old Delhi. Every now and then, he received big sacks full of dried stems, roots, leaves and other plant parts arriving straight from Delhi. On one occasion, Hakim Sadiq found out that the herbs sent were not those he had played for. He got very angry and immediately made a phone call, shouting to the responsible never ever to attempt to fool him again. This episode gave shape to the claims of many hakims and manufacturers who had spoken about the problem of adulteration and substitution. At the same time, it was a reminder about the enormous value of knowledge of *shināḵẖat-i adviyah* ('identification of medicines'). Hakim Sadiq relied on his experience and knowledge of raw materials instead of on pharmacological standards, as he was skilled enough to assess the quality of the single drugs he purchased trusting his senses. A researcher from a department of *ʿilm al-adviyah* explained that before standardization, it was the hakims who conducted the quality control of the drugs. They knew for example that the medicinal properties of certain plants varied from the location where they were collected, hence some ingredients still bear the name of geographic regions, because it was known that the soil of that area made the medicinal plants better for medical purposes. In this way, he claimed, hakims were already aware of the fluctuations present in medicinal plants and recommended the use of those growing in a specific region.

The inclusion of Unani and other forms of traditional medicine in the Drugs and Cosmetics Act followed the recommendations made in the Mudalier Report, which promoted the emulation of standards used in biomedicine for traditional medicine. As a consequence, the production of Unani drugs was influenced by the adoption of standard procedures of production that have been imposed to the manufacturing of Unani products without taking into consideration the specificities of Unani drug production, which remained safeguarded only through hakims producing medicines at small-scale in their own *davāḵẖānahs*. The manufacturing standards employed in the large-scale production of Unani pharmaceuticals were introduced emulating biomedical standards, using biochemical parameters to define acceptable ranges that ensure the quality of the single drugs and classical compound formulations. In this way, pH levels or the exact amount of time that each ingredient takes to be digested are measured in order to meet the requirements of GMP. The NFUM sets the pharmacopoeial standards for

Unani medicines in India, and as such it has not only contributed to obtain a certain homogeneity in terms of quality of Unani medicines, but it has also served the purposes of Unani pharmaceutical companies seeking to manufacture classical formulas using cheap substitution ingredients, as discussed in the previous chapter. Standards, thus, do not always fulfil the purpose of raising the quality of medicines, on the contrary: they can also actually lower their quality and, with it, the reputation of Unani medicine, as feared by some informants.

The shelf life established in the Drugs and Cosmetics Act 1940 (rule 161-B, iii) for Unani medicines is a particularly interesting case. The director of a RRIUMs told me in a conversation that the 'best before' or expiry date concept was problematic when applied to Unani medicines. According to him, it was a new concept that did not exist when hakims or their family members used to prepare the medicines by themselves. It was the other way around, he argued, as hakims would say 'I have a very special medicine, it is very old!' In this sense, medicines were like wine: the older the medicine, the better. Today, he claimed, the idea that old medicines are more powerful was still in the minds of some old people in India. He regretted that hakims were compelled to throw away the medicines after the 'best before' date, although the medicines may not have expired yet and, depending on the formula, they may even be more potent than before. Also, those practicing privately have to do the same, he went on, as they could not convince some of the young patients anymore that the medicine may still be good, or even better. 'Best before', he vehemently argued, was not the same as 'date of expiry'. According to him, some of the medicines which did not improve with time did not lose their properties completely, only their effect was reduced to the extent that to obtain the desired results, larger quantities were required. He claimed that neither 'best before' nor the 'date of expiry' of Unani medicines could be compared with allopathic medicines, which could be harmful if administered after expiration.

Interestingly, the Drugs and Cosmetics Act exempts certain Ayurvedic and Siddha drugs from the 'best before' regulation, arguing that their efficacy increases with time (Rule 161-B, i). Although some Unani preparations also become 'even better' with the passage of time, no such exception applied for any Unani medicine: the act established a date of expiry ranging from one to five years for all Unani drugs (Government of India 1940: Rule 161-B, iii). Products whose date of manufacture goes back beyond the established shelf life 'shall not be in circulation' (ibid.). A producer of Unani drugs explained that to deal with this legal situation, the concerned products were packaged only after they had been 'ripening' in containers in the production units for some time ranging from weeks to years. The date of manufacturing printed on the label, thus, did not necessarily correspond to the actual date of manufacturing but could refer to the date of packaging instead. In this way, this producer had found a suitable way to stick to the regulations without compromising the quality of his Unani products. It is significant that in spite of the commonality of this practice—I heard of several manufacturers who proceeded in a similar way—, the regulations have not been adjusted to meet the requirements specific to Unani medicines, as in the case of Siddha and Ayurveda. This leads to a situation where regulations aiming to ensure the quality and safety of Unani medicines, which assumed that standards used for biomedical pharmaceuticals have a universal application, turn out to minder their efficacy.

Because hakims making medicines in their own *davāk̲h̲ānahs* were exempted from the regulations of the Drugs and Cosmetics Act, it could be argued that the traditional forms of drug production and storage are considered by authorities to be safe enough not to be prohibited. Hence, the introduction of standards for the regulation of Unani pharmaceuticals is not only explained by external pressure such as that of the WHO or the global market of CAM, but also by a necessity to protect the public against unscrupulous producers of fake or low-quality products who do not care about 'defaming' the name of Unani medicine in order to make money. Unani producers complaining about this kind of producers explained that the problem of low-quality Unani products could not be solved through the regulations alone. They demanded more control and law enforcement from the authorities to curb adulteration and ensure safety through the implementation of GMP. While the regulations exemplify how the production of Unani medicines was modernized emulating biomedical pharmaceutical principles, these examples reveal how Unani resists biomedicalization as producers manage to defy standards in order to ensure the quality of their products.

Variations of Medicine and Multiplicity

Differences in medicine do not constitute a temporary disruption or anomaly, but should be seen as an intrinsic part of it (Mol and Berg 1998). Diversity is often considered problematic in biomedicine by those involved in its practice, and coordination work is done in order to align the variations (ibid.). The case of Unani medicine is different, as variations seem to have always been on the agenda. In Graeco-Islamic medical encyclopaedias and handbooks, the descriptions of diseases and their treatments follow a standardized scheme that seems characteristic of Persian medical literature

(Kurz and Reichmuth 2012). Yet the texts did not go into details regarding the patients, the environment and other aspects considered therapeutically vital according to theoretical works (ibid.). This omission presupposes an individual application of the standards: 'Anamnesis and treatment laid on the expertise of each practicing physician and did not have to or could not be presented in a standard or general way' (Kurz and Reichmuth 2012: 240, my translation). This argument can be applied to contemporary Unani medicine, as hakims adapt therapies to patients' responses. Further, exclusive knowledge continues to be an important source of professional authority among private practitioners of Unani in spite—or perhaps precisely because—of the introduction of medical degrees and registration. As Guy Attewell aptly pointed out, Unani was never a homogeneous system of medicine, hence its newly organized profession could never constitute a single authoritative group (2007). This aspect continues to characterize the professional Unani landscape, where claims of authority, legitimacy and authenticity by different Unani professionals enact Unani in multiple, yet not always contradictory or mutually exclusive, ways. Because variations in Unani are not just tolerated but are—moreover—expected, we may argue that multiplicity is inherent to Unani.

The pursuit for treatment originality followed by hakims on a small scale continued to operate under the logic that the medical practitioner was the authority capable to discern between benefit and detriment and what was best for patients. The practice of the private hakims I observed continues to be more 'eminence-based' than evidence-based (Schmidt Stiedenroth 2019a). In contrast, the standardization of Unani practice in institutional settings through a common teaching curriculum and a limited number of available drugs in the clinics leaves little room for physicians' innovation. Moreover, the nature of institutionalized settings itself makes the physicians' pursuit of originality redundant: as government employees, their income does not depend upon their reputation, hence they do not require to satisfy their patients as private practicing hakims do.

While the institutionalization of training and practice sought to systematize Unani in search for its acceptance and recognition, it has failed to establish itself as an exclusive source of Unani medical authority. As college training alone cannot produce good hakims, old sources of professional recognition remain in place, being peers and patients often more important than recognized degrees and legal status. Because *tajribah* remains an important legitimating factor, even those hakims without a family background can build up a reputation on their own, and many *k̲h̲āndānī* hakims today do not belong to a centuries-old lineage of physicians, but are rather third, second, or even the first generation to practice Unani thanks to self-study and experimentation.

The idea of uniqueness and variation in medical practice has been thought to contradict the notion that medicine, as a science, should not leave room for variations as it should be, instead, a coherent and standardized unit (Mol and Berg 1998: 7). But as Gananath Obeyesekere argued for the case of clinical falsification in Ayurveda, 'the generation of new medical prescriptions is possible because Āyurveda is a science of medicine' (1992: 172). The same applies for Unani, where the creation of new knowledge by practitioners through clinical experimentation at an individual level not only characterizes its practice, but it is considered its virtue. The art of Unani is as important as its science.

The situation in contemporary India suggests that either the government authorities were sensitive enough to recognize the value of an individualized approach in Unani medicine by not interfering in the imposition of standards at all levels, or that they failed to implement regulations such as those pertaining to registration. Whatever the case may be, there is room left for variations, allowing for different forms of knowledge production and legitimation to coexist, each enacting a different Unani.

The apparent ontological tension between the cohesiveness enacted through systematization and the multiplicity of practices of Unani medicine is defused when examined though Mol's theoretical framework (2002). As discussed in the previous chapter, Unani is construed as a coherent system of medicine by unifying efforts that establish what it is through coordination work, while at the same time allowing it to remain flexible in practice. Unani's inherent multiplicity, as discussed in this chapter, defies any efforts of standardization, and even in times of standardized packed medicines and college degrees, some Unani practitioners manage to create their own singular knowledge and, with it, to establish their own professional authority based on individual practice. It is through distribution in Mol's sense, i.e. the coexistence of multiple, incompatible realities but the enactment of only one of them at a particular time and place (2002: 96ff.), that Unani medicine can be a system of medicine characterized by multiple practices that defy some of the standards that define it in other contexts.

3. Beyond Humouralism

During a long conversation with Hakim Zillurrahman at his residence in Aligarh in 2012, I asked him to define Unani medicine in one single sentence. He began talking about the temperaments and the four humours and their importance as they constitute the basis of Unani. He explained that they are central because through their observation, a physician can establish the cause of the disease, and knowing the cause is crucial for the selection of appropriate treatment. Hakim Zillurrahman argued that excess of one humour caused imbalance and that, when there is imbalance, the human body becomes susceptible to disease. Unlike in allopathy, he went on, in Unani medicine there is the idea that disease is caused by the dominance of one humour. Therefore, the line of treatment has to address that excess humour. Medicines give the body *ṭ̤āqat* ('strenght') to heal itself. Therefore, he stressed, the cause of disease has a central role in Unani, and this is the main idea on which the system is based. Now, if Unani had to be defined in one sentence, he would say temperaments, humours, and *arkān* ('elements'), as the system is based on them. 'That is Unani identity, because there is no other system based on the four humours and addressing the issue of cause of disease', he concluded.

Hakim Zillurrahman's emphasis on elements, temperaments, and especially humours as Unani's identity reflected the answers given by hakims and Unani graduates when asked what Unani medicine is. Similarly, the scholarly study of Unani medicine has been characterized by representing Unani as a humoural form of medicine. In their study of Medieval Graeco-Islamic medicine, Peter Pormann & Emilie Savage-Smith argued that '[t]he single most pervasive explanatory medical principle was that of humoral pathology inherited from the Greeks' (2007: 43). The understanding of humoural balance in the body as a healthy state and that of humoural imbalance as disease was attributed to Hippocrates (Pormann and Savage-Smith 2007: 9) and embodied the ambivalent relationship between Unani medicine and Western science: on the one hand, humouralism stood as evidence of a common origin and, as such, of a strong historical connection between both. On the other hand, it materialized the breach between Unani and Western science from the nineteenth and twentieth centuries based on the rejection of humouralism through the emergence of modern science and the discovery of the germ theory.

While humouralism has been widely accepted as the epistemological framework of Unani and other forms of medicine, a recent publication has challenged the centrality of this theory in so-called humoural medical traditions (Horden and Hsu 2013). It may be asked, then, if these claims can be extended to the current practice of Unani medicine and, if yes, what the implications could be. The present chapter focuses on the role of humoural (im)balance in the practice of Unani physicians and its theoretical underpinnings. Here, I focus on hakims practicing privately and not in institutionalized settings. I start by exploring the concept of medicine and the fundamental principles of human physiology presented in textual sources and by hakims themselves, to conclude with a discussion about humouralism and looping effects.

Fundamental Principles of Unani Medicine

The Concept of Medicine and the Principles of Human Physiology

In his book *Uṣūl-i Ṭibb* ('Principles of Medicine'), which was conceived for Unani college students, Said Kamaluddin Hussain Hamdani defined *'ilm-i ṭibb* ('medical knowledge' or 'medical science') as:

> That knowledge that discusses health and lack of health with regard to the human body, or where the decline of health is discussed so that if health has been acquired it can be protected, and if health has been extinguished, meaning that disease has arisen, then it can try to recover health (Hamdānī 2011 [1998]: 29).

This definition of medicine as a science of health and its decline as well as its preservation and restoration clearly reflects the definition of medicine provided by Ibn Sina in his *Qānūn,*[40] which remains the accepted definition in contemporary Unani medicine. Both cure and prevention, or *ḥifāẓat-i ṣiḥḥat* ('preservation of health'), are considered central aspects of medical science. In this context, the *asbāb-i sittah ẓarūriyah* ('six essential factors') play an important role. These factors are considered to necessarily influence the human body, because humans cannot live without them: air and environment, food and drinks, physical activity and rest, mental activity and rest,

40 '*Ṭibb* (Medicine) is the science by which the states of the human body, regarding health and decline of health, are identified: its purpose is to preserve health if its already attained and to restore it when it is lost' (Ibn Sīnā 1993: 1). Ibn Sina's definition of medicine, in turn, derived from Galen's treatise *On [medical] Sects for Beginners* (Pormann and Savage-Smith 2007: 41).

sleep and wakefulness, as well as evacuation and retention. The importance of these factors for the preservation of health is reflected in sayings such as 'Let food be thy medicine and let thy medicine be food', a famous quote attributed to Hippocrates. Apart from the six-essential factors, Unani books also address the *asbāb g̠hair ẓarūriyah* ('non-essential causes') which may, or may not, influence the body and thus health. These include geographical conditions, housing, occupation, habits, age, and gender (Ahmed 2009 [1980]).

Hakims consider the human body as capable of healing itself thanks to a self-preservation power or faculty. This concept of *quvvat-i mudabbirah* ('self-preservation') is the equivalent of the concept of *medicatrix naturae* attributed to Hippocrates. Its Greek legacy is centered on the idea of *ṭabīʿat* ('physis' or 'nature'). In everyday Urdu usage, *ṭabīʿat* refers to temperament and mind disposition and is related to health and well-being. Asking someone about his *ṭabīʿat* is a common greeting set phrase in Urdu-speaking contexts. Hakim Faruqi from Lucknow asserted that to understand Unani medicine one had to understand that 'nature itself is the physician.' As an example, he explained that if someone cuts his finger and it bleeds, the blood will come like the 'military' (he used the English word). He would tell the patient to press the finger and hold it high, in this way the patient would prevent the 'military' from coming. Similarly, he went on, cough is not a disease. It is a bodily reaction to expel phlegm when there is an excess of it, or a natural reaction when there is itching in the throat. We can scratch other body parts with our fingers, he argued, but we cannot scratch our throat, and this is why we cough. In this way, *ṭabīʿat* ('nature') is the *ṭabīb* ('physician'): the body itself knows what to do. As a further example, the hakim mentioned what happens when a person gets an upset stomach when he did not check the food before ingesting it. It is no coincidence, he stated, that the nose is just above the mouth. A person is supposed to check (smell) the food before eating it. But supposing that a person did not do it and gets an upset stomach, what does the *ṭabīʿat* do? It causes vomiting. The vomiting is good, because the person will be expelling the poisoning food. And what will the *ṭabīb* do? He would give water to the patient. Water will induce vomiting, which should continue until all the bad food has been expelled. Water would also prevent dehydration caused by vomiting. A physician has to twist nature ('*ṭabīb ṭabīʿat ko mūṛnā hai*'), in this case the physician would give chili to the patient. Through this, the next time that the patient drinks water the *ṭabīʿat* ('bodily nature') will not induce vomit because the stomach will need the water to neutralize the hot chili. Through this measure, the physician would curb dehydration. The body, he concluded, heals itself, the hakim helps but, ultimately, healing is in god's hands.

Unani literature classifies medical knowledge (or medical science) under theory (i.e. the knowledge about the fundamental principles) and practice (i.e. knowledge about health, diseases and their treatments). Canonical texts such as Ibn Sina's *Qānūn* or Jurjani's *Ẕakẖīrah* (which was influenced by the *Qānūn*) further classify medical knowledge under the following sections: a) *Kulliyāt- i umūr- i ṭabī'īyah* ('Works on the principles of physiology'), b) *Kulliyāt-i asbābo amrāẕo agẖarāẕ* ('Works on the causes of diseases and necessities'), c) *Kulliyāt nabẕ baul o barāz* ('Works on pulse, urine and motions'), d) *Kulliyāt-i adviyah* ('Works on drugs'), and e) *Kulliyāt-i 'ilāj yā uṣūl-i 'ilāj* ('Works on treatment or principles of treatment') (Hamdānī 2011 [1998]: 27). The principles of human physiology encompass the understanding of the *bunyādī uṣūl* ('fundamental principles'),[41] including what constitutes the human body (microcosm) and how the body stands in relation to the universe (macrocosm). As for the body, the fundamental principles include *arkān* or *'anāṣir* ('the four elements'), i.e. earth, water, fire, and air; and their *kaifiyyat* ('qualities'), i.e. *garam* or *ḥār* ('hot'), *sard* or *bārid* ('cold'), *kẖushk* or *yābis* ('dry') and *tar* or *raṭb* ('moist') which determine the *mizāj* ('temperament') of individuals as well as of substances like drugs and objects like the organs of the human body. The *kaifiyyat* ('qualities') mentioned above play a crucial role when it comes to establish the cause of disease, and hence, its treatment. The four humours are considered particular of the human body, they are characterized by the four qualities, too: the temperament of blood (*dam* or *kẖūn*) is hot and moist, that of phlegm (*balgẖam*) is cold and moist, yellow bile (*ṣafrā'*) is hot and dry, and black bile (*saudā*) is cold and dry. Apart from these, *a'ẕā'* ('tissues' or 'organs'), *arvāḥ* ('pneumata', also referred to as 'soul' or 'vital spirits'), *quvvā'e* ('faculties' or 'powers'), and *af'āl* ('functions') are components of the human body and are considered to be part of the fundamental principles of Unani medicine (Ahmed 2009 [1980]; Azmi 1995; Kabīruddīn 1934). The human body and its parts are directly connected to the outer world, hakims consider health and disease to be the product of the interactions between them, as elaborated below.

'What is First'

In concordance to Graeco-Islamic textual sources, modern textbooks on Unani medical theory consider health and disease as the product of four

41 Sometimes also called *kulliyāt*. Attewell referred to them as 'the so-called "foundational principles" (*usul al-tibb* or *usul-i tibb*, or *kullyat*)' (2013: 129). *Kulliyāt* refers to the subject that includes basic sciences such as philosophy and logic, history of medicine, and the fundamentals of Unani medicine (Aligarh Muslim University 2014b).

kinds of causes following Aristotelian philosophy. Hamdani explained them as follows: the *asbāb māddiyah* ('material causes') 'are the causes in which health and disease are present, i.e. the elements, humours, organs and pneumas', the *asbāb fāʿiliyah* ('efficient causes') 'are the causes which create alterations or changes in the human body, or which preserve it. For instance, the essential and non-essential causes', the *asbāb ẓarūriyah* ('necessary' or 'formal causes') 'for instance temperament and faculties and composition', and the *asbāb tamāmiyah* ('final causes') 'whose example are the functions' (Hamdānī 2011 [1998]: 145). According to Hamdani, if the causes of the human body (*asbāb badan-i insān*) mentioned above are maintained in moderation, then health is preserved (ibid.).

Unani literature discusses the causes of disease under the subject *Kulliyāt-i asbāb o amrāẓ o ag͟harāẓ* ('works on the causes of diseases and necessities'). As the name suggests, failure to meet the necessities of the body leads to diseases. The causes of disease are complex, and it is beyond the scope of this book to discuss their theory in detail.[42] However, it is important for us to know that they influence one another. For example, the faculties may become impaired influenced by a negative environment, bad dietary habits, or high levels of stress, all of which influence a person's humoral balance and, thus, the restorative nature. An impairment of the faculties may influence the organs, creating problems for their proper functioning. Hence, a person gets sick because her *ṭabīʿat* ('nature') cannot function properly due to disorders or imbalances rooted in the causes, among which the six-essential and the non-essential factors, as efficient and thus primary causes for change, were central. When *ṭabīʿat* is impaired, other diseases (secondary diseases) may arise as the body makes efforts to restore or cope with an impaired bodily function or any state affected by a primary disease, creating further deficiencies or excesses.

In the Urdu version of *Kulliyāt-i Nafīsī*, Hakim Kabiruddin explained the *asbāb* ('causes') of health and disease as *'jo pehle ho'* ('what is first') (1934: 184). Unlike many representations of Unani medicine, the theory of causation of health and disease, which also corresponds to the one presented by Ibn Sina, is not centred on the balance of the humours, but it is rather based on complex entanglements between responses to causes inside the body (such as the organs and their functioning) as well as outside of it (environment, climate, food, etc). These, in turn, are intimately connected to the humours and their temperaments and hence, with their balance (see Ibn Sīnā 1993). When dealing with a disease and explaining its cause,

42 For a detailed overview see Kabīruddīn (1934).

however, textual sources like the *Aksīr-i Aʿẓ am* dealing with the practical aspects of medicine often refer to humoral imbalances as the cause of disease (Kabīruddīn n.d.). For example, *yarqān* ('jaundice') is said to be caused by a flow of non-putrefied bilious and melancholic humours towards the skin and its connected parts (Kabīruddīn n.d.: 542). Here, it is important to note that this kind of practical text takes theoretical knowledge of Unani medicine for granted. In this way, the author addresses the material cause of disease only, as he expects the reader to know that material causes represent manifestations of diseases and are, in turn, connected to efficient, formal and final causes as well. This becomes clear when we examine how hakims arrange treatments.

Diseases

A *k̲h̲āndānī* hakim who formerly directed a reputed Unani college in North India and still practiced privately stated that the treatments given in Unani were all about whirling the humours. He explained that different diseases arose from humoral changes which could be caused by external forces that cannot be controlled ('*g̲h̲air marẓī*'), for example when there is sunshine or it gets cold, or by things that can be controlled, for example food. According to him, all diseases are initially *damavī* ('sanguine'), *balg̲h̲amī* ('phlegmatic') or even *ṣafrāvī* ('choleric'), but when they become chronic, their temperament turns *saudāvī* ('melancholic'). When that stage has arrived, he explained, the physician should focus on treating the excess of black bile (*saudā*).

When talking to patients, hakims occasionally refer to the temperament or quality of a disease. For instance, calculi of any sort are considered to be hot diseases (*garmī*), one hakim explained that renal calculi (*gurde kī pathrī*) is a *ṣafrāvī* disease, i.e. caused by excess of yellow bile. Liver diseases are considered to be caused by cold, and so are paralysis, joint pain (often referred to as rheumatoid arthritis), and sinus problems. These are linked to an excess of phlegm produced by cold. A prominent phlegmatic disease is *ṣudāʿ* ('migraine'), Hakim Ahmad explained that it is caused when phlegm dries up and gets stuck in the head, producing blockages that cause headaches. He also held excess phlegm responsible for hair loss and grey hair at an early age.

Hakim Sadiq often told his patients that they do not have a disease, but a disorder. When asked what he means by that, he explained that a disorder cannot be cured by a doctor. This is the case for example when someone has a running nose, but it does not go away with the doctor's treatment. As another example he mentioned menstrual complaints which, according to him, are not a disease but a disorder related to black bile. If this disorder is not treated, he argued, it becomes a disease, like for example polycystic disease. Thus, following Hakim Sadiq, a disorder is an impairment of normal bodily functions related to humoural imbalance which could cause disease if not corrected. Following this logic, for Hakim Sadiq there is not such a thing as mental illness (*nafsyātī marẓ*), as he once explained to a patient. 'Depression, tension, emotion, these are not diseases, these are disorders!' The patient insisted about having 'trouble' (*pareshān*), but the hakim was emphatic: 'What? You are a mental patient, you don't have any disease, it's a disorder. There is no cure for that in the whole world.' He advised the patient to abstain from sour and cold foods and said that as long as he keeps the regimen, he will be fine.[43] By saying that there was no cure, the hakim did not mean that the patient could not be treated. Rather, he was insisting that the condition has to be managed and cannot be eliminated with drugs only, requiring a constant effort from the patient's side to maintain the regime instead. Hakim Sadiq's concept of mental health (and disease) reflected Galen's idea that 'the faculties of the soul depend on the mixtures of the body and we derive a good mixture from our food and drink and other daily activities and this mixture is the basis on which we build the virtue of the soul' (cit. in Farage 2008: 23), whereby mental problems arise as a consequence of disorders caused by external factors (including essential and non-essential causes) which in turn affect humoral balance and the soul. It should be noted here that the Arabic *nafs* means psyche, i.e. mind, soul or spirit. Consequently, translating *nafsyatī* as 'mental' or even 'psychological' does not constitute a Westernizing exercise. However, one should be cautious as not to assume that approaches to treatment in Unani follow the exact same logic as in biomedicine, especially in the case of a shared etymology of Greek origin.

Most of the patients came to the *Shifa Mahal* after having received biomedical treatment and not being satisfied with its results. This was the case for most Unani practitioners as well as other practitioners of indigenous medicine in India (cf. Naraindas 2014b: 114). Hakim Sadiq often complained that biomedical doctors do not address the disorders, which he termed the actual cause (*sabab*) of the disease. He accused biomedical doctors for treating only secondary diseases and not the primary ones that caused them. Because of this, patients did not get well in spite of being under biomedical treatment, which was either based on a wrong diagnosis or was symptomatic,

43 The patient had been diagnosed by a biomedical doctor with a brain hematoma.

neglecting the actual cause of the disease. To make this point, he told me to present a case of hyperthyroidism as a special case in my thesis:

> The patient had been in the *maṭabb* a couple of days before. Hakim Sadiq asked her to approach the desk and told me to note down the details of this case. The patient was a ten-year-old girl, she was wearing an *anārkalī*[44] and fancy earrings. Her cheeks and throat were swollen. Her face seemed like the face of a fat person, but the rest of her body was slim, with a complexion that looked normal for her age. I smiled at her several times but every time she looked away, apathetic. Hakim Sadiq told me to write:
> 'Zeenat Ji – 10 years old
> Hyperthyroidism
> Patient is on tablet Thyroden 75mg per day
> Swelling of cheeks'
> The hakim told me that the patient had been under his treatment for two days and asked her: 'How much improvement?' The mother of the patient, who was standing beside her, said that she was much better as she touched her own cheeks. Hakim Sadiq asked: 'Fifty per cent relief?' and the mother answered yes. He turned to me and said: 'The doctor gave her medicines for thyroid, but thyroid is the secondary disease. That... What am I doing? Sinus is her primary disease, it is because of sinus that there is thyroid.[45]

This case exemplifies that, for Hakim Sadiq, the biomedical treatment for hyperthyroidism was not working for this patient because it was not addressing the primary disease identified by him as 'sinus', a term commonly used in India to refer to a blockage of the sinus cavity which can range from a running nose to sinusitis. To be effective, the treatment had to address the causes of the sinus problem. In the *Qānūn*, Ibn Sina explained that primary diseases are often not noticed until the secondary disease appears, and that a primary disease is that which still persists even after the disappearance of the other (1993: 189). Further, he argued that knowledge of anatomy and how the organs are related to each other is crucial for discerning if a disease is primary or secondary (ibid.). Hakim Sadiq shared this view. He often argued that biomedical doctors failed to distinguish between primary and

44 A women's long dress worn over tights-like trousers.

45 'Thyroid' was a colloquial term commonly used in Urdu to address both hypo- and hyperthyroidism, similarly to the usage of 'BP' ('blood pressure') to address hypo- and hypertension.

secondary diseases, addressing only the latter. In doing so they provided relief—if at all—to the symptoms only, and as a consequence the problems of the patients continued.

Hakim Sadiq compared biomedicine to Unani arguing that biomedicine considered each organ separately, while Unani looked for the cause of disease. Once he told a patient: 'What is Unani? In modern medicine, the organs are separate from each other. The way we see it, there are no diseases of the organs, it is humoral causes. Black bile, yellow bile, phlegm and blood, it is a thing of four humours.' Diseases, he argued, were caused by humoural imbalances and, consequently, the treatments should address these as well as the causes producing those imbalances.

Unani physicians did not always communicate aetiologies to their patients. Most of the time, patients received a diagnosis and recommendations related to them but not a complete explanation of the causes of the complaints. The causation of diseases was often identified tacitly, often I could only find out more about it when I directly asked the practitioners. In a moment when there were no patients in his *maṭabb*, Hakim Ahmad and I discussed the causes of calculi and fibroids. He told me about gallbladder stones, which in Unani are called *ḥiṣāt-i mas̱ānah,* explaining that the disease is *ṣafrā'ī* ('bilious') and *damī* ('sanguine'). Not only that: 'If phlegm dries up, it can also happen.' I asked him if the phlegm dries because of dryness and he said yes. He showed me an article that he had written for the newspaper, it read that the incidence of gallbladder stones was higher in the North-Indian belt. 'Also, kidney stones are caused by dryness, migraine also.' I asked what about fibroids? He said: 'Not fibroids. Fibroids are abnormal tissues. They develop from soft tissues [...] There are blood fillings in the internal [uterine] walls, from the menses, abnormal tissue develops from them.' Hakim Ahmad told me that he treated them with medicines that expelled the blood and the abnormal tissue through contractions along with the menstrual fluid. He said that women were prone to them 'after pregnancy or during puberty' and that fibroids were just earth and water, which gets hard when it dries up. 'Tissues adopt the form of fibroids, and in this way a cyst appears also.' He said that lifestyle, especially diet, has a big influence on the formation of this problem. Hence, while Hakim Ahmad identified the formation of stones with the dominance of certain humours (*ṣafrā* and *dam*), he articulated the causes of uterine fibroids in relation to specific periods in life, lifestyle and diet. Also, the influence of the climate was implied through the notion that the disease was more common in the North-Indian belt, a region considered to be drier than Mumbai.

Treatments and Prevention

Hakim Faruqi distinguished two categories of treatment: *ʿilāj bi-l misl* ('treatment through like') and *ʿilāj bi-ẓ ẓidd* ('treatment through opposites'). While the first is translated as homeopathy (*similia similibus curantur*), the latter corresponds to the principle of *contraria contrariis curantur* which is attributed to Hippocrates and refers to curing with the opposites.[46] This hakim explained that Unani uses the latter. The medicines used by hakims either increase or decrease the heat in the inner body, their use depends on the quality of the disease. Since diseases are characterized by bodily imbalance due to the prevalence of specific qualities, Unani therapies operate within this framework in order to counterbalance the action of an excessively dominant quality in the human body. According to most hakims, the first step in the treatment of a disease consists in neutralizing its temperament following the principle of *ʿilāj bi-ẓ ẓidd*. Therefore, if a person suffers from a disease considered to be hot, hakims would prescribe cold medicines in order to neutralize the heat affecting the humoral balance and causing the disease. For long term results and as a preventive measure, hakims would additionally recommend *parhez* ('abstinence') from food having the same quality as the disease.

Hakims classify drugs and food according to their qualities and temperaments: *garam* ('hot'), *sard* or *ṭhanḍā* ('cold'), *khaṭṭā* ('sour'), and *mīṭhā* ('sweet'), each being either cooling or heating. In Unani medical texts we find a classification of single drugs—including herbs and spices as well as fruits and vegetables commonly used in South Asian cuisine—according to the four qualities hot, cold, moist and dry (see Table 1). These qualities are used to manage disease following the concept of *ʿilāj bi-ẓ ẓidd*, whereby diseases considered cold are treated with warm producing food and medicines, whereas cold diseases with warm producing ones, or through abstinence of foods depending on the temperament of the disease.

In practice, the application of this principle is not as simple as it may appear. Malaria, for example, is considered a hot disease. However, patients may suffer from shivering and actually feel cold in phases when the body temperature drops. A patient suffering from malaria and feeling cold once asked a hakim if he could eat cold foods, but the hakim scolded him, pointing out that it was common sense to avoid cold foods when one feels cold.

46 While this may be translated as allopathy—in contrast to homeopathy—, such translation is not used among the Unani fraternity because in the South Asian context the term allopathy is reserved for biomedicine.

However, he prescribed antipyretics (of cold temperament) for this patient. The treatment, thus, is not necessarily guided by the symptoms, but by the quality attributed to the disease.

Hakims emphasize that Unani treatments are effective in the long term. This is regarded as one of the most important assets of Unani medicine vis-à-vis biomedicine. Hakim Ahmad and I discussed the case of a patient with haemorrhoids. He told me that the patient suffered from constipation and this is why piles appeared, the reason being *k̲h̲ushkī* ('dryness'). He explained: 'in the case of piles, the muscles of the anal canal have to endure for a long term, a tumour-like structure emerges.' He addressed the problem through dietary changes, the reduction of meat consumption in particular, to normalize the motions. Hakim Ahmad asserted that in Unani piles are removed using drugs, whereas in allopathy the patients are subjected to surgery, whereby the piles are removed but tend to come back, thus failing to provide a long-term cure. Hakims often stressed that their treatments take time, and compared Unani with biomedicine to make this point clear to their patients: while biomedicine can offer quick relief through surgery or symptomatic treatment, they claimed that being patient in Unani is worth it, as the disease will be eradicated from its root. Hakim Sadiq once said: 'The patient wants it to happen quickly, but an accident happens if the car runs fast!' Addressing the root cause of diseases, which is often related to lifestyle changes, bears the disadvantage of taking a long time to yield results. However, once recovered, patients are said to be cured once and for all, or at least as long as they adhere to the recommended measures.

Finding the Root Cause of Disease

Observation and Questioning

The first thing a good hakim should do when a patient sets foot into the *maṭabb*, so I was often told, is to observe. Physicians claimed to gain information about the patients' *taklīf* ('complaint'), their *ṭabīʿat*, and *mizāj* primarily through observation. For example, one hakim explained, a patient of choleric temperament would move from one chair to another and would not be able to sit quietly, whereas a phlegmatic person would be very quiet and only rarely get angry. Observation, however, is almost always complemented with questioning. In spite of common representations of Unani stressing the role of pulse and even uroscopy, observation and questioning constitute the most important forms of diagnosis in Unani clinical practices. It is often on the basis of them that physicians decide if further diagnostic procedures are required. When new patients came, Unani physicians usually asked them first of all to state the reason for their visit. Very often, however, it was the patients themselves who started the conversations inside the *maṭabb* after sitting down on the chair set for them, close to the hakims, listing their complaints before the physician had even a chance to ask about them.

Practitioners rely primarily on questioning, this was evident when they wrote the prescriptions before taking the pulse, which is not an uncommon practice. Apart from the symptoms or complaints, questions often address the patient's sleep, how she passes urine or stool, what tastes she prefers, and how she reacts to foods of certain qualities, for example hot or cold. The importance of questioning is mentioned in influential classical texts. According to Ibn Sina, for example, questioning about the symptoms is necessary in order to find out if a disease is secondary or primary (1993: 190). While the narratives of skilled hakims emphasize the ability of being able to make a diagnosis without asking questions, questioning constitutes a very important method of diagnosis both in theory and practice. However, a few hakims show their skills not by not asking questions to their patients, but rather by anticipating their complaints. Hakim Azim told me that, thanks to his experience, after listening to one or two complaints mentioned by the patient, he was able to guess further complaints accompanying those. A good physician shall tell the patient what he has, and not the other way around, he said. This was commonly the case of patients coming with urine tract infections or women with gynaecological problems. Most patients were impressed when physicians asked them about the presence of certain complaints before they even mentioned them. This, however, was generally speaking rather the exception than the rule, as not all physicians could anticipate complaints. Hence, most of the time, hakims finished the questioning by asking patients: 'Anything else?'

In practice, observation does not only comprise paying attention to the patients' expression or behaviour, it also includes clinical examinations such as auscultation and palpation, depending on the case. Hakims commonly use a stethoscope when dealing with respiratory problems, and would palpate a patient in case of swelling—like that caused by hyperthyroidism, oedema or trauma—or pain—especially abdominal and back pain—, for example. One hakim routinely examined the eyes and tongue of patients. Differently, Hakim Sadiq often checked the throat and nose of his patients. Through these examinations, he often found diseases which patients did not complain about, but whose treatment was of primary importance to tackle the actual disease.

For example, he often diagnosed patients with *bavāsīr-i anaf* ('nasal polyps') which, according to him, blocked the oxygen supply and affected other organs and functions of the body, including vision. The following case illustrates how Hakim Sadiq combined different diagnostic methods in his consultations:

> Two men approached the hakim, one of them was a new patient. The patient was 37 years old. Hakim Sadiq checked his pulse in both arms, then he got up and touched the patient's cheeks and examined his throat and nose while I held the torchlight. The throat was reddened and seemed to have inflammation. The nose was reddened, too, and looked almost entirely blocked. The hakim said: 'It's all blocked, look at this!' and asked the patient about his job, he was a driver. Hakim Sadiq told him that he could get *fālij* ('paralysis') or 'thyroid'. He explained that the patient's blood had phlegm and told him not to eat cold, nor acidic foods, nor oil. Incredulous, the patient asked: 'Oil?' and the hakim answered 'Yes. Phlegm has increased in the blood, it comes from the cold, it has to be taken out.' Hakim Sadiq told them that with the medicines and *parhez* ('dietary restrictions') he will get better.
> Hakim Sadiq: Did you have a [blood] sugar test done?
> Patient: No
> Hakim Sadiq: You have to do a sugar test.
> The hakim told the patient that the sugar level was measured in fasting state and after eating. He explained that the test was important to see if he had or if he would get diabetes in the future.
> Hakim Sadiq: There is research going on in Unani, if you have to keep a dietary restriction then you have to follow it. […] You should eat without oil.
> The patient's companion asked the hakim to note down the dietary advice so that they would not forget. The hakim wrote a prescription.
> Hakim Sadiq: Is your stool clean?
> Patient: It is clean
> Hakim Sadiq: It [phlegm] also came to his liver. [To the patient] Do you go to sleep after eating? I will give you a decoction 'number seven', it is very necessary to drink the decoction.
> Hakim Sadiq noted down the ingredients for the *joshāndah* 'number seven' (his own formula) and its dosage. He explained to the patient how to prepare it and when to drink it. He prescribed medicines for four days, charging Rs. 110/- for each day. He noted the dietary advice on the backside of the decoction recipe: 'Lentils, mung beans, without oil, without sour.' Hakim Sadiq received the payment and said 'You should come back in four days and bring your urine.'

It is worth noting that in no moment the patient uttered his complaint: it was the hakim who told the patient what his problem was. This consultation shows that, for a first assessment, questioning and observation are very important, but before that this hakim examined the patient's pulse. Through pulse, questioning and observation, Hakim Sadiq identified excess of phlegm as the patient's problem. What mattered for him was that (excess) phlegm was circulating in the blood, this is why he advised to avoid foods classified as sour and cold, which are considered to be cold producing and hence to increase the amount of phlegm in the body. After four days of treatment and dietary restrictions, Hakim Sadiq would assess the patient's condition and reaction to the treatment following the clinical falsification method described in the previous chapter. He would also conduct an examination of the patient's urine. Still, further investigations (uroscopy and a blood sugar test) were required to obtain a better picture of the patient's state as well as of how the excess phlegm in the blood has further affected the patient.

Another *k̲h̲āndānī* hakim argued that questioning was essential to find out the root cause of disease, as the occupation of a patient or his dietary habits could sometimes easily explain the cause of disease. A patient working on the fields and being constantly exposed to sunlight would react differently to cold foods than a washerman who was in constant contact with water. In this way, eating cold foods could be beneficial for the farmer, but detrimental for the dhobi. Diagnosis, however, is not only about the root cause of disease, but also about the present condition and prognosis. Pulse examination is said to be among the best methods to obtain precisely this information.

Pulse Examination

Nabẓ ('pulse') is considered Unani's diagnostic method *per excellence*, even though nowadays very few hakims claim to be well versed in it. Its significance for medical practice is reflected in the numerous works dedicated to it. Galen is said to have composed 'eighteen books and eighty-nine small treatises on the causes of pulses, the distinction between pulses, and the art of prognosis from listening to pulses' (Farage 2008: 22), whereas Ibn Sina dedicated whole nineteen sections to the discussion of the pulse in his *Qānūn* (1993: 203ff.). Pulse, he stated, is to be felt at the wrist for reasons of accessibility and for being close to the heart. Pulse has many varieties—even normal pulse has—, some of them are linked to its frequency, similarity of strokes, degree of expansion, or strength.

Although in Urdu hakims spoke of pulse diagnosis as *nabẓ dekhnā* ('to see the pulse'), the pulse is felt through touch as physicians place two to four fingers over the radial artery on a patient's wrist in order to feel its contractive movement.[47] 'Seeing' the pulse is considered one of the most important practices in Unani medicine and it is argued that only a few excellent hakims could achieve its mastery. Some even spoke of seeing the pulse not as a practical skill to be learned through practice, but as a revelation that only seers, i.e. those close to god, could attain.[48] The idea of 'seeing' the pulse, thus, may derive from this understanding of pulse as a revelation to chosen ones. It is perhaps because of its elusive nature that narratives related to pulse diagnosis and *nabbāẓ* (hakims skilled in it) abound in representations of Unani.

In one of those rare moments where no patient was around, I asked Hakim Sadiq, who routinely felt his patients' pulse, what does he 'see' in it. He laughed and said 'Do I have to teach you the pulse also? Good!' Placing four fingers over my wrist, he explained: the first finger (index) was for the head and neck, he showed me with the other hand the area of the face and around his check while telling me this. The second (middle) finger was for the chest, he told me as he moved his hand around his chest to show me. The third (ring) finger was for the belly, while the fourth (little) finger was for the kidneys and the lower part of the body. As one of his staff members spoke to Hakim Sadiq and he immediately got up and left, I could not ask him how he related what he 'sees' to the diseases or complaints of the patients.

Neither Hakim Sadiq nor any of the physicians whose practice I observed diagnosed using the pulse only. As discussed above, questioning and observing patients are also important aspects of the diagnostic routine, and so is the use of pathological examination reports. From the clinics I observed, the examination of *qārūrah* ('the first morning urine') was only practiced in the *Shifa Mahal*. This diagnostic method was used in combination with the others:

> Hakim Sadiq was seeing a patient who had not brought any urine sample. The hakim told the young man that he cannot tell him what he has because

47 Tamil language uses the same idiom to describe the practice of pulse reading in vital spots and Siddha medicine (Sieler 2014: 325; 2015: 143).

48 According to Susanne Kurz, this notion was also present in Persian medical treatises of the Mughal period (personal communication, November 2014). For a discussion around the magical aura of pulse diagnosis in Ayurveda and related practices see Langford (1999).

> he had not seen his urine yet. The patient, then, extended his arm over the pile of reports he had brought and were scattered over Hakim Sadiq's desk, smiling. Hakim Sadiq, instead of checking his pulse, said: 'After checking the pulse, [I know] there is an infection, but I tell you what infection it is after I have seen the urine. Is your stool clean?

Many patients, especially old ones, believed that hakims could or should diagnose from the pulse only. In practice, however, asking for the stool, i.e. questioning, was as important as the pulse and the examination reports brought by the patient. However, unless he saw his urine, Hakim Sadiq could not tell the exact nature of the disease and, hence, he could not treat it specifically. Similarly, Hakim Ahmad complemented pulse examination with other diagnostic methods. According to him, and this was reflected in his practice, pulse examination was the first step in any clinical examination. Hakim Ahmad claimed that a patient's pulse gave him a rough idea of the complaints, and through it he could make a diagnosis close to fifty percent certainty. However, to be hundred percent sure he required the help of pathology. Hence, he asked patients to get different tests done when necessary.

The literature provides concrete details about what is supposed to be 'seen' in the pulse. The *Kitāb an-Nabẓ* ('Book of the Pulse')—an Urdu translation by Hakim Ajmal Khan of sections of Ibn Sina's *Qānūn* dealing with pulse, edited by Hakim Kabiruddin—, describes different kinds of pulses as well as the reason for specific characteristics such as a pulse's weakness or power (Kabīruddīn 2012). This book not only provides illustrations on the kinds of pulse and how to identify them, it also discusses the influence of weather, age, and even country on the pulse (ibid.). Similarly, an Urdu textbook on pulse and urine diagnosis used in a Unani college in Lucknow describes the causes for different kinds of pulses (*asbāb-i nabẓ*) in relation to the bodily need for regulating heat and coolness (Idrīsī n.d. 21). It describes the causes for the existence of different kinds of pulses and for their alteration in accordance with the Aristotelian causes described above (ibid.). Changes in the pulse, for example, are caused by essential (*lāzim*) causes such as the *asbāb-i sittah ẓarūriyah* and non-essential causes such as exercise or bathing (ibid.). This suggests that knowledge in pulse examination is not only useful to assess the condition of a patient and its prognosis. Importantly, sound knowledge and skill on *nabẓ*, ideally, also makes it possible to identify the causes underlying those changes, and as such to find the root causes of disease. However, because pulse diagnosis is never used on its own, it is difficult to establish to what extent this is possible in practice.

'It is Written in the Books that Urine Speaks to the Hakims'

Qārūrah ('urine', lit. the flask used for urine diagnosis) or *baul* ('urine', as commonly mentioned in the literature) are denominations to one of the least practiced traditional diagnostic methods in contemporary Unani medical practice: uroscopy. Most Unani practitioners rely on urine reports based on laboratory analyses. The inspection of a patient's *qārūrah* with the mere eyes has become an extravagant practice that only a few old hakims and their trainees cared to maintain. While most patients expected hakims to check their pulse, some patients reacted with surprise when Hakim Sadiq asked them if they brought their *peshāb* ('urine'). Hakim Sadiq, his son Hakim Sabir, and their trainees were the only Unani physicians I could observe using uroscopy for diagnostic purposes, although I also heard about a few other hakims who also did. Dr. Farzanah and Sakinah were avid trainees in this skill; fascinated by the accuracy in which certain conditions could be diagnosed, or at least suspected, they wanted to know how this was done. After taking a look at a urine sample, Dr. Farzanah explained to me that urine diagnosis is a skill that requires experience. When I asked her if she did not learn this during her training at the Unani college, she laughed: 'Only in theory, not in practice. The practice [in college] is mostly allopathic.' Although the diagnosis through urine and stool (*baul o barāz*) is a component part of the BUMS training under the subject *Kulliyāt nabẓ baul o barāz* ('Works on pulse, urine, and stool [diagnosis]'), students argued that they were not practically trained in uroscopy. In contemporary Unani practice, stool and urine probes are most commonly examined in the laboratory by trained personnel who do not necessarily have training in Unani medicine but in biomedical pathology. This was the case in one of the CCRIUM branch offices. Although hakims routinely asked their patients for their motions (for example their frequency, if they were 'clean', or if they had difficulties when passing), I never witnessed an examination of faeces outside a pathological laboratory or heard about any hakim doing so.

Unani medical theory considers the examination *qārūrah* ('urine') to be one of the most important tools for medical diagnosis. For an adequate urine diagnosis, the first morning urine, still in fasting state, is required (Ibn Sīnā 1993: 224). Ibn Sina listed seven aspects to be taken into consideration during urine diagnosis (1993: 226). The same ones are presented in a student's book authored by the lecturer in a private Unani Medical College in Lucknow: its *rang* ('colour'), *qivām* ('substance or texture'), *ṣafā'ī o kadūrat* ('clarity and turbidity'), *rasūb* or *talchiṭ* ('sediments or residues'), *miqdār balḥāẓ qillat o kaṣ̱ rat* ('quantity in terms of scarcity and frequency'), and *kaf* or *jhāg* ('foam') (Idrīsī n.d. 39). According to this textbook, these aspects are associated with the presence of different humours. For example, a yellow colour in urine is attributed to yellow bile, red colour to blood, black to black bile, and white to phlegm (ibid.). A greenish colour is also possible, Idrīsī quoted the *Shaiḵẖ* (Ibn Sina) arguing that green is the product of the mixture of blue and yellow, hence greenish urine is classified as yellow (ibid.).

I never observed Hakim Sadiq or his team looking explicitly for traces of one of the four humours in the urine, nor commenting about their presence in any of the samples. When I asked Dr. Farzanah why, she refuted my suggestion and explained that black bile can in fact be found in urine, but it was a very bad sign: persons having black bile in urine were about to die. I did not see such a case during my stay, but she assured me that she has had. In his monograph examining the medical history of black urine, particularly in Western contexts including the Hippocratic tradition, Voswinckel argued that black urine was considered a deadly sign (1993: 48) and suggested that it was such a rarity that only few significant practitioners came to see it (1993: 2f.). Black bile in urine as a sign of imminent death resonated with the idea that diseases in an advanced stage have a *saudāvī* temperament. Although black urine was for centuries considered a clinical picture of its own, descriptions of it in Western medical books began to fade in the middle of the twentieth century (Voswinckel 1993: 1). Voswinckel explained its disappearance from biomedicine as the consequence of the development of urine analysis around 1850, which replaced the description of urine colour by the chemical identification of pigments (1993: 6).

For centuries, uroscopy remained a respected form of medical diagnosis. It was practiced in European medicine from the middle ages, influenced by the same textual tradition that Unani medicine was a part of (Büttner 1991; Fangerau and Martin 2012). It was routinely used until its decline in the nineteenth century and some traditional practitioners in Germany still use it (Stolberg 2009). Its decay in Western medicine was not so much grounded on the lack of accuracy in establishing a suspicion or diagnosis, but rather on the increased appropriation of this practice by non-qualified medical practitioners. This created a need for professionalized doctors to establish their medical authority through distancing themselves from whom they considered to be quacks (Stolberg 2009: 167ff.). Also, its potential to be used by patients to test physicians' knowledge (especially when it was not combined with other diagnostic methods), as well as an increased rejection towards urine grounded on hygienic aspects and its incompatibility with the respectable figure of the physician were other reasons for its decay in the European context (ibid.). When asked for reasons for not conducting urine examinations, hakims often gave explanations based on hygienic reasons or the patients' feelings, saying that it would be shameful for the patients to bring their own urine in a bottle. Other practitioners explained that pathological examinations of urine were equally reliable, hence there was no need to conduct *qārūrah* observations, as patients often came with these reports during their first consultation anyways.

Some patients were surprised when asked to bring their urine, a few were even reluctant to do so, this was especially the case with upper-middle class patients. But Hakim Sadiq insisted, and to convince his patients he explained the necessity to combine different diagnostic methods with urine examination. He also legitimized the practice with the textual tradition. While convincing such an apprehensive patient, he once remarked: 'It is written in the books that urine speaks to the hakims.' The examination of the *qārūrah*, however, was not always necessary. Hakim Sadiq and his team asked primarily patients complaining of a burning sensation when passing urine, or lower back pain, or of feeling an urge to urinate but being unable to do so to bring their *qārūrah*. Also, patients with sinus, diabetes, kidney, and liver problems were requested to do so.

One time, a patient did not know that the *qārūrah* examination was conducted traditionally, and brought her urine sample in a small plastic container like those used for pathological urine and stool exams. Hakim Sadiq complained to the patient: 'The bottle is not clean [transparent], I use eyes, not a microscope!' The container had to be big enough and not totally full so that the liquid had enough space to move inside. It was also important to bring the urine early in the morning. Hakim Sadiq turned away samples of patients coming after 11am because, according to him, urine brought late was not reliable. Sometimes, when the urine samples presented abnormal qualities (i.e. a very dark colour, particles, turbidity, etc.), Hakim Sadiq asked the patients at what time they ate dinner in order to ensure that the urine samples were not corrupted. When presented with an anomaly, he asked patients if this was really the first morning urine. A few times it was not the case, and the hakim told the patients to come back another day.

Hakim Sadiq would often check the urine of various patients at once, in this way he did not need to get up every time and walk to the veranda for each patient. Patients who brought their urine samples kept them outside the house in the veranda, often wrapped in plastic bags. Hakim Sadiq and his team conducted urine examinations in a routinized, even ritualized way. None of the physicians touched the bottles containing the urine samples, they asked the patients to hold them from the top instead. They would in turn hold the patients' wrists and move them in such a way that the urine inside the bottles whirled, revealing a different consistency, clearness or turbidity, as well as particles or sediment that were not visible previous to this movement:

> Once, a man in white shalwar *qamīẓ* and topi announced to Hakim Sadiq that he had brought his *peshāb* ('urine'). Hakim Sadiq got up from his chair and told me to come along. I walked behind him, passing the men's waiting room towards the veranda. There were three bottles with urine inside plastic bags hanging on the house's fence. Hakim Sadiq examined them one by one. He asked, as he always did, whose urine it was, pointing to one of the bottles. Once the owner was identified, Hakim Sadiq asked the patient to hold the bottle, loosely, from its neck. He then grabbed the patient's arm and moved it in such a way that the liquid inside began spinning. While the urine whirled inside the glass, a lot of particles became visible. The patient said 'there is also a burning sensation' and the hakim remained silent. He then asked the second patient to grab his urine bottle. The liquid showed no particles inside, but it was not as clear as the previous one; the urine looked turbid. Hakim Sadiq asked this patient if he had 'BP' (blood pressure problems), the patient said yes. Then he examined the third sample. The urine looked like pineapple juice, though it was more greyish than yellow. It had no particles, but it was very turbid. Hakim Sadiq nodded and walked inside, without uttering a further comment.

The observation of urine helped Hakim Sadiq and his apprentices to establish a concrete suspicion of a certain disease. He could easily identify diabetes, for example. Also, urine easily revealed possible urinary infections as well as renal problems. In this way, the practitioners combined the anamnesis with the findings of the pulse and the urine diagnosis. If the urine strongly suggested serious problems like kidney diseases or diabetes, the physicians asked the patients to get examinations from a laboratory. The second use of urine examination was to check if the patients were really healed after the course of treatment. Sometimes, patients assured the physicians that they felt better, and even the examination reports showed favourable figures. However, the physicians only stopped the treatment when the urine showed that the infection or whatever problem they were suffering from was gone. Through uroscopy, Hakim Sadiq and his team would know that the treatments have worked and were no longer required, or if treatment had to be continued.

According to Hakim Sadiq, the examination of the *qārūrah* brought about information that could not always be obtained from high-tech examinations. Instead of looking for traces of humours, what Hakim Sadiq saw in the urine ranged from 'fungus' and 'pus cells' to 'albumin'. Hakim Sadiq sometimes referred to these just as *kacrā* ('trash'). The presence of sediments always meant an infection for him, the more sediments the urine had, the more acute the infection. Also, the colour of the urine as well as its consistency was considered. A patient with an almost transparent and clear urine was said to be 'very weak'. Very turbid urine was often a sign of diabetes, an orange-reddish colour was caused by bilirubin, whose presence in urine indicated an impaired function of the kidneys. Once, a patient's urine presented fine powder-like particles, Hakim Sadiq stated that it was albumin. Albumin, a protein produced in the liver, was commonly taken into consideration in the pathological urine examinations and blood examinations (for serum albumin) that he and his team ordered their patients to conduct. Albumin levels are closely associated with the function of the liver in biomedicine, and its appearance in the urine was related to kidney problems. Judging from the *qārūrah*, Hakim Sadiq would ask patients to get pathological urine examinations or vice-versa. The case of urine diagnosis provides a vivid example of how a technique considered to be 'traditional' or even outdated is used today in combination with modern urine and blood analyses, being by no means incompatible with them.

Therapeutic Practices

'Ilāj ('treatment' or 'cure') is crucial for the reputation of hakims: much of their patients' satisfaction, and hence their source of income, depended on the perceived success of the therapies. The therapeutic landscape of Unani medicine offers hakims a wide array of treatments which are commonly classified into *'ilāj bi-l ghiẕā* ('dietotherapy'), *'ilāj bi-t tadbīr* ('regimental therapy'), *'ilāj bi-d davā* ('pharmacotheraphy'), and *'ilāj bi-l yad* ('surgical treatment'). Some of these therapeutic categories overlap, Ibn Sina for example considered dietotherapy as part of the regimental therapies (1993: 318), and so did the *Kulliyāt-i Nafīsī* (Kabīruddīn 1934: 454). Different textbooks or departments in Unani public facilities classify techniques such as venesection or cupping as regimental therapies or surgical treatments, depending on the case. Although surgery is included in the BUMS curriculum, surgical treatment in Unani practice corresponds, broadly speaking, to simple manual or operative methods and not to complex surgical procedures. The surgery departments of some Unani hospitals conduct minor operations such as circumcisions

or therapies which some classify under the regimental therapies, such as wet cupping. While in theory changes in the diet are ideally the first step in any medical treatment, and drugs are only to be prescribed if dietary and other regimental adjustments provide no results, in practice drugs have become almost inseparable from Unani practice. Diet still remains an important aspect, but medicines have become so important that patients were disappointed in the rare cases when a hakim sent them home without a drug prescription, only with dietary advice and exercise instructions.

Food and Health

Food plays a very important role in Unani medical practice, hakims consider certain medicines to be like food (*khānā jaise*), and also food itself is considered to be intrinsically related to health and disease. Medicines are 'eaten' in Urdu language (*davā khā jātā hai*), perhaps a linguistic proof that in South Asia food and medicine are closely connected. Not only are medicines sometimes cooked in the kitchen (Bode 2008; Bright 1998), food is also considered medicine because of its qualities and actions on the body. It has been proposed that among Muslims in Hyderabad, food practices are embedded in a medico-culinary discourse which considers culinary pleasure as well as the health impact of the qualities of food, as laid down by Unani theory (Roger 1991). In that context, recipes take care of appropriate combinations of hot and cold qualities and they also have to consider the influences of the season of the year (ibid.).

Parhez ('abstinence') is an Urdu word of Persian origin which can also be translated as 'regimen'. Urdu sayings such as *sau 'ilāj ek parhez* ('hundred treatments one abstinence', better translated as 'prevention is better than cure') or *parhez sab se acchā nusk̲h̲ah hai* ('abstinence is the best prescription') encapsulate an understanding of Unani as preventive medicine. But while *parhez* in these sayings is associated with prevention and the preservation of health, in the *maṭabbs* it is frequently articulated as the temporary abstinence of certain foods with the aim of restoring health. Hence, in Unani medical practice diet does not play only a preventive role, but also a therapeutic one.

According to Ibn Sina, the diet of a patient has to be adjusted according to the nature of his problem. Depending on it, food intake has to be reduced so that no energy is wasted in the process of digestion and the body can employ most of it on self-healing (1993: 318f.). When a patient is very weak, food—either its quality or its amount, depending on the case—should be increased, so that a sick person can gain energy from it (ibid.). As in

Ayurveda, in Unani digestion is discussed in analogy to mixing and cooking processes (Bode 2008: 30; Roger 1991: 14; Speziale 2010b: 188), a legacy from the Hippocratic works (Zimmermann 2011 [1982]: 129). Digestion is considered to affect not only the production of bodily humours, but also their circulation in the human body. It is for this reason that digestion itself is seen as a central process influencing health. While commenting on a case of a patient with nasal congestion, Hakim Ahmad said: 'Inshallah, the sinusitis, the congestion will get better. Amoxicillin… potassium dries the phlegm and as long as it remains dry it does not do its work. The nose also gets blocked, the patient cannot sleep, snorting appears.' He paused shortly and then added: 'The proper functioning of digestion is necessary. If the digestion is not alright, then phlegm comes into the blood, causing blockage.' Here, digestion was held responsible for keeping the humours in the right place, avoiding disease. If digestion functions properly, other bodily processes are also more likely to maintain a proper function. Conversely, if the function of the organs is not impaired, then the body has energy to digest properly and health can be maintained.

Although Ibn Sina classified foods not only in the cold and hot binary but also in light/heavy, rich/poor, and healthy/unhealthy, it is the hot and cold producing qualities which seem most important in medical practice, perhaps because not all of these categories were reproduced in later treatises, as stated by Roger (1991: 14). These hot and cold classifications are present in popular concepts, too. For example, I heard in conversations with acquaintances and also Hakim Ahmad told me that men should not eat acid foods (which are considered to be cold producing) because they cause sexual problems, as they produce 'hormonal imbalance'. Conversely, he explained that it was the progesterone in pregnant women which 'asked' the body for acid foods, causing cravings in pregnant women.[49] Acid foods are considered to be cooling (for example citrus fruits are classified as moist in the first and third degree and cold in the second degree, see Table 1), abstention from them is recommended to patients suffering from 'cold' diseases, like for example a common cold characterized by a running nose. Patients with haemorrhoids and constipation are advised to avoid wheat rotis and better eat those made of sorghum flour instead. However, patients are cautioned that roti should not be eaten continuously, as it produces heat, which in excess can be noxious.

Although *parhez* was an important aspect during the observed consultations, it was not always prescribed. And yet, almost every patient

49 The craving for pickles (*acār*) is popularly considered to be a sign of pregnancy in India.

expected Unani treatment to include dietary restrictions. Sometimes when a hakim did not mention it the patients asked about it. On some occasions the hakims had just forgotten to tell the patient the banned items, but other times—although rarely—they said that there was no *parhez*. Dietary restrictions, thus, always depended on the affliction and its cause, and were very often, but not always, relevant for the treatment. They were usually prescribed along with medications.

Many patients, especially women, visited hakims for weight loss. They complained that their bellies had grown and asked the hakims for remedies for weight reduction. Hakim Sadiq explained to a female patient who asked him about weight loss during the consultation: 'We will also take care of weight loss, but you should not go for dieting. If you have to reduce weight you should not do dieting, it is dangerous.' Hakim Azim was often consulted by female patients who wanted to reduce weight, he claimed to have medicines for that. However, he also prescribed exercise, commonly walking or simple exercises, as part of the weight loss regime.

Apart from the role of foods and their heating or cooling effects in the restoration and preservation of health, the quality of foods in terms of their nutritious value, adulteration of natural qualities, as well as contamination with pesticides in the case of vegetables or hormones in the case of meat are considered to affect health. Several hakims regretted that the quality of food has diminished during the last decades. Processed food was considered a big problem among informants and, in the case of meat, they blamed hormones as the cause of many hormonal disorders, especially among women (Solomon 2016). Hakim Sadiq usually warned patients about the problems of processed (i.e. adulterated) honey. He was an advocate of honey consumption, and many of his medicines contained honey as an ingredient. However, he would always stress that his medicines were prepared with hundred percent pure honey with no added sugar. Once a patient asked him on the phone if he could eat roti with honey. He answered: 'You can eat roti with honey. Eat as much honey as you like, but do not eat honey if it is processed!' The hakim hung up and turned to a patient sitting in front of him: 'You can get processed honey all over the world! It causes diseases!'

Honey is a very important ingredient in Unani medicine, and as part of *ṭibb-i nabavī* ('prophetic medicine') it is also important in Muslim contexts. Hakim Ahmad used neem honey for patients with diabetes. He explained that 'fructose is transformed directly into carbohydrate, and the sugar level goes up.' In the case of neem honey, the fructose was mixed with the components of the neem and because it was not converted quickly into carbohydrates in the body, it could be used for diabetes. He further explained that there was no machine to test the honey in order to find out which kind of honey it was (neem, saffron, etc). For this, it has to be tasted, meaning that whoever did it must know the different kinds of honey very well. He regretted that nowadays only few people knew how to identify different kinds of honey. The health of diabetic patients especially was considered to be at stake in case of honey adulteration, and it was for this reason that the quality of the honey was of utmost importance.

Several practitioners shared the impression that the temperament of the patients has been shifting due to lifestyle changes. According to Hakim Ahmad's brother, who was a BUMS student, the increased ingestion of fast food has led to a change in the temperament of Indians in general. He argued that in India we could find a lot of people with phlegmatic and choleric temperaments. This could be specifically observed in the cities, where the hectic life had contributed to this shift and was reflected, according to him, in the increase of liver diseases among the urban population. He stated that 'melancholic temperament is less in India.' Also, Hakim Azim considered fast food and soft drink consumption as problematic. He linked these with the lifestyle of Mumbai, meaning a fast life characterized by 'tension' of different sorts, including sexual tensions. As he explained, many people living in Mumbai had left their villages in the pursuit of better job opportunities in the city. Instead of nutritious meals prepared by their relatives at home, they ate *bāhar kā khānā* ('food from outside'). This was commonly considered to be not only of lower nutritious value, but also dangerous as it could produce gastro-intestinal diseases due to poor hygienic conditions in the places where the foods were stored, prepared, and served. Apart from that, some hakims argued that fast food was 'not suitable' for the Indian population. While Americans and Europeans were supposedly used to drinks such as cola and foods like pizza and pasta, hakims shared the view that for Indian people the best food was home-cooked Indian food, and that fast food consumption made the Indian population sick on the long term.

Food is such an important part of health management that even Dr. Hussain gave dietary advice to his patients. When I asked him why he instructed some patients not to eat rice, I was surprised when he explained the reason in humoral terms, saying that in allopathy the disease was caused when the immune system was not strong enough to fight the disease, while 'in Unani system, there are *balg̠ham, ṣafrā', dam* and *saudā*, these are the four items of the body, four parts, four things. *Saudā, ṣafrā', dam* and *balg̠ham* should be in a proper concentration, if they lose their proper concentration, then disease arises in the body. Out of these four, if their level becomes imbalanced, disease arises'. He further added that in diet, many items produce *saudā, dam, balg̱ẖam,* and *ṣafrā'*. 'That is the principle. Many items influence the *k̲h̲ilṭ*, four *k̲h̲ilṭ*[50] are there, they are influenced by our diet, by our environment. If so many of these items are eaten, then they will produce *balg̱ẖam*, it will induce a *balg̱ẖamī* disease.' While giving an injection to a patient and preparing the next one, he added: 'Accordingly, we diagnose which *k̲h̲ilṭ* is pronounced, that we have to decrease. Then we will get to the disease.'

Lifestyle and Regimen

In the opening of a medical camp on the occasion of World Health Day in Hyderabad in April 2013, Dr. Wahid, then director of the Central Council for Research in Unani Medicine (CCRUM) in the same city, held a speech about high blood pressure, an affliction which the WHO chose as the topic of that day (WHO 2013). He spoke about modern research that demonstrated that regular exercise can help to keep the blood pressure levels within normal ranges. Centuries before any of the studies he mentioned were published, the importance of exercise and lifestyle for the preservation of health had been already recognized by physicians. Regimen, according to Ibn Sina, is the 'management of the essential factors' (1993: 318). Following the principle of the *asbāb-i sittah ẓarūriyah*, adequate and balanced rest and activity, both physical and mental, are required for the maintenance of health in the human body. Diabetes (*ẕayābeṭus*) and blood pressure problems (*fishār ad-dam*), commonly referred by patients and hakims as 'sugar' and 'BP', were both linked to changes or disruptions in lifestyle including exercise and dietary habits. Many of the diseases that afflicted patients in contemporary India are considered to be caused by changes in the lifestyle of the population, as discussed above. Following Hakim Sadiq, the timings for food ingestion, sleeping and waking up are relevant for the production of 'juices' or 'secretions' in the body, as they affect the function of the liver and other important organs and glands. These timings were of central importance in his clinical practice and that of his team, while the other practitioners hardly paid attention to them, focusing on the quality of the food only, as discussed above.

Differently, exercise was more often recommended among hakims when deemed necessary. Walking was among the most commonly prescribed forms of exercise, especially for women. Hakims acknowledged the difficulties for women to conduct exercise like walking outside home because of purdah. If jogging was not possible, Hakim Sadiq recommended brisk walking instead.

50 The plural of *k̲h̲ilṭ* is actually *ak̲h̲lāṭ*.

He also suggested two specific exercises which patients could practice at home, laying on their bellies. For the first, patients had to hold their heads with the hands, elbows resting on the surface, and then to lift each foot towards the buttocks, alternating legs. For the second, patients had to lift their upper body, resting their palms on the surface and bringing their shoulder-plates together, just like in the cobra practiced in hatha yoga. However, he did not use that name. He considered both exercises to be part of Unani medicine. Hakim Sadiq also recommended breathing exercises which resembled pranayama.[51] He would show his patients how to breath, closing the left and right nostrils alternatively and instructing them to do that ten to fifteen minutes daily. He claimed that many of the problems that patients came with were caused because the patient 'does not get oxygen'. According to the hakim, the regular practice of this breathing exercise had a very positive influence on overall health, including the reduction of vision problems because 'from it you get full strength. The waste material behind [the eyes] goes away completely'.

Sport was seen as a positive activity and Hakim Sadiq encouraged his patients, especially young ones, to practice sports. Once, a seventeen-year-old patient narrated that he practiced swimming and the hakim nodded approvingly, suggesting that he swim freestyle. In this way, the patient could reduce his belly, which was important because 'diabetes is coming.' The hakim touched the belly of the patient. The boy was heavily built, but not fat. However, he had a prominent belly and Hakim Sadiq predicted that he would become diabetic if he did not change his lifestyle.

On another occasion, a female patient came with an ultrasound of the abdomen and the pelvis. The reports read 'mild hepatomegaly with fatty infiltration of liver', 'P.C.O.S., advice for hormonal'[52] and 'mild increase in size and parenchymal echotexture is increased + multiple tiny cysts in both ovaries.' The patient also brought the report of an ultrasound of the neck, it read 'evidence of multiple small cervical nodes on both sides, largest one is 19x9mm on the right side, 16x7mm on the left side.' Hakim Sadiq explained to the patient that she should walk in the morning, every day, four kilometres until sweating. Four kilometres was a standard distance prescribed by Hakim Sadiq. Exercise was recommended because sweating was considered necessary to ensure proper bodily functioning; it was for this reason that the four practitioners I spent time with recommended exercise until sweating. The regimental therapies address the idea that

51 For a study on meditation and breathing manuals of Sufis and yogis in the late Colonial Period and a brief discussion on Muslim Yoga see Green (2008).

52 P.C.O.S. is the acronym of polycystic ovarian syndrome.

digestion always produces residues, some of which cannot be evacuated by the physis alone. The accumulation of these residues can be harmful for the human body, especially when they undergo putrefaction and affect the temperament (Ibn Sīnā 1993: 264f.). While drugs can aid the excretion of residues, they can also evacuate good humours in the process, thus reducing the strength of auxiliary organs (ibid.). Hence, exercise is considered to be better suited for evacuating digestion residues without affecting negatively the function of organs. This idea is applied in practice, as in the following case where the patient received no drug prescriptions:

> A chubby seventeen-years-old patient came with a report of cholesterol and blood sugar levels. The young man, who was dressed in jeans and T-shirt, looked rather wealthy. Hakim Sadiq showed the case to his granddaughter, an MBBS student. The hakim explained to his granddaughter that in 25 years, the red line would go up to 'here', while lifting his finger from the red line on the paper up to the air. He said: 'Right now there is no treatment for him. What is it? He has to walk four kilometres every morning. He should eat home-made food. There is no drug.' While pressing holes in the reports for filing, Hakim Sadiq asked the young man if he felt dizziness, the patient said no. The hakim filed the report and wrote on the folder 'OVEREATING IS CRIME' in English, using capital letters. He showed it to the patient and said: 'Look, this is your medicine.' He told the patient to come again in four months, and wrote no prescription for him. At first, it seemed that the patient thought that the hakim was joking, but his expression changed rapidly to ashamed and disappointed once he realized that Hakim Sadiq was serious about it.

This was not an isolated case. On another occasion, a man brought a teenage boy and asked Hakim Sadiq to check him. The hakim, who had greeted the man with utmost respect and arranged an extra chair for him to sit,[53] explained: 'First of all a diagnosis has to be made!' He then immediately asked the boy for the times of his meals and when he usually wakes up. The boy said that he wakes up at eight in the morning. The hakim said: 'this disease will go on its own if you wake up one hour earlier to eat'. He explained further that there was no treatment for this, since the patient actually did not suffer from any disease. 'The system works from five in the morning', said Hakim Sadiq, and explained that if one keeps the timings 'intelligence comes'. Before saying goodbye, Hakim Sadiq warned the boy:

53 This deferential treatment indicated that the man was considered important by the hakim.

'You should get up before eight! Hormonal changes happen [if you don't], it can be dangerous.' He gave him no prescription.

Hakim Sadiq's understanding of health took into consideration the circadian rhythm of the human body. For example, once he told a diabetic patient that the pancreas was the insulin producing gland and that it started working early, this is why he should get up before sunrise. Waking up and eating at the appropriate times was considered essential for the maintenance of health (*hifāẓat-i ṣiḥḥat*). The imbalances caused by not respecting the proper timings for waking up and sleeping as well as eating were not considered as diseases themselves, but were seen as potential causes of disease, the actual roots or primary diseases. The 'correction of the system', as hakims named it, was central in Unani practice. While here Hakim Sadiq did not necessarily name the humoral categories explicitly, the imbalances caused by living a lifestyle contrary to the metabolic rhythm were a central aspect of his practice. Once, a young woman consulted Hakim Sadiq. He told her to remove the veil and checked her pulse, then he asked her at what time she usually gets up. The woman uttered an answer I could not hear and Hakim Sadiq asked Faridah (his granddaughter, the MBBS student): 'Which juices are produced?' Faridah answered: 'Pepsin, and so on'. The hakim turned to the patient and told her that those juices are produced in the morning and this is why one has to get up early. He spoke about tuberculosis and how it is transmitted, saying that if her body had strength, she would not get sick. Similarly, Hakim Sadiq explained to another patient whose ultrasound report diagnosed renal calculi that albumin increases over night and the joints hurt, therefore he should not eat meat before going to sleep.

Respecting orderly times for eating and sleeping is also important to support the excretion of waste material of the human body, as in the following case:

> A male patient came, Hakim Sadiq had examined his urine a few minutes before. It had a yellow, slightly orange colour, it was turbid and with particles. While seeing the urine, Hakim Sadiq had told the patient that 'it has a lot of problems.' Sitting at his desk, the hakim asked the patient for his occupation, the man said that he had a government job. He complained of haemorrhoids and Hakim Sadiq explained that haemorrhoids are caused by constipation. The diagnosis on the *ciṭṭhī* read *qabẓ shadīd* (+) ('severe constipation')' and *bavasīr* (+) ('piles'). The hakim asked the patient for the timings at which he normally ate breakfast and lunch. The man said that he ate lunch before two in the afternoon. 'Excellent! What about dinner?' The patient answered that he eats dinner late, and Hakim Sadiq

> told him to eat earlier: 'Take your food at seven in the evening and you'll get no BP, no sugar, you'll get nothing at all. [...] Haemorrhoids are not a disease, it is a disorder. As long as you stick to the timings for drinking and eating you will have no haemorrhoids. It is written in the books that constipation is the mother of the greatest diseases!'

The idea of constipation as the mother of the greatest diseases (*qabẓ sab se baṛī bīmāryon̲ kī ammā hai*) is based on the concept of excretion and retention (*istifrāg̲h̲ o iḥtibās*), one of the six essential factors. Eating at the right times, thus, not only helps regulate the fluids of the body, it also avoids constipation and, thus, ensures the proper evacuation of waste material from the human body together with sweating through exercise. The evacuation of waste material is considered essential to prevent the corruption or putrefaction (*ʿufūnat*) of the humours.

Apart from food, exercise, and habits, the regimental therapies include a myriad of other practices such as *ḥijāmah* ('cupping'), *ḥammām* ('Turkish bath'), or *taʿlīq al-ʿalaq* ('leeching'). At the time of fieldwork, only a handful of Unani practitioners included these in their practice. These therapies were confined mostly to government settings such as the Nizamia College Hospital in Hyderabad or the Centre of Excellence for Regimental Therapies in Puduvoyal, Tamil Nadu (see Chapter 6). This can be explained by a general neglect of non-pharmacological therapies other than exercise and diet, as well as for practical reasons such as lack of space and infrastructure in the case of hammams or baths or access and facilities to keep leeches, for example. Hakim Azim prescribed no regimental therapies except for dietary advice and exercises. Apologetically, he explained that lack of space was an issue. Indeed, the tiny *maṭabbs* where his consultations took place did not offer the possibility to add some of these practices into his therapeutic repertoire. However, a few private practitioners were making efforts to revive some of these practices, particularly cupping and leeching.

A regimental therapy which was gaining increased popularity at the time of my fieldwork was *ḥijāmah* ('cupping therapy'). The technique consists of the application of glass or plastic cups in order to create local suction on the skin. Hakim Ahmad had introduced cupping to his therapeutic repertoire recently when I visited for the first time in 2013. According to him, *ḥijāmah* evacuated corrupted matter (*k̲h̲arāb hūʾe māddah*) and recommended its practice for various ailments, including skin diseases and migraine, problems that were caused by an excess of humours or by them 'being stuck' in the body (Schmidt Stiedenroth 2019b).

Unani Medicines

The walls of the *davākẖānahs* I visited were usually covered with shelves full of glass bottles, plastic containers and paper boxes filled with Unani drugs, either branded or self-produced. Unani medicines are manufactured in different formats such as capsules, round and flat pills (*ḥabb* and *qurṣ*) powder (*safūf*), syrup (*sharbat*), distillate (*ʿarq*), electuary (*maʿjūn*), and stomachic (*javārish*). Most patients expect hakims to prescribe some of these medicines as part of the treatment. While the knowledge on materia medica and its properties is also imparted in the classrooms of Unani colleges, it is generally agreed that its mastering requires an enormous deal of exposure: a good hakim should not only know the properties and qualities of materia medica, but he should also be able to identify plants and other ingredients in different forms, from the living plant in the mountains, desert or jungle, to the dried roots, leaves, flowers, bark, seeds, and stems as found in the market. Hakim Faruqi claimed to know the name of more than ten thousand medicinal plants in Arabic, Persian, and English; that he could recognize each of them; and that he knew which part is used for what. I asked him how he learned all this. He laughed and told me that when he was a little boy, every time his family went somewhere, his father, who was a hakim, would tell him: 'look at that plant, its name is so and so and it is used for this and that' or 'look at that tree!' and so on. Once back home, he would sit and work with some parts of the plants, look them up in books and write down everything he could find out about them.

Materia medica and formulations, in Unani literature referred to as *mufradāt* ('single drugs')[54] and *murakkābāt* ('compound drugs'), comprise an important part of Unani's textual corpus. Physicians compiled their recipes in their *bayāẓ*, *qarābādīns* ('pharmacopoeias') were compiled with formulae addressing specific diseases. There are two main subjects that deal with medicines in the literature: *ʿIlm al-adviyah* ('Pharmacology'), and *ʿIlm aṣ ṣaidlah* ('Pharmacy'). While the first is dedicated to the knowledge of Unani materia medica, its identification and uses, the latter is related to the modes of preparation of compound medicines in Unani. Medicines, be them simple or compound, have their own temperament, which is crucial

54 The recognition of *mufradāt* ('single drugs') and their medical properties in Unani stands in contrast with classical Ayurveda, where—according to Pordié—single plants are not considered medicinal objects *per se* (2014b: 67). However, Ayurvedic companies have reformulated medicines in the context of the global pharmaceutical market, and nowadays we find single plants marketed as Ayurvedic medicines (ibid.).

Table 1: Classification of some single drugs based on the table 'Groups of medicines with regard to their degree of temperament' presented in a textbook of Unani pharmacology (Laṭīf, Tajuddīn and Āfāq 2004: 16).

First degree	Second degree	Third degree	Fourth degree
	Hot medicines		
Lavender, fig, sweet almond, pistachio, borage and its flower	Walnut, afsantin (*artemisa absinthium*), peppermint, cinnamon	Chamomile, ajowan, babchi (*psoralea corylifolia*), dried ginger	Copper sulphate, aconite
	Cold medicines		
Guava, plum, papaya	Amla (*phyllanthus emblica*), common violet, spinach, citrus fruit (*turunj*)	Psyllium (*ispaghula*), ice, anjabar (*polygonum bistorta*) seeds	Ajowan from Khorasan, opium, devil's trumpet (*datura metel*)
	Dry medicines		
Amla (*phyllanthus emblica*), walnut, silk worm (*bombix mori*), lavender, mung bean	Ajowan from Khorasan, anjabar (*polygonum bistorta*), cardamon, *indar jau* (the seeds of *neru antidysentricum*)	Babchi (*psoralea corylifolia*), resin, mustard seed	Opium, copper sulphate, devil's trumpet (*datura metel*), aconite
	Moist medicines		
Guava, grapes, fig, sweet almond, borage, spinach, citrus fruit (*turunj*), common violet	Psyllium (*ispaghula*), apricot	Peach, citrus fruit (*turunj*)	*Lūbyā* [soy bean?]

for their therapeutic application, as it defines their quality and, hence, action. Medicines are classified according to their qualities and degrees of action, from the first degree or lesser action—which includes food items which are commonly ingested without a specific therapeutic intention—to the fourth degree—which denotes poisonous items that can be lethal if not administered with precaution (see Table 1). This classification, and in particular the fourth degree contradicts the common claim that Unani medicines have no side-effects. In reality, some hakims argue, any drug that has an effect has a side-effect, too. The *fann-i ṭibb* ('art of medicine') consists precisely in combining drugs in such a way that the beneficial effects outweigh the negative ones. The principle of *'ilāj bi-ẓ ẓidd* ('healing with the opposites') is very important when it comes to medicines, as administering a patient a medicine of his own temperament might—following Hakim Ahmad, who held an MD in *'Ilm al-advīyah*—, result in the patient vomiting or in another bodily reaction aiming at the expulsion of the medicine.

Hakims routinely prescribed medicines in accordance to this principle, especially taking into consideration the temperament of the disease, as in the following case:

> A male patient, roughly 50 years old, suffering from erectile problems and 'anxiety feeling' came for a control consultation after having started the course of treatment. As I would learn later from the words of Hakim Ahmad, the patient was an engineer who had a lot of family and job-related problems. The first time he came to the *maṭabb,* the patient did not have children, which caused him a lot of 'tension' according to the hakim. After Hakim Ahmad's treated him, the patient got a son and since then 'the brain tension subsided.' The man greeted the hakim with familiarity as he sat next to him. Hakim Ahmad asked him how he was doing and the patient complained of excessive heat and dried eyes since he started the treatment.
> Hakim: Use oats as well. Because your eyes are getting dry
> Patient: What is the reason for it?
> Hakim: Some of the medicines you are taking dry the fluid
> Patient: What should I do now? During the day I eat cold things, watermelon... it does not cause me much problems. But at night...
> The patient went on explaining his choice of cold foods because it had been hot during the previous days, but since the weather cooled down 'my immunity went down and I am taking strong medicines...'
> Hakim: The brain is a very sensitive issue. Phlegm appears from the cold and [with it] a sinus problem...
> Patient: My eyes are dry and [...] there are a lot of problems. After the operation... allopathic medicines do not give me much strength. Now the issue is that I don't have strength, my muscles are weak. The semen became less, before it was a hundred percent content, now it became seventy percent. Erection... this has been happening for six or seven months.
> The hakim felt the pulse of the patient and while doing so he took a look at the patient's file. The patient asked if he should change his diet. The hakim advised him to mix fennel [hot and dry both in second degree], coriander powder [cold and dry both in second degree], and black caraway [*nigella sativa*, hot and dry in third degree]—with ajowan [hot in second degree] if desired— and to add it to the meals. The patient said that one powder caused him a lot of problems, the hakim told him to reduce the dosage of it by half. Additionally, he prescribed *k̲h̲amīrah munaqqá-i dimāg̲h̲* ('brain purgative electuary') and *qurṣ mumsik o muqavvī* ('retentive and strengthening pill') 'for the testis.'

> Hakim: Take these, one is a Unani [medicine] with calcium. The brain and other vital organs will benefit a lot from it.
> Patient: What does it do, to support the metabolism?
> Hakim: In direct form, the metabolism… it's like a tonic. It gives the brain the things it needs.
> P: Are they hot?
> Hakim: You will not get much heat from them, they are second degree, the previous one was fourth degree […].

While the hakim did not explicitly acknowledge neither the temperament of the patient nor that of the disease, the production of phlegm due to the cold weather was mentioned. The prescriptions and dietary advice suggested that the patient was affected by cold and moist disease which had to be treated with heating and drying medicines, whereby the excessive heat and dryness of the previous medicines had to be tackled to reduce the side effect (dry eyes) caused by the treatment.

Apart from the intrinsic qualities of medicines (cooling, heating, moisturizing or drying) and their degrees as explained above, medicines and food are also classified according to their *afʿāl* ('actions')[55] and their *istʿimāl* ('use'), as found in numerous treatises on single and compound drugs and in the NFUM. Examples of *afʿāl* include *muharrik dimāg̱ẖ* ('brain stimulating', e.g. tea and *arthemisa absinthium*), *musak̲h̲k̲h̲in* ('heating', e.g. onion and garlic), *muddir* ('diuretic', e.g. rhubarb and *k̲h̲yārain*, cucumber or musk-melon seeds), and *musakkin* ('sedative', e.g. opium and devil's trumpet) (Laṭīf et al. 2004: 8ff.), whereas *istʿimāl* addresses the indications of a medicine for particular diseases or symptoms.

The patients' response towards the medicines are said to depend on their format. A hakim explained that *aqrāṣ* ('pills') are more powerful than capsules, which contain only the powder. He said that one would need five capsules and only one tablet to equal the content. I asked if he sometimes uses the powder alone, he said yes, but that is not suitable for all patients. Especially women are sensitive, some of them vomit because of the bad taste of the powders. This is why he advises patients to take the powders mixed with honey. Another good technique is to slice a banana and put the powders in the middle, close it and eat it. He saw this as an effective way to ensure that the whole content of the medications reached the digestive system.

55 The Ferozson's Urdu-English dictionary translates *afʿāl al-adviyah* as 'pharmacology' (afʿāl al-adviyah n.d.).

The environment also plays a role in the action of drugs. While discussing a book on Unani medical treatment, Hakim Ahmad explained that 'each state has its own environment.' At first, I did not understand what he meant, so I asked him if he meant the climate? He said no, what he meant was that medicines are like food. Like for me, coming from another country, I might have problems with the food in India. I nodded. He said that the same happens with medicines, their effect varies according to the place. Like in Mumbai the climate is dry and in Uttar Pradesh (UP) the effect of certain medicines is stronger than in Mumbai. As an example, he told me about a patient with fibroids who did not react very well to the medicines until she left for UP. There, the effect of the medicines was greater and she got better results. Although the influence of the environment is considered relevant for the causation of diseases, not all practitioners applied this principle in practice. Unani drugs were often prescribed like biomedical drugs, i.e. considering their action as encapsulated in the active components of the drugs only, instead of taking into consideration the framework within which their actions and qualities are supposed to take effect. This was often the case in institutionalized settings, as discussed in the previous chapter.

Unani pharmaceuticals deserve special attention because they appeal to and create common values (Bode 2002, 2006, 2008; Bright 1998; Whyte et al. 2002). It has been observed that pharmaceutical products in form of tablets or capsules—which constitute new forms of preparation similar but not equal to traditional ones—, have their own charm, as they are 'often believed to contain the power of healing in themselves' (van der Geest and Whyte 1989: 346). Indeed, as observed during medical consultations, tonics, capsules, and pills had a special allure among patients. While it has been reported in the past that patients would be confused if practitioners did not recommend any *parhez* (Taylor 1976: 290), patients in most Unani consultations were confused when they were sent home without any drug prescription. Patients seemed used to leaving a clinic with at least one prescription. The clinics I observed for longer periods had all a dispensary attached to them. The consultations were for free, but the medicines were not. This drug-centred approach made the prescription and retail of pharmaceuticals—either self-produced or branded—a must for the sustainability of the business model. Although, as seen above, patients were occasionally sent away with lifestyle recommendations only, these cases were exceptions and not the rule.

Medications have become a symbol for the Unani system as sometimes practitioners went as far as to differentiate which system they practiced depending on the medicines prescribed, even though concepts of disease causation and health recovery were mixed. This was the case of Dr. Hussain, who used dietary restrictions to support biomedical treatments. In Dr. Hussain's practice *parhez* was an added value which, according to him, did not interfere with biomedical treatment. Interestingly, although Dr. Hussain included the humoral paradigm in his medical practice, he still claimed to practice 'allopathic medicine' because the medications he prescribed were mostly biomedical. He did not see himself as a hakim because, according to him, he lacked much knowledge about medicinal herbs and their preparation. We can conclude from this that he followed an integrative approach in practice, whereby the Unani concepts of disease causation were integrated into the management of disease along with allopathic therapies. However, he defined his practice according to the medicines he mainly used and not according to underlying ideas of disease causation and management. Dr. Hussain often said: 'I take the best of the two systems. What is important is the patient. I can use Ayurveda, Unani, all I use.'

Humoralism and Looping Effects

It is remarkable that while contemporary representations of Unani medicine tend to emphasize the role of the four humours and their balance, the definitions of medicine introduced at the beginning of this chapter did not mention them as distinctive features of Unani. Definitions of *ṭ̤ibb* as the science of health, its preservation and recovery can be understood as universal definitions applying to all forms of medicine, as they do not focus on the specific ideas underlying medical practice, but rather on the aim of medical science. As discussed in Chapter 1, *ṭ̤ibb* was 'just' medicine, as no distinction between Unani and other forms of medicine was done in precolonial texts attributed to the Graeco-Islamic textual tradition since *ṭ̤ibb* was understood as global medicine in those times (Kurz 2014). However, when we take a look at contemporary definitions and descriptions of Unani medicine, the four humours are ubiquitous and even dominant to the extent that even I caught myself introducing Unani medicine as humoral medicine in academic talks and in the classroom.

The enactment of Unani as humoral medicine was, until very recently, hardly questioned by scholars studying Unani. Attewell convincingly argued that the epistemological framework of Unani medicine encompasses much more than its humoral theory, and that in representations 'the humoral theory and its related concepts have been largely assumed to be central to practice, and the place of its theory is often assumed to exist outside time and socio-political context as a cornerstone of aetiology, diagnosis, and therapeutics' (Attewell 2013: 129). This development arose from the necessity to attribute the humoral theory as the distinguished feature of indigenous medicines during the late Colonial Period. This was an agenda pursued by Hakim Ajmal Khan in his struggle for attainment of recognition for Unani medicine (Attewell 2013: 137). In this way, the four humours were essentialized as the theoretical basis of Unani medicine, constituting often the core of its representations (Quaiser 2013). The emphasis on the humoral bodily constitution and its capacity to heal itself was used to contrast Unani with the germ theory of Western medicine, which was in turn employed as a metaphor for external agents attacking the inside (Quaiser 2013: 30). The fundamentals of Unani were instrumental 'as distinct markers to essentialise the body by Unani, in opposition to the colonial and communal politics of western medicine and Ayurveda respectively' (ibid.). This later point is interesting: contrary to what is commonly assumed, the humoral theory was not necessarily seen as the common ground shared with Ayurveda, but as a distinct feature of each form of medicine. Fabrizio Speziale (2014b) analysed how different authors of the Graeco-Islamic tradition discussed the *tridosa* in analogy to the four humours of the Graeco-Islamic tradition from the sixteenth century, not without confronting conceptual problems and proposing strategies to deal with them. There were even attempts to combine the Avicennian with the Ayurvedic humoral theories in order to update medical knowledge and adapt it to its new context, a notable example is Nagawri's model discussed by Speziale (2018: 90ff.). Although different paradigms coexisted, the combined approach never really competed against the Avicennian one, and combined models failed to establish themselves in the postcolonial context, where the differences between the systems were emphasized (Speziale 2014a; 2018: 98). In this way, the four humours may also be interpreted as an identity marker for Unani medicine not only against biomedicine, but also against Ayurveda.

Regarding medical practice, we cannot assume that the epistemologies present in the texts of the Graeco-Islamic medical tradition were always applied (Savage-Smith 2013). For example, case studies recorded by students of Razi (d. 925) explained the causes of illness on humoral terms, but 'the therapy is never couched in humoral terms' (Savage-Smith 2013: 92). Importantly, imbalances were not considered to be based on humours but rather on the four primary qualities, which in turn stand in direct connection to the environment and the *asbāb-i sittah ẓarūriyah* (Savage-Smith 2013: 101f.). This is significant, because the practices of hakims described above suggest the same. Not being explicit about the role of the humours, however, does not necessarily mean that they are irrelevant.

At this point it should be clarified that I have no intention to argue that the fundamental principles still have a prominent role in institutionalized practices. When faced with a long queue of patients and short time to see them all, practitioners acted pragmatically, seeking to satisfy the patients' more pressing needs and neglecting the search for the root cause of disease. Long-term treatments were often substituted by immediate symptomatic treatment in such cases. The skills and knowledge of a physician as well as his own interest and training, together with the expectations of the patients, they all played a role in Unani clinical practices.

In the introduction to his book *Basic Principles of Unani Medicine*, which sought to reconcile Unani with modern science, Azmi referred to the humoral theory as follows:

> It appears from this definition that the real cause of disease lies in the imbalance of humors, but it is not so. In fact, the four humors are the seat (maḥal) of diseases, not their cause. [...] It is probably the first time that the real cause of diseases has been associated with the aṣbāb-i sittah ḍarūriyah [...], and compared with modern concept of the etiology of diseases. I have proved that there is no basic difference between the two concepts [biomedicine and Unani] and that the difference is only in the mode of treatment (1995: xi).

The examples discussed above also point out to humoural imbalance as the seat of diseases and not as their cause, which rests ultimately in the essential and non-essential factors. However, the statement that the only difference between Unani and biomedicine lays on the mode of treatment is a dangerous simplification. The clinical interactions discussed in this chapter suggest that the theories behind disease causation cannot be separated from the treatments, their correspondence being a legacy of the Aristotelian theory of causality. The idea of treating with the opposites as well as the mechanical expulsion of excess in the body are all related to the fundamental principles whose most central aspect appears to be the primary qualities or *kaifiyyat* and with them, their effects on the human body. Savage-Smith, who came to the same conclusion in her study of medieval Graeco-Islamic sources, proposed to use the adjective 'humoral' to address 'the nosology and etiology of the period' and suggested to search for another word 'to designate the qualitative balance that dominated therapeutic care' (Savage-Smith 2013: 104).

The term 'humoral pathology', which was used to describe medieval therapeutics, has a Western origin and was spread in the European historiography of medicine in the nineteenth century (Savage-Smith 2013: 103f.).[56] Following her and the authors mentioned above, the descriptions of Unani medicine as humoural medicine are largely a product of representations and reification efforts. Once again, we are confronted with looping effects: European historiography mingling with the processes whereby Unani medicine had to find distinctive features and create its own identity for purposes of legitimation. The observations presented in this chapter suggest that the description of Unani as a humoral-based medical practice, although not entirely wrong, is biased. Even though humoural imbalance is not considered to be the root cause of diseases in Unani medicine, practitioners talked about the four humours as being the most important aspect of Unani. This can be interpreted as the product of looping effects and dynamic nominalism, whereby practices of naming interact with what its named (Hacking 2002: 26). While Unani is referred to as a humoral form of medicine, the analysis of the private clinical practices of hakims corroborate the claims made by Attewell (2013) and Savage-Smith (2013) suggesting that this denomination does not do justice to the broadness of its scope. This aspect is of vital importance in order to understand processes of appropriation of modern concepts and technologies into Unani medicine.

56 For the case of Ayurveda, it has been similarly suggested that the idea of health as bodily balance is a product of colonial modernity (Mukharji 2016: 142).

4. The Appropriation of Modern Scientific Advances and Concepts

The adoption of modern concepts and techniques seem ubiquitous in the theory and practice of contemporary Unani medicine, from Unani textbooks in Urdu including biomedical terminology to the use of modern diagnostic techniques by hakims. BUMS graduates are trained to read examination reports and to understand the names of the most common allopathic drugs prescribed to patients, they are further familiarized with diseases as described both in Unani as well as in biomedical textbooks. Even the most seemingly conservative hakims argued that the use of modern diagnostic methods per se did not present a threat to Unani as a system of medicine, as long as they were used as diagnostic aids and physicians did not rely solely on them.

As argued in the previous chapter, Unani medicine should not be understood simply as a 'humoural medicine,' because its fundamental concepts are based on complex understandings of causation of health and disease among which the humours constitute only one—albeit important—part. Building on this argument, this chapter analyses the integration of modern concepts and technologies in the private practice of hakims, proposing that the ideas of conflicting epistemologies and biomedicalization of traditional medicine necessitate a revision if they are to be applied to the case of Unani.

A Case of Biomedicalization?

The Unani fraternity generally accepts the integration of modern science into Unani as a positive and natural development. In contrast, social science and humanities scholars studying traditional forms of medicine have been far less enthusiastic about the phenomenon. Criticism of the integration of modern advances into traditional medical practices has addressed several aspects, focusing on the gaps between humoral-based pathology and biomedicine, and the attempts to bridge them (Bode 2008: 145ff.). The adoption of modern concepts by practitioners of traditional medicine has been considered a capitulation to biomedicine which, at best, simplifies the complexity of traditional forms of medicine by neglecting their fundamental principles, and at worst separates them completely from their epistemologies. This process, critics argued, may lead to the rationalization of traditional forms of medicine to the extent that they may no longer provide the added value that currently makes them so important and even necessary (Janes 1999). Further critiques have been concerned with the risk of absolute subordination of traditional medicine to the dominant paradigm of biomedicine through the adoption of modern technologies and concepts as well as research methods (Pordié 2010; Speziale 2010a), and with problems of matching or validating indigenous aetiologies and nosologies with modern scientific concepts (Adams and Li 2008; Naraindas 2014b).

The problematic aspects of the use of modern diagnostic techniques in traditional medicine in South Asia have received particular attention. For the case of Ayurveda, the use of methods seeking to visualize the interior body and represent it as 'truth' were said to conflict with the epistemological humoural basis of traditional Ayurvedic practice (Langford 2002: 155ff.). For Unani, institutionalized training, policies towards indigenous medicines in colonial and postcolonial India, and the demands and expectations of the public, caused the displacement of traditional diagnostic methods such as urine and pulse diagnosis, leading practitioners to reorient 'their traditions towards the technology and concepts at the core of western medicine' (Attewell 2005: 415ff.). In a similar vein, Hamdard's Elementology project, which sought to reconcile the four elements with modern chemistry, was approached very critically, as it was concluded that '[m]erely re-labelling classical ideas and concepts will not turn Indian medicine into a modern scientific undertaking and will not gain Indian medicine prestige within the arena of modern science' (Bode 2008: 151). These critics share the assumption that modern concepts and techniques underlie a biomedical epistemology, and that this epistemic framework is incommensurable with that of traditional forms of medicine. Further, the adoption of modern advances and concepts by practitioners of traditional medicine is seen as indicative of the dominant position of biomedicine over other forms of medicine.

Informed by this literature, I could not understand why so many Unani hakims and researchers I had spoken to during my first stay in the field seemed oblivious to such problems when discussing the integration of modern concepts and technologies into Unani practices. They saw neither a risk of biomedicalization, nor a potential danger that the epistemological bases of Unani would become superfluous and unnecessary, leading eventually to the extinction of Unani medicine.

While the dominance of biomedicine cannot be denied, this dominance is not necessarily absolute or even existent at all times (Baer et al. 1997). Claims about the superiority of Unani medicine vis-à-vis biomedicine abound among the fraternity. These are not just empty claims about herbal medicines having no side-effects. What makes Unani superior to biomedicine, according to the fraternity, is that it addresses the root cause of diseases, and not just their symptoms. As long as this core characteristic of Unani remains intact, the fraternity sees no risk of biomedicalization in the use of modern technologies or concepts.

The BUMS curriculum covers anatomy, gynaecology and obstetrics, clinical methods, and other subjects, drawing on biomedical textbooks such as Grey's Anatomy and Hutchinson & Hunter's Clinical Methods (CCIM n.d.: 168ff.). Through the study of books like these, students should integrate modern medical knowledge into the practice of Unani, leading to new forms of Unani medical practice and a widened understanding of what Unani medicine is. This development was the product of an inclusive understanding of Indian medicine regarding 'modern advances' as defined in The Indian Medicine Central Council Act of 1970, which stipulated the regulations regarding the training and registration of practitioners of Indian Medicine. The Act defines Indian Medicine as 'the system of Indian Medicine commonly known as Ashtang Ayurveda, Siddha or Unani Tibb, whether supplemented or not by such modern advances as the Central Council may declare by notification from time to time' (Government of India 1970). The CCIM gave a more precise definition of 'modern advances' in March 2003:

> 'Modern Advances' be read as advances made in the various branches of Modern Scientific medicine in all its branches of Internal medicine, Surgery, Gynaecology and Obstetrics, Anaesthesiology, diagnostic procedures and other technological innovation made from time to time and declare that the courses and curriculum conducted and recognized by the Central Council of Indian Medicine are supplemented with such modern advances (CCIM 2004).

Although this definition sought to clarify what is meant by 'modern advances' in the law, the term remains broad and open for interpretation. Notably, the advances are not attributed to biomedicine but to 'Modern Scientific medicine', a broad category itself. The inclusion of modern scientific advancements in terms of knowledge, diagnostic methods and technologies, thus, is sanctioned by the Indian government and reflected in the BUMS curriculum. As discussed in Chapter 2, institutionalized training and practice does not adequately transmit Unani medical knowledge in the way that long-time training with an established physician does. In the case of Unani, the diagnostic usage of pulse and urine examinations has declined remarkably as the inclusion of modern diagnostic methods has spread to the extent that they are often the diagnostic method of choice. Arguably, BUMS graduates can more easily interpret a blood test examination report than 'see' the pulse of a patient.

The widespread use of modern diagnostic methods attracted my research interest from the outset. I was fascinated by how they could be combined with the fundamental principles of Unani, because the four humours were not directly manifested in ultrasound reports, nor in blood or urine parameters. I asked informants how they reconcile the use of modern diagnostic methods or modern scientific research with the fundamental principles of Unani. This question often produced a confused reaction in interlocutors, who did not see what had to be reconciled. When talking about research and asking about the problem of incompatible epistemologies, an old hakim who had a high rank post at the CCIM at the time of the interview cautioned me to rethink my stance:

> You should be very careful and see that allopathic medicine is not the same as scientific advancements. Unani should not mingle with allopathy, but it should make use of technology as much as possible [...] [Modern diagnostic techniques] are not exclusive of allopathy, and it is important that the practitioners use them only as confirmation tools and not as the only sources of information.

This statement made me realize that modern diagnostic methods or artefacts are not considered to be biomedical, but are—in line with the regulations—seen as modern advances that no system of medicine could claim for itself. Modern diagnostic techniques as well as modern scientific research are understood as epistemologically neutral and hence compatible with Unani or, for instance, with any form of medicine. Implicit in my question was the assumption that modern diagnostic methods encapsulated biomedical understandings that conflicted with those underlying Unani practice. The hakim explained that modern diagnostic methods had been integrated into the BUMS curriculum with the aim of confirming diagnoses established by Unani physicians, not to replace them. He saw this replacement as a main problem, but he saw no incompatibility on the epistemological level as I did at that time.

Similarly, the principal of a Unani medical college in South India gave a very instructive answer to my question about the compatibility of diagnostic techniques and Unani practice:

> College principal: See, allopathic sciences are very different from the modern, other scientific technologies, they are different ones. Because X-rays were not invented by allopathic doctors. X-rays were invented by

some chemists, some physicists [laughed]. Also, ultrasound, they were all developed by biotechnologists. Those technologies have been adapted in medicine by allopathic people.
KS: So, you separate between the modern technologies and...
College principal: Definitely! Definitely these are technologies, not allopathic drugs, ehh! Doctors, they adapted it. So, first, the X-ray films were developed by the physicists, OK? Then the rays also, the X-rays were invented by Roentgen. Roentgen was a scientist, a physicist, not an allopathic doctor [...] Then ultrasound, it's the sound waves that produce a picture. That science also they have adopted, put it on the abdomen, now it is established. Instruments, science is always developed by somebody, they [allopathic doctors] are adopting it. Even we, Indian medicine doctors, are adopting these: we have an X-ray department in [the college's] hospital, an ultrasound, pathological lab, that is TC [total count], DC [differential count], RBC [red blood cells], haemoglobin, all we are seeing... urine, albumin, sugar deposits, motions.... everything! And in our syllabus, there are modern books also, we are keeping in the syllabus [...]. So, day by day, the Unani medicine is enriched by adopting the sciences or modern developments. What is happening outside we are adopting in to our system, and we are becoming enriched. [...] What I am telling, why can we take that development? Why can't we incorporate it? Make it easier, it doesn't do any of these things, and it is not a religious book like Bible or Quran that deviating from it will become heresy! [laughed]. No, in our medicine books are not like that. Even we can say Avicenna, what he has written, in one way he has given this definition, agree or not agree with him, but for that simply saying is not sufficient, I should prove it. Where Avicenna has been wrong, what is there, and what is the possible error thing which has prompted him to go in that way. Because at that time there was no microscope, there was no biochemistry [...] so limited sources [were] available to Avicenna, he was thinking and he has written the books. So more than 90 per cent is correct, but even 10 per cent might be wrong. He is a human being, it is not theological science.
KS: And what happens to the humours, the elements in the body? Like it is said that it has not been proved that black bile actually exists.
College principal: See, that theory, no one can deny, nobody can disprove. Such a strong base it is having.
KS: What is the base?
College principal: Yes. Human body is the base, human body is the base. Whatever our ancestors have written about, the temperament, and the criteria for assessing a person, it is crystal clear, you can see even now, you can assess.

Unani practitioners often argued about the scientificity of Unani and the constant integration of new knowledge throughout its history. The college principal's contrasting of Unani's classical texts with the Bible or Quran reflects an anti-dogmatic stance which welcomes the integration of modern technological advances and the development of new branches of knowledge, such as biochemistry. However, he remained firm regarding the existence of the humours and the concept of temperaments. For him, scientific advances may bring new knowledge, but they do not refute the obvious: as long as a physician is able to draw on his experience in order to assess a patient's temperament, it has to be accepted as existent. For him, the humours are 'crystal clear' and, as such, cannot be questioned. But how clear are they? The following sections examine how modern advances are integrated into Unani clinical practices without requiring an epistemological reconciliation.

Using Modern Diagnostic Methods

The advance of technology had a profound impact on medicine, revolutionizing the way in which diagnoses were reached. Unani medicine was no exception. Stethoscopes and sphygmomanometers belong to the basic equipment in almost every *maṭabb.* Some practitioners use them routinely and some use them rarely. BUMS students learned how to use these tools and how to interpret pathological examination reports, practicing these skills during their internships in biomedical facilities. In this way, Unani practitioners were not only allowed to make use of modern diagnostic methods, but were moreover encouraged to do so.

Anecdotes of physicians confirming diagnoses through modern diagnostic methods during the Colonial Period suggest that they were introduced in Unani practice as soon as they were available. One of these anecdotes narrates how Hakim Ajmal Khan diagnosed a uterine cyst or tumour through pulse diagnosis, and how the diagnosis was confirmed by an exam report obtained in a hospital by a 'lady doctor' (Fārūqī 1995: 161). This anecdote extolls the pulse reading skill of Hakim Ajmal Khan, as the examination report confirmed what he had already 'seen' through the pulse.

Anecdotes like this abound; they suggest not only that diagnostic technologies are not incompatible with Unani practice, but also reveal how they can be used to grant legitimacy to a physician's prowess in particular and to Unani medicine in general. While the use of modern diagnostic methods in their earliest days seemed to have been mainly for confirmation purposes, nowadays most hakims employ them as diagnostic aids. A minority of hakims order exams in order to satisfy patients who, they claimed, would otherwise think that they were not examined thoroughly. Other hakims use examination reports as proof of effectiveness of their medical treatments.

Private practicing hakims do not only make use of the test results brought by their patients, but often ask patients to get certain tests done, depending on the case. Hakim Ahmad, for example, would not hesitate to instruct his patients to get laboratory tests. He was familiar with the most common blood and urine test parameters. He would look at the reports, analyse them, and integrate the information provided into his reasoning as a Unani physician in order to arrive to a diagnosis and find the cause of the disease. But how do hakims combine the information provided by modern diagnostic methods with the fundamental framework discussed in the previous chapter? Does the use of medical technologies lead to a biomedicalization of Unani medical practice? I address these questions through an examination of two common uses of modern diagnostic technologies in Unani: as diagnostic aids, and as proof of effectiveness.

Diagnostic Aids

Diagnoses and therapies in the private practice of hakims that I observed commonly followed the framework of the fundamental principles of Unani medicine: diseases were considered to be caused by humoural imbalances which, in turn, were linked to the four qualities and the essential and non-essential factors. Modern diagnostic methods were integrated into this framework. Instead of imposing biomedical parameters and providing simplified disease categories, hakims made use of figures and images in ways that suited their understanding of health and disease. Let us take reproductive tract infections as an example, as these were very common among female patients consulting the *Shifa Mahal*. Radiographs and ultrasound are useful to identify this condition, because they can indicate inflammation of the pelvis or uterus. A blood test report can indicate an infection, for example if the white blood cell count is high. These results alone, however, cannot lead to a final diagnosis. Hence, they are combined with clinical examinations such as urine and pulse diagnosis and observation through a cervical examination using a vaginal speculum. The questioning of the patient is very important too, as the physician should know, for example, if there is white discharge, itching, or pain. If a reproductive tract infection is clinically confirmed, a cervical swab test is prescribed in order to find out which organism is responsible for the infection. This information is necessary in order to prescribe adequate supportive treatment, for instance, antibiotics, antivirals, or fungicides.[57] Most importantly, however, the hakim focuses on strengthening the patient's *ṭabīʿat* in order to support the healing process and avoid complications, among which liver problems are considered common, as patients had often been exposed to painkillers or antibiotics for long periods following the advice of previous doctors.

The following consultation illustrates how Hakim Sadiq integrated examination reports in his clinical consultations:

> A woman wearing a black abaya sat next to me, from the other room a young man or boy approached the desk with clear difficulty. His face was showing signs of pain as he walked towards us, he was very thin. [...] The young man said that he had brought urine, and Hakim Sadiq said: 'First see the urine!' We walked towards the porch, two patients were holding bottles with urine ready for examination. Hakim Sadiq instructed the young man to hold his own urine. The patient grabbed the plastic bottle with his left hand from above, keeping his wrist soft; his fingers looked like a spider catching prey. The hakim came forward, held the young man's wrist and shook it softly in a way that the bottle started shaking, too, the liquid swirling inside. The hakim controlled the movement of the urine sample without even touching the bottle by himself. The clear urine had a bright yellow colour, which the hakim considered normal. However, through the swirling, many small particles appeared as they began floating in the liquid. Hakim Sadiq turned to the patient, saying: 'See, before it was a lot, the thick ones are going away now', suggesting that the patient had been there before. The hakim made a dismissive gesture with his hand, which the patient understood: He went to empty the plastic bottle in a cement sink used for this purpose. [...] We walked back to the desk and I took the patient's folder to study his file, following the hakim's instructions. He was talking to the patient while I was trying to understand the meaning of the medical terminology inscribed in the examination reports. One of them said that the rheumatoid factor was negative. Meanwhile, Hakim Sadiq explained to the boy—according to the reports he was only 13 years old, but he looked older—and to his mother, who was the woman sitting next

57 Hakims usually prescribed antibiotics or antifungals in case of acute conditions if the patients were not already taking them, but they would complement this therapy with dietary advice and other measures in order to strengthen the patient's *ṭabīʿat*. The sole use of drugs targeting the infections, they argued, did not address the root cause of the disease but only one of its manifestations.

to me, that the *lo'āb* ('fluid') from among the bones was finished, and that he should eat goat's meat to change that. Hakim Sadiq asked the patient's mother what the boy had eaten, and the mother answered with another question: 'What should I give him?' The hakim said: 'Give him mung beans, give him sweet fruits. You shall give him strength, you can give him clarified butter with roti.' Hakim Sadiq examined the boy's throat and nose, one of the compounders held a torchlight, illuminating the interiors of the patient's nose and mouth. The throat looked swollen and Hakim Sadiq asked the boy if he ate mangoes, the boy said no. The hakim told him that he should eat vegetables. Hakim Sadiq sat down and grabbed the folder that I had just placed on his desk. He flipped through its pages and, as I glanced again over it, I noticed that the ESR (erythrocyte sedimentation rate) was high. Hakim Sadiq begun writing a new prescription sheet (the previous one was almost a month old), saying aloud:

Hakim Sadiq: Diagnosis... joint pain, nasal polyps. Do you have headaches, son?

Patient: Yes

Hakim Sadiq: Head... ache.

As the hakim wrote the prescription the patient explained that he had some problems with a *puṛyā* ('powder medicine'). Hakim Sadiq turned to me shaking his head and said that the boy had been wrongly given antibiotics for three whole years.

Patient: I ate idli two or three days

Hakim Sadiq: You can eat idli

The patient said that he had a lot of pain. Hakim Sadiq explained that he has been taking medicines for four days now, but he should think that he will be taking medicines for the next forty days. He glanced at the big calendar hanging on the wall in front of his desk, and calculated when the patient shall come again, writing the date on the sheet.

Hakim Sadiq: Are your bowels coming clean?

Patient: They haven't been clean for two or three days, less was coming

Hakim Sadiq: What else?

The patient touched his shoulders, saying that he had pain. Hakim Sadiq told him that his problem is a bone problem while he simulated the movements of the joints rubbing his knuckles. He turned to me: 'His liver is weak, the SGPT [serum glutamic pyruvic transaminase][58] is in the upper normal limit. That increases with cold food. Liver disorders are caused by cold, write that down!'

58 The SGPT is an enzyme whose elevation in blood indicates liver or heart disease.

> The hakim showed me the reports (SGPT 40,000/IU/litre), and told the patient and his mother that he should not eat anything cold. He told the boy to walk because the movement stimulates the production of joint lubrication. Hakim Sadiq studied the previous prescription while one compounder brought a spoon full of a reddish *maʿjūn*. The hakim told the boy to say 'Bismillah' before eating it, after doing so the patient swallowed the paste. Hakim Sadiq instructed the mother to give him mangoes at night, and not to eat cucumbers. They chatted in a jovial manner, laughing also. The hakim said that the boy should not eat two kilos at once when he says that he should eat these foods, but he should eat some.
> Mother: Cumin seed?
> Hakim Sadiq: Yes, cumin, and you can also give him garlic.
> Hakim Sadiq explained to them that other physicians only give pain killers, but he does not. He said that he has prescribed a medicine 'that decreases the pain and that also clears the stool.' He asked the patient 'do you feel cold right now?', the boy said no. Hakim Sadiq explained that one of the medicines he prescribed contains saffron, and that saffron is very expensive. He asked one of the compounders to bring the saffron, after a few seconds the young pharmacist came with a big transparent plastic container full of the red, precious stigmas. Hakim Sadiq opened the container and extracted a hand full of saffron, allowing the tiny threads to drop softly down through his fingers. He then looked at the boy and said: 'The weight will increase after doing weight lifting, don't worry!' The three of them laughed.

This consultation demonstrates how examination reports complemented other diagnostic methods. While the big particles had diminished in the urine, sediments indicated that the patient was not healed yet, even though the rheumatoid factor was negative in the newest test result.[59] Hence, the hakim did not consider the patient to be healed and warned him that the treatment may take another forty days. From the SGTP level in the patient's blood, as well as through the known history of long-term intake of antibiotics, the hakim inferred that the patient's liver was weak, and consequently advised him to avoid cold foods (cucumber), and to favour hot ones (garlic, cumin, mangoes). He also prescribed a medicine containing saffron, which is also considered to be of hot temperament. Clinically, there was no epistemological gap between the understanding of Hakim Sadiq and the findings

59 Negative results in a rheumatoid factor exam do not rule out the disease in biomedicine either.

presented by the test results. These merely provided information on the signs of disease (e.g. problems in the liver) and were combined with other signs of disease provided by other sources in order to arrive at conclusions about the health state of the patient. SGPT levels, ESR and the rheumatoid factor were integrated into the consultation without producing a conflict with the fundamental principles of Unani medicine. Unani principles were used to address the root cause of disease, as suggested by the treatment and the dietary advice prescribed.

Apart from complementing other diagnostic methods as in the case above, pathological examinations could also provide crucial insights into a patient's condition which may not otherwise have been suspected by a hakim:

> A woman wearing a niqab came to sit at the desk, she was accompanied by a man wearing a shalwar *qamīẓ*, a topi and glasses. He had a long beard which seemed made out of thin wires, their clothes suggested that they were a pious Muslim couple. Hakim Sadiq told her to remove her veil. As she lifted the cloth covering her face, her double-chin was revealed. The hakim asked her to remove everything [i.e. the cloth covering her neck, too]: 'You have to show the thyroid [gland]'. Dr. Farzanah palpated the patient's neck after the cloth was removed.
> Hakim Sadiq: [To Dr. Farzanah] Is it? Is it not?
> Dr. Farzanah shook her head in negation and Hakim Sadiq reached for the patient's wrist to feel her pulse.
> Hakim Sadiq: Are you from outside India?
> Patient: No
> Hakim Sadiq: Did you eat breakfast?
> Patient: No.
> Hakim Sadiq spoke to the man who was accompanying the patient (most probably her husband) and told him that she has something in the kidneys. The man extracted several examination reports from a plastic bag and the hakim took a look at them while Dr. Farzanah examined two X-ray images that the patient had just given to her.
> Hakim Sadiq: How many children?
> Patient: Two
> Hakim Sadiq: Small?
> Patient: Four [years old, meaning the youngest child]
> Hakim Sadiq: Have you taken contraceptive pills?
> Patient: No—and she explained that she had a miscarriage after the birth of the youngest child.
> Hakim Sadiq: [Looking at the radiographs] The reports are good.

He highlighted with a yellow text-marker the text in the ultrasound report saying:
'– Liver increased in size with incr. Parenchymal echotexture
– Calculus in gall bladder 18x11mm
– Uterus: Anteverted, increased in size; cervix appear hypertrophied
Impression: Hepatomegaly, diffuse fatty infiltration, cholelithiasis, bulky uterus, hypotrophied cervix'.
Hakim Sadiq explained to the patient and the man about the proper timings for meals and for waking up in the morning: 'It is a system, it is Sunna. Doing it is great Sunna'. Hakim Sadiq told his granddaughter [the MBBS student], who was sitting next to us, to explain 'the exercises' to the patient. The three of us took the patient to the examination room. Dr. Farzanah wanted to do an internal pelvic examination, but the patient said she was on her period, so she did not check her. As we walked back to the desk, Hakim Sadiq was talking to the man:
Hakim Sadiq: ...then yellow bile remains and then one gets hungry. [To his granddaughter] Can't it be regulated, kid?
Granddaughter: It is self-regulating.
I asked the hakim' granddaughter, discreetly, what was he talking about, she said 'secretions of gall-bladder.' Meanwhile, Hakim Sadiq explained to the man that the patient will have to come every day for medicines. He gave her instructions to come and ask for a token, a common procedure in the *Shifa Mahal* for women who get intravaginal medicines: they would ask for a token after payment and then they would wait for any of the two female physiotherapists trained by Hakim Sadiq to take them to the examination room and apply the medicines in private. Hakim Sadiq asked Dr. Farzanah to write down a *joshāndah* recipe he dictated. The diagnosis in the patient sheet he had just finished writing read:
'Gall bladder calculi (+)
18×11mm
Abdominal pain (+)
Inflamed uterus (+)
Bulky ut (+)
Accumulation of fluid in the cervix (+)
(History) Miscarriage
Diabetes (+)'

In this consultation, the hakim established the gall-bladder calculi diagnosis mainly as the result of the ultrasound report. He also made use of other examination reports brought in by the patient, as well as questions to the patient and pulse reading. He explained the cause of the problems to the patient and her companion following the fundamental principles of Unani. The advice given to the patient fits within the notion of gall-bladder stones being a *ṣafrāvī* disease. An interesting aspect here was how the hakim's granddaughter, an MBBS student, translated *ṣafrā'* as gall-bladder secretions to me. This constituted not just a translation into English, but moreover a translation into the language of biomedicine which she was more familiar with. However, Hakim Sadiq's question about its regulation suggests that he actually meant *ṣafrā'*. Judging from other consultations, as seen in the previous chapter, it appears that the hakim asked this question in order to tell the patient about the importance of respecting appropriate timings for sleeping and eating, as he considered that these lifestyle factors influenced bodily secretions which, in turn, had a decisive effect on health on the long term.

The problems in the patient's reproductive tract, which lead to a miscarriage in the past, required local medication. Exercises, together with eating and sleeping at regular times, formed a regimen to support the *ṭabīʿat* and facilitate the healing process as well as to avoid any relapse in the future. This consultation exemplifies how modern diagnostic methods may inform a physician about the exact problem of the patient, but not about its cause. The ultrasound clearly showed the gall-bladder stone and uterine problems, but could not reveal why the patient was affected by these health problems. And since, as exposed in the previous chapter, it is the causation of the disease which is explained mostly through the fundamental principles of Unani medicine, the use of modern diagnostic methods did not contradict the framework used by Hakim Sadiq to identify and treat the health problems of this patient.

This case further illustrates how different diagnostic methods were combined by Hakim Sadiq and Dr. Farzanah in their clinical practice: First, through observation and palpation, a thyroid disorder was discarded.[60] This was followed by a pulse examination. Before he saw the examination reports, Hakim Sadiq suggested a kidney problem. After that he questioned the patient and examined the test results brought by her: two radiographs and an ultrasound. An internal examination would have been conducted to confirm clinically the diagnosis of the ultrasound report, but that was not possible because the patient was menstruating. No urine diagnosis was used during this consultation, perhaps because the reports matched with the findings of the other methods used. In any case, the suggestion

60 For this hakim, thyroid problems were considered to be a secondary disease (see Chapter 3).

of a kidney problem was discarded after Hakim Sadiq saw the ultrasound report and was not included in his final diagnosis.

Although hakims often stress that modern diagnostic techniques should not substitute other diagnostic practices, many agree that certain important information can only be obtained through them. For example, traditional diagnostic methods cannot reveal the exact size of stones, which hakims considered to be very important to decide if a patient should be referred for surgery or if she could be treated with Unani medications. Dr. Hussain explained the necessity of this information during the consultation with a patient complaining of lower back pain:

> Dr. Hussain: Does the pain come from above or below? [He examined the patient, palpating his belly].
> Patient: I get a burning sensation when passing urine.
> The doctor turned to me and said: 'He has the classical signs of liver stone. The pain on the sides which goes until the urethra [pointing with his hands the genital area], and also the report says that he has renal calculi. The two signs are very important: what the patient says, and what the report says. With both together, as we have now, we can diagnose hundred per cent [renal] stones. Now, what is important is the size of the stones. If they are up to six or seven [mm] in size we can treat, sometimes even up to eight or nine we can treat with herbal medicine. But if the size is more, we risk causing hydronephrosis, or we would obstruct the tract, this is why knowing the size [of the stones] is important, because we do not want to cause complications for the patient. The size we can know only with an ultrasound, a sonography.'

Although Dr. Hussain admittedly practiced allopathic medicine, he would try to use Unani medicines whenever he considered that patients would benefit from them. In this case, establishing if the stones were manageable with herbal medicines was only possible through an ultrasound examination revealing their size. This kind of information, however, served practical purposes only and did not interfere with the framework of disease causation used by hakims. When using herbal medicines, Dr. Hussain switched to the fundamental framework of Unani, explaining the action of the therapies through its logic. However, because he lacked deep knowledge about most Unani drugs and their use, he would mostly prescribe biomedical drugs. This approach provided quick relief to his patients, most of whom presented infection-related complaints, unlike the clientele of Hakim Azim, Hakim Ahmad, and Hakim Sadiq, who were sought after mostly for the treatment of so-called lifestyle diseases.

A common argument employed for the justification of the use of modern diagnostic techniques in Unani medicine is their higher accuracy in terms of establishing the actual health state of a patient. However, many hakims opine that modern diagnostic tools are only reliable if combined with traditional diagnostic methods. Machines are not perfect, they argue, hence examination reports are not always to be trusted. Hakims are cautious about the quality of the examination reports produced by different laboratories, and would often suggest to their patients to get tests from laboratories they trusted. Hakim Sadiq sometimes requested patients to get new examination reports when these did not seem to be accurate (for example when fasting sugar tests results suggested that the exam was not done in a fasting state) or when the tests were too old to be used to assess the current situation of a patient.

Patients often come with pathological examinations in hand, sometimes expensive ones such as CT (computerized tomography) scans. Judging from their complaints, these examinations were not necessarily required for establishing a diagnosis. Medical practice is influenced by the economic interests of pathological laboratories that offer a 'cut' from the laboratory's fee to the physicians recommending them. In cases when the treating doctor ordered unnecessary tests that were expensive but gave no insight into the patient's condition, hakims ignored the reports. While examining a patient's inconsistent blood reports regarding the rheumatoid factor, Hakim Sadiq explained once to a patient: 'The reactive protein was positive, then it was negative. Hence, I do not trust the report, the drug therapy shall be continued.' The judgment of a good physician, thus, is considered superior to any report alone.

Proof of Effectiveness

When I first visited Hakim Sadiq in the Summer of 2012, I was brought to him by a relative of his who also practiced Unani in Hyderabad. Dr. Rashid had brought me to several *k͟hāndānī* hakims in the city, helping me to fulfil my wish to visit experienced private practitioners of Unani. When we arrived, the clinic was full of people. Still, Hakim Sadiq gave us a warm welcome and invited us to sit in a separate room while his son Sabir continued attending patients. Sweet mangoes and gulab jamun were brought to us and we talked about Unani as we ate. The old hakim explained that he had knowledge and practice on many drugs which were all prepared right there, in his house. He told me that he used urine and pulse diagnosis, complemented by blood and urine tests, ultrasound, and X-ray images. He asked someone to bring the files of some of his patients and he showed me the 'before' and 'after' positive changes in the blood levels of, for example, serum creatinine. Serum creatinine is an important indicator of renal health or disease in biomedicine and, as I would find out a year later when I came back to conduct participant observation at the *Shifa Mahal*, it was also a central parameter in his medical practice.

During my first visit, Hakim Sadiq took me for a tour and showed me how the medicines were produced by his staff and where their ingredients were stored. He extracted some of his most precious single drugs from locked cupboards and drawers around the house: pearls and ambergris, lapis lazuli from Afghanistan, saffron from Kashmir. His staff produced medicines under his supervision, and his treatments consisted not only of these self-produced drugs, but also of dietary advice, exercises, massages, and other manual techniques such as the application of heat. He diagnosed with the pulse and was the only hakim I saw routinely using uroscopy as a diagnostic tool. When I returned to Hakim Sadiq's clinic more than a year after my first visit, he smiled friendly and said that he recognized me. He told me to sit next to him at the desk where he conducted patient consultations. It was there that I would spend the next three months. The first thing he did was to ask one of his staff to bring the files of certain patients. He instructed me to read them and to ask questions. As I sat reading blood and urine test reports and ultrasound examinations, a few patients started arriving. At that moment I felt frustrated: I had the chance to sit with an experienced and reputed hakim and observe how he practiced, but instead I had to go through a pile of files with biomedical examination reports. It was not until later that this situation, uncomfortable as it was for me at first, unfolded as a deeply interesting one. Hakim Sadiq knew that I was conducting research on Unani medicine. He also knew that I was interested in his practice. Aware that I was going to write about him, he was keen to show me—and not just tell me—that his therapies worked. I realized that the reports were proof of effectiveness, evidence of the success of his practice as a hakim (Schmidt Stiedenroth 2019a). The reports were not fulfilling a diagnostic purpose, but a legitimating one instead. This is not a recent phenomenon in Unani medicine, as suggested by various anecdotes of famous hakims. One of them narrates:

> The son of Mr. Charles, the additional commissioner of Lucknow, who was a doctor, was affected by a big renal stone through which he suffered from problems and uneasiness at all times. The doctors advised him to undergo surgery [...]. One day, Mr. Charles showed the X-ray of the gentleman to Hakim Abdulmuid. After seeing the X-ray, the hakim forbade

> surgery, he would give common drugs used for stones from his own clinic instead. [...] After a month, another X-ray of the kidney was taken, and this one showed no signs of the stone. The problems of the patient were also completely gone. The hakim relieved the patient from his troubles and danger without any operation. Mr. Charles was touched and happy after seeing the accomplishment of the hakim (Fārūqī 1995: 213f.).

This anecdote exemplifies that the success of Unani therapies can be demonstrated through modern diagnostic methods and not only through the patient's relief. Further, the fact that the patient who was successfully treated was a Westerner and, on top of that, a practitioner of Western medicine extols the success of the hakim's skill—and of Unani medicine—even more by proving that no surgical procedure was required to heal the patient. Here, X-rays were used to demonstrate the superiority of Unani against Western medicine.

Hakim Sadiq kept folders with 'before' and 'after' reports which he and his son would show to patients with similar problems in order to convince them not only to get treated by them, but also to follow their advice and remain patient. This helped make the point that a treatment may take a long time, but brings results on the long term (Schmidt Stiedenroth 2019a). Hakim Sadiq used examination reports as proof of therapeutic success, employing the files of other patients to convince new patients to pursue his treatment (ibid.). When looking at these files and the different examination reports, which were ordered chronologically from 'before treatment' to 'during treatment' and 'after treatment', some reports showed increased levels of serum creatinine during the course of the therapies. This, Hakim Sadiq and his team would explain, was caused by the patient's *badparhezī* ('non-compliance') with the dietary and lifestyle advice. We may compare this notion with the anecdote presented above, where compliance was explicitly mentioned in connection to the success of the therapy. Hakim Sadiq and his team also used modern diagnostic methods to keep track of the patients' improvements and compliance.

Hakim Sadiq was not the only hakim presenting proofs about the success of his treatments through modern diagnostic methods. As discussed in Chapter 2, a family hakim from Hyderabad, who was well known for a heart-disease family recipe, also kept records of the effects of his treatment in folders containing 'before' and 'after' examination reports (ibid.). The first were blood tests reports showing high cholesterol levels and ultrasound pictures of blocked arteries or aortic stenosis cases, while the latter showed normal cholesterol levels, open arteries and no stenosis. His son showed these files to me, arguing that they prove that the family recipe works. Their clinic seemed to be well known, the hakim and his son told me that many patients consulted them after finding no relief with allopathic medicine (ibid.).

These hakims' use of modern diagnostic techniques to attest treatment success is similar to the use of radiographs documented among bonesetters in the Southern May Highlands (Hinojosa 2004) and in Hyderabad (Attewell 2016), as well as among *ācāns* (practitioners of vital spots medicine) in South India (Sieler 2015: 150). Neither the bonesetters nor the *ācāns* would use X-rays only for diagnostic purposes; they were employed also for their 'confirmatory power' (Hinojosa 2004: 275) and 'as documents of proof of their medical legitimacy' (Sieler 2015: 150). Bonesetters in Hyderabad used X-rays 'in order to produce evidence that "proves" the effectiveness of the treatment' and to 'challenge the stigmatization of this form of therapeutics as ineffective or indeed iatrogenic' (Attewell 2016: 5). The introduction of radiography to the practice of bonesetters appears to be a recent phenomenon as described by these authors. In contrast, the anecdote presented above suggests that X-rays have been used by hakims since the Colonial Period.

Among medical technologies, those involving the visualization of the interior body have been particularly interesting for social science scholars. In his analysis of French medicine in the nineteenth century, Foucault analysed how the clinical gaze changed with the advent of pathology, privileging the visual into what counts as possible knowledge (2005). Indeed, the development of technologies of visualization was instrumental in the development of 'objectivity' as epistemic virtue (Daston and Galison 2010 [2007]). When instrumentalized, ultrasound images can be very powerful because visualization is privileged over experience in terms of evidence, even though the visual is always subject to the interpretation and gaze of the observer (Petchesky 1987). This point has been convincingly demonstrated in a comparative study of Chinese and ancient Greek anatomy (Kuriyama 2002 [1999]).

While Hakim Sadiq trusted urine observation or a patient's expression, he equally acknowledged that unhealthy states were also manifested in ways that escape the gaze and needed to be identified using other senses. Pain, for example, could not always be assessed visually in clinical practice, yet it was an important sign of disease. While, as seen in the previous chapter, even though Unani literature suggests that the predominance of certain humours may be visualized, for example, through urine having different colours, the practice of hakims had not totally undergone the shift from body-centred to image-centred diagnostics which is considered a marker of biomedical practice (Hinojosa 2004: 281). Hakims remain instrumental in interpreting the results provided by technology, and those results are considered one among various diagnostic methods, which together usually require a sort of triangulation in order to provide reliable information.

The use of diagnostic reports as evidence of treatment effectiveness rests on the perception of them as being objective. However, their 'objectivity' is not so much based on their visual as it is based on their scientific nature, as science is considered a universal and neutral realm by hakims. Hence, many hakims sustain that claims of success can be made universally through modern diagnostic technologies. Exam reports showing improvements in the levels of blood sugar or serum creatinine are considered to speak for themselves to patients in a 'language of science' whose authority is hard to deny.

Biomedical Technologies?

Medical anthropological literature tends to treat medical tools and technologies as biomedical, even though they have been appropriated by other professional groups (Hildebrand 2012; Langford 2002; Naraindas 2006). These tools and technologies are considered to embody modernity in a way that is often connected to the biomedical profession in terms of medical knowledge or institutions, mainly because biomedical professionals claim authority over their use for themselves (Hildebrand 2012). It has been argued that biomedicine's ownership claims over the X-ray technology 'restricts the legitimate exercise of authority to those using the approved technology' (Hinojosa 2004: 270f.).

While such claims of ownership may apply in the Guatemalan context, in India the regulations pertaining to the AYUSH systems of medicine legitimate the use of modern scientific advances by Unani physicians, thus neutralizing any exclusive authority claims over 'modern advances' by biomedical practitioners. As discussed above, medical technologies are considered by both the Indian state and the Unani fraternity to be the product of scientific advances that no form of medicine can claim for itself. State regulations sanctioning the use of medical technologies by different professionals contribute to defining which professional group can make legitimate use of them. Unlike the Maya bonesetters, who 'acknowledge the powerful presence of biomedical institutions' through speaking about X-rays (Hinojosa 2004: 280), most hakims do not identify X-rays or for instance any medical technology with biomedicine. Hence, analysing medical technologies as biomedical per se—even though their development and usage may, at least initially, underlie a biomedical framework—, can be misleading. Like any form of technology, medical technologies do not exist in a vacuum. As argued by David Arnold, 'the "social life" of mechanical objects needs to be understood in context and cannot be presumed to be uniform and universal.' (2013: 5). The adaptation of (diagnostic) technologies into Unani practice illustrates this.

In the case of Tibetan medicine, ultrasound could be useful to confirm diagnoses, but they are not considered as reliable as traditional diagnostic methods (Adams 2002a: 203). This seemingly contradictory approach 'was a good indicator of the complicated cultural negotiations undertaken by traditional Tibetan medical practitioners in order to awkwardly both accommodate and distinguish their medicine from its "modern medical" counterpart' (ibid.). The ways in which examination reports are used to demonstrate effectiveness cannot only be understood through an examination of epistemologies, but requires an examination of multiple forces including history and manifold globalization fields (Adams 2002a: 217). This observation applies for the Unani case as well, because the state support granted to traditional forms of medicine provides a legal framework that detaches medical technologies from biomedicine and allows hakims, as well as other so-called AYUSH practitioners, to officially appropriate them.

The appropriation of biomedical technologies has been defined as 'the ways in which biomedical techniques are (made) fit to specific local worlds, and consequently are changed and simultaneously bring about sociotechnical changes' (Hadolt et al. 2012: 186). Guy Attewell rejected the notion of appropriation for being linked with ownership, suggesting instead an examination in terms of 'a technology-in-practice assemblage' dealing with how X-rays and other technologies 'have been diverted, or re-routed' to present evidence of efficacy instead of being used as diagnostic methods (2016: 5f.). In the context of Unani, appropriation, rather than diversion, appears to be more useful. Modern diagnostic techniques were embedded by hakims into their conceptual frameworks and adapted to their practical needs in a process of 'braiding knowledge', a metaphor used by Projit Mukharji to understand how the use of technologies made Ayurveda 'modern'. According to Mukherji, '[n]either Ayurveda nor "Western" science are static or fully defined entities in this crossing. They are multi-stranded spools selectively braided together by the presence of the "entangled objects."' (2016: 27). In the process, the entangled objects are themselves transformed, having the capacity to 'give rise to new identities and figures' (ibid.). Hakims practising privately use modern diagnostic methods to convince patients about treatment success or in order to obtain useful diagnostic information which was consequently used following the framework laid down by the fundamental principles of Unani medicine, transforming the technologies in the process.

As discussed in Chapter 2, while modern techniques seem to have replaced traditional methods for diagnostic purposes in institutionalized settings, the reason for this does not rest on the modern technologies themselves, but on the institutional framework of knowledge transmission that has led to a 'fracturing of medical knowledge' (Attewell 2005). However, when Unani practitioners paid attention to its fundamental principles in practice, as done by Hakim Sadiq and other hakims practicing privately, they claimed that the use of modern diagnostic methods not only did not interfere with the Unani understanding of disease causation, but even sustained this paradigm. Instead of imposing biomedical parameters or different epistemologies, the use of modern technologies was transformed by hakims to demonstrate the broad scope of Unani medicine and even its superiority vis-à-vis biomedicine. This, however, was not the case in all Unani settings, particularly not in institutional ones.

Unani practitioners do not attach medical technologies to any particular framework, biomedical or otherwise. For example, the biochemistry parameters revealed in blood or urine tests reports are regarded as part of a general anatomical knowledge which does not stand in opposition to the Unani body. The added dimensions of materiality are not considered to concur with Unani knowledge, but to complement it. As stated by Prohit Mukharji based on Stacey Langwick, 'to take materiality seriously we cannot assume that any one epistemic regime has the monopoly in defining it' (Mukharji 2016: 151). Contrary to biomedical drugs or surgery, which hakims consider to encapsulate a distinct, biomedical understanding of disease causation, modern technologies are considered compatible with Unani's understanding of disease causation, because they are seen as the product of science, which in turn is regarded by hakims as neutral. This understanding allows hakims to appropriate modern technologies within the Unani configuration in order to establish diagnoses and causes of disease, to prescribe treatments accordingly, and to present evidence of therapeutic success to prospective patients. Unani medicine has traditionally incorporated new advances and knowledge, and modern diagnostic methods—for whatever purpose—are no exception.

Modernizing Concepts

On Matter and Qualities

The existence of the elements (*arkān,* lit. pillars, fundamentals or *ʿanāṣir,* lit. elements) is commonly accepted in Unani medicine. Both terms *arkān* and *ʿanāṣir* are used interchangeably in contemporary Unani literature, even though their meaning is different. Although they are commonly described as the four classical elements—fire (*nār* or *āg*), water (*mā'* or *pānī*), air (*havā*), and earth (*arẓ* or *miṭṭī*)—, their understanding in contemporary Unani medicine is broad and contested. Many Unani practitioners argued that nowadays it is clear that there are more than just four elements; most of them interpreted *arkān* as the chemical elements of the periodic table. This interpretation was promoted by Hakim Abdulhamid, who, from the 1970s onwards, engaged in a project called 'Elementology' which sought to 'bridge the "communication gap" between traditional and modern medicine' (Bode 2008: 147f.). The Medical Elementology project brought together international scientists, including from outside the Indian subcontinent, who met in a WHO-sponsored conference in 1983 which lead to the foundation of an 'International Union of Elementologists' (Vohora and Dobrowolski 1990; Vohora and Khan 1983). Although this project was said to have remained mostly 'an academic exercise and did not bring unani tibb the international recognition Hakim Abdul Hamid was hoping for' (Bode 2008: 147), its influence has been deep and is still traceable in contemporary Unani medicine. According to Bode, while the Elementology project sought to vindicate Unani knowledge as established in the classical texts, it failed to convince and to fulfil its aim to validate Unani as compatible with modern, scientific research standards (ibid.).

While this project has been dismissed by some members of the fraternity, its influence is still present in recent Unani research. For example, a practitioner in Hyderabad showed me his Unani postgraduate thesis on men's sexual diseases in which he discussed the influence of the elements on health. He referred to magnesium and calcium in particular. In this way, he integrated modern concepts as a reinterpretation of the ancient principle of the elements. The aim to reconcile Unani (or, for instance, concepts of ancient Greek philosophy) with modern chemistry is taken for granted by most BUMS students and graduates, and the elements of modern chemistry have found their way in contemporary practices of Unani. Hakim Sadiq, for example, would tell patients that their problems were caused by the fact that 'oxygen does not come'. He also drew from chemistry to explain *parhez* ('dietary restrictions') to one of his patients, as when he told him to eat vegetables that contain *shorah*. The patient asked what *shorah* meant and the hakim pressed his eyes as if trying to remember, saying: 'Potassium chloride... alkaloid. It has cold in it, it is in citrus [fruits]. Don't eat spinach, tomatoes, squash. What should you eat? Mung beans. There is too much acidity in yoghurt.' 'Which one has magnesium?', asked the patient, and Hakim Sadiq answered: 'The temperament gets cold from magnesium.'

It is tempting to suggest that Elementology cemented the path for integrating biochemical aspects of human physiology into Unani medicine, offering a common ground with biomedicine. However, it is not clear if the role of potassium and magnesium in the practice of Hakim Sadiq corresponded to the influence of Elementology or if it was a product of his readings of general literature—including newspaper articles—on medicine, diet, and health. Regardless of whether these elements were considered by the hakim to correspond to the *arkān* in the Elementology sense or not, they were still part of his practice and, hence, part of contemporary Unani. Their integration into the Unani framework through the attribution of qualities that affect the temperament corresponds to the classical concept of *arkān*. This made their integration plausible. In this way, they did not seem to be a substitution of the fundamental principles of Unani. Instead, they could be seen as an extension of them. As the explanation of Hakim Sadiq above suggests, it is not the elements themselves which are of paramount importance for the physician, but rather their qualities and, hence, their influence on the human body. Thus, the quality of an element, and not its material composition, seems to be the most relevant aspect for clinical practice.

Not everyone agreed with the interpretation of *arkān* as chemical elements. Hakim Syed Zillurrahman, one of the most important Unani scholars in contemporary India, explained in conversation that *arkān* was often wrongly translated as 'elements' because it meant liquids, gases, solids, and heat in the human body. He explained the connection between the *arkān* and the temperaments: the qualities dry, moist, hot, and cold correspond to the four humours, and the most essential humour in the human body, he explained, is blood. The most essential *rukn* (sg. of *arkān*) is liquid, because without liquid neither humans nor animals nor plants could live. This was why the humour blood (*dam*) is liquid as well. Even though this hakim rejected the interpretation of *arkān* as the chemical elements, his interpretation is still centred on the qualities of the elements.

The association of the four elements with the four primary qualities goes back to Aristotle and it was later on adopted in mediaeval Islamic philosophy and science (Belo 2018). Ibn Sina expanded this model arguing that elements transform themselves into one another, as the primary qualities effect changes (ibid.). The focus on the qualities could be extended to the humours, too. Establishing the nature of the three *dosas* of Ayurveda in relation to the four qualities (hot, cold, wet and dry) of the Graeco-Islamic tradition was one of the main concerns of Muslim physicians translating Indian medical texts (Speziale 2014b: 793), accounting for their importance. The relevance of the qualities for treatment in the Graeco-Islamic tradition has also been documented. The achievement of balance was not centred on the humours, as often assumed, but instead on the four primary qualities via environmental factors (Savage-Smith 2013: 101f.), much in line with the clinical practices analysed above.

In his book on the principles of Unani medicine, Hakim Syed Ishtiaq Ahmed dedicated several pages to a discussion of the different interpretations of the elements (2009). His own position corresponded to a synthesis of Elementology with Hakim Zillurrahman's ideas. The *arkān,* he argued, correspond to the chemical elements, but they are still four because four is the number in which they can be classified according to their qualities which he, in turn, interpreted as the three states of matter (solid, liquid and gas) plus heat, which he understood in a relative way, i.e. not necessarily as hot but as heat producing (Ahmed 2009: 5ff.). With this interpretation, Ahmed argued that accepting the number of elements proposed by modern chemistry today represents no challenge to the basic concepts of Unani. It is worth mentioning that Ahmed's book, which was first published in 1980, was re-printed by the CCRUM in 2009 due to its success as a teaching book for BUMS students. In the preface of its reprint, Mohammed Khalid Siddiqui—then director general of the CCRUM—wrote that the book was considered 'an important addition to the contemporary Unani medical literature' and that students and scholars received it with such enthusiasm, emphasizing that the first edition 'sold like a hot cake' and soon became rare as the demand for the book kept increasing (Ahmed 2009 [1980]: i). This book is an interesting example of efforts of reinterpretation of the fundamentals of Unani through modern concepts. It epitomizes the enormous influence—or even dominance—of such an approach in contemporary Unani medicine, especially in institutionalized settings, a legacy from Hakim Kabiruddin, as Ahmed himself acknowledged (2009). This approach was characterized by the interpretations of Unani concepts in accordance to biochemical and anatomical understandings of the body as in biomedicine, like for example the interpretation of *rūḥ* (pneuma, vital spirit or soul) as oxygen or the *ak̲h̲lāṭ* (humors) as any fluid in the body, including intracellular fluids, trans-cellular fluids and vascular fluids (Ahmed 2009 [1980]).

Such efforts of harmonization, however, are not accepted by the whole Unani fraternity. In conversation, Kunvar Muhammad Yusuf Amin—a medical pharmacologist working at the *'Ilm al-adviyah* department of the Ajmal Khan Tibbiya College in Aligarh—pointed out that the holism of Unani medicine was dependent on its understanding of what he called levels of being (*darjāt-i vojūd,* lit. degrees of existence), which include a supra-corporeal (metaphysical) level. For him, the interpretation of *rūḥ* as oxygen creates confusion, because it assumes that *rūḥ* is a corporeal entity when it actually belongs to 'the subtle level', meaning that it is not physical.[61] Prof. Amin, himself not a BUMS but an MBBS graduate with a personal interest in logic, philosophy and Sufism, argued that the metaphysical nature of certain fundamentals of Unani, like *arvāḥ* (pl. of *rūḥ*) did not create problems for modern research, as they could be studied through their physical correlates. As an example, he mentioned increase of heat, which according to him manifested itself in the body through an increase in temperature and also through curly hair. By measuring these physical correlates, he stated, it was possible to integrate metaphysical aspects of Unani into modern research, in his case the pharmacological and clinical research of Unani drugs.[62]

This explanation is crucial for two reasons. First, it is an example of how metaphysics has not been rejected in the epistemic framework of Unani, and how causality is still considered a valid scientific method. Secondly, and linked to that, it points towards the importance of the qualities (i.e. hot, cold, dry and wet) and their effect on the human body. Hakims and scholars such as Prof. Amin suggest that, as long as the focus remains on the qualities, for example heating or cooling, the different interpretations about the physical or metaphysical nature of the fundamentals of Unani does not affect their application in medical practice.

Different interpretations coexisted in contemporary Unani medicine, but they all seemed to share the understanding that the qualities, and not matter, were the relevant characteristics of elements, pneuma and even the humours. It is not the substance itself, but rather the action and effect it has on the body that is clinically relevant for Unani practitioners. In this way, the multiple interpretations of the elements—as chemical elements, as states of matter, or both—coexist without leading to a conflict in practice because the underlying idea of qualities is shared by them.

The case of the elements exemplifies how ancient understandings of health and healing are harmonized with modern Western science without challenging their central idea in practice. In this sense, talking about a 'modernization' or 'biomedicalization' of Unani concepts, like in the case of the Elementology project, should be done only carefully. While Bode dismissed such an attempt to reconcile the fundamentals with modern

61 For a discussion on different interpretations of *rūḥ, nafs* and *'aql* as soul and as material and non-material bodily entities in Islamic thought see Tritton (1971).

62 For similar views of metaphysical entities having no form but qualities among practitioners of Ayurveda see Bode (2012).

science as 'less convincing' (2008: 145), I would rather suggest that looking at the core ideas behind the surface through an analysis of the interpretations of the elements or, for instance, of humours, pneuma, etc. in descriptions as well as in practice makes it possible to get closer to the heart of the matter and to understand that hakims are primarily concerned not with form or substance, but rather with quality in terms of action.

Combining Unani and Biomedical Knowledge

The institutionalization of Unani training and practice, which fostered the integration of modern diagnostic methods and subjects like anatomy and biochemistry as well as methods of scientific research into Unani, has led to new forms of medical practice where the fundamental principles were often neglected and, in some cases, not even considered at all. It is well known that most AYUSH graduates practice biomedicine, or at least a mixed form where the fundamental principles of Unani hardly play a role at all. But what about private practitioners like Hakim Sadiq, who practice in more traditional ways and could certainly not be said to practice allopathy? How do they combine Unani and biomedical concepts in their seemingly traditional practice?

Although the fundamental concepts of Unani may seem very different from biomedical ones, the Unani theories of causation of diseases do not necessarily conflict with biomedical understandings in practice. Because, as discussed in the previous chapter, humoral imbalance is considered to be the consequence of other factors, biomedical aetiologies fit to a certain extent the framework used by Unani physicians. The example most commonly mentioned by hakims to make this point combines germ theory and the response of the immune system with the concept of *ṭabīʿat*. Since a healthy body should be capable of healing itself, hakims argue that viruses or bacteria do not always make people sick. Hence, disease could not be solely explained by the presence of pathogens. Only when there is a humoral imbalance—caused by an imbalance of qualities which, in turn, is attributed to changes in the essential and non-essential factors—does disease arise, because the immune system would not be able to fight the disease on its own. Here, the causation of disease is articulated in the idiom of a weakness of the physis (*ṭabīʿat*) and its impaired ability to maintain health.

During my last two weeks in the *Shifa Mahal*, Faridah, Hakim Sadiq's granddaughter, also spent time in the clinic. She was an MBBS student and her grandfather wanted her to gain exposure to clinical practice during her summer break. Hakim Sadiq wanted her to be in the clinic from early

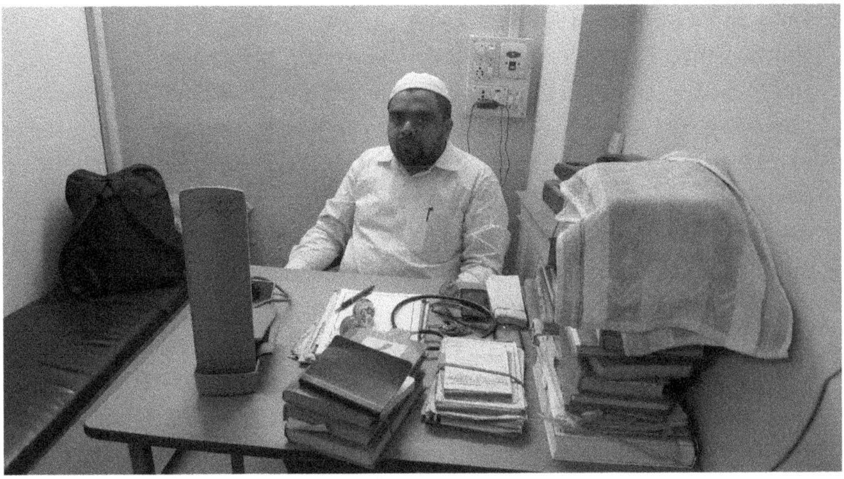

3. Hakim Muhammad Islahi in his clinic in Mumbai (2013).

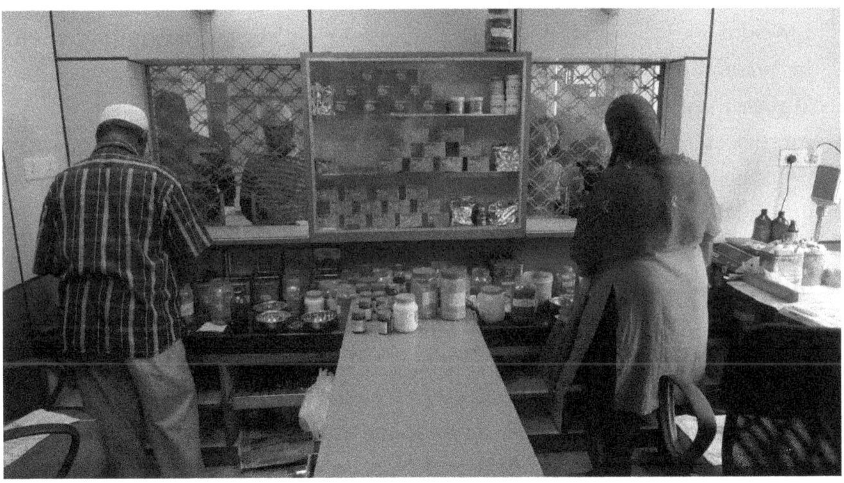

4. The dispensary of the Research Institute of Unani Medicine in Chennai (2012).

morning until noon. Her presence was a unique opportunity not only to observe how Hakim Sadiq transmitted his knowledge, but also because the conversations between the two revealed how transactions between biomedical and Unani knowledge took place, as in the following case:

> A female patient came, she touched Hakim Sadiq's feet when greeting him, a sign of great respect. The hakim turned to me and explained her case.
> Hakim Sadiq: She had Bell's palsy one and a half years ago. Now it comes and goes. [Turning to his granddaughter] Now how does it come?

Farzanah: From infection
Hakim Sadiq: That's wrong. An oedema forms in the nerves.
Hakim Sadiq examined the patient and asked one of his physiotherapists to massage the patient's ear with *rog̱han-i bābūnah* ('chamomile oil'). He explained to us that chamomile oil has anti-inflammatory and antibiotic properties as he showed me how to do the massage, from behind the ear downwards with vibrating finger pressure. Hakim Sadiq said to his granddaughter that this information could be found in any Unani book and that she should go sit and read about it to remember. Farzanah did as her grandfather said and fetched an anatomy teaching book from a desk's drawer; the book was an illustrated biomedical text entitled *Dr. Chandra Sia's Human Anatomy*. She was searching for the section on the anatomy of the nerves, but when her grandfather returned to the desk and saw what she was doing, he told her to search for the anatomy of the ear first of all. He turned to me and said, in English: 'Everything is possible in medical life!' His granddaughter found the ear section in the book and the explanation of the nerve supply, the communication between the ears and the facial nerve was mentioned. Hakim Sadiq said 'did you see?' She nodded and said that in her book it is explained in more detail. She went upstairs to get her own book and came back a few moments later with *Diseases of the Ear, Nose, and Throat* by P.L. Dhingra and S. Dhingra, fifth edition. The hakim said: 'Catarrh, an oedema forms and there is no blood supply.' As she found the section on the ear in the book, both of them observed the illustration of the internal anatomy of the ear and he explained: 'Phlegm comes out from here, a condition arises.' He then told his granddaughter to highlight the text in the book saying 'oedema or inflammation can easily compress the nerve and cause paralysis.' He pointed to the image of the ear and explained that the nerves were compromised in the process, telling her to remember that. He asked her for the name of the book and then asked his son to order it for himself.

In this example, biomedical knowledge as presented in the biomedical textbooks did not contradict, but rather sustained the theory of causation of Bell's palsy (*laqvah*) as understood by Hakim Sadiq: phlegm, through catarrh, obstructs the blood supply and compresses the nerve causing paralysis. We may note that for Hakim Sadiq it was excess of phlegm that caused this particular kind of paralysis when it blocked the nerve. His treatment therefore consisted of massage with chamomile oil and medications that facilitated the expulsion of the phlegm causing inflammation and nerve blockage. Patients with *laqvah* were often sitting in a corridor of the *Shifa Mahal* spitting phlegm in a plastic bag after having taken a powder that facilitated its expulsion. Usually, a staff member would come and massage their face from the ear downwards towards the nose with vibrant movements after the patients had spitted enough phlegm. They had to come regularly to the clinic in order to receive the facial massage. *Parhez* is very important in the treatment of *laqvah* patients; they have to avoid cooling foods (*ṭhanḍā* and *khaṭṭā*) which are considered to promote the production of phlegm. The temperament of chamomile is described as warm in second degree and dry in the first degree (Aʿvān n.d. 106), thus opposing the coolness and moisture of phlegm, following the principle of healing with opposites described in the previous chapter. Also, Hakim Sadiq advised patients of Bell's palsy not to use air conditioners nor to sleep with fans on, as the cold wind may affect their condition negatively.

Hakim Sadiq had an excellent reputation for the treatment of Bell's palsy. One of his former patients told me about his own case. One day he could not move half of his face and could not speak properly. The doctors told him that there was no treatment for this condition. An acquaintance recommended Hakim Sadiq. When he got to the clinic, he had been suffering for three days. The hakim told him that he was lucky that he got there relatively quickly, as the later the treatment starts, the longer it takes and the less are the chances for therapeutic success. The therapy had begun a few years before we met. Now, he said, he sticks to the *parhez*. He was fine and thankful: not being able to move half his face had been a very frightening experience which he did not want to repeat.

The aetiology and treatment of *laqvah* followed by Hakim Sadiq resonates with the explanation of this condition given in the *Aksīr-i Aʿẓam*, a book on diseases, their symptoms and treatments whose Urdu translation by Hakim Kabiruddin (n.d., ca. 1940) is very popular among hakims and BUMS students. The *Aksīr-i Aʿẓam* states that *laqvah* is caused by the descent of a humour (*k̲h̲ilṭ*) from the brain into the jaws and its nerves, causing the muscle tissue of the face and eyes to immobilize or convulse, resulting in two possible forms of *laqvah* which have been described by Galen (Kabīruddīn n.d. 196). Regarding its treatment, the book recommends a regimen whereby the patient is kept in a house protected from darkness and wind and sits with nutmeg, cloves or dried ginger in his mouth in front of a fire of burning *jhā'ū* wood (*tamarix indica*). Further, the regimen prescribes the avoidance of a cold home or anything that produces phlegm or winds, abstinence from all food and drinks except for honey water, enemas to expel the phlegm, and medicines of warm temperament during the first days (Kabīruddīn n.d.

197ff.). All the drugs mentioned, including honey, are considered to have hot and dry temperaments of varying degrees (Aʿvān n.d.).[63]

This case illustrates that it is misleading to assume that biomedical and Unani aetiologies are always incompatible. Biomedical knowledge may not only not oppose, but it may even support, to a certain extent, the aetiologies as addressed by hakims. Hakim Sadiq did not consider the disease itself as exclusive of Unani; for him, the cause was explained in part through anatomical knowledge, using the same understanding of the human body as currently shared by biomedicine and Unani (i.e. that paralysis can be caused by oedema or inflammation when a nerve is compressed) and the history of the patient's complaints (i.e. catarrh and its characteristic increased production of phlegm, exposure to cold, etc.), two aspects that may be considered as facts by any biomedical or Unani physician. It is not surprising, thus, that most Unani practitioners and students do not see a problem in the introduction of subjects such as anatomy in the BUMS course, because the human body is considered the same, irrespective of any system of medicine being practiced.[64]

While differences between Unani and biomedicine were established, these are not based on anatomical knowledge: as previously discussed, the clinical relevance of humours and elements does not reside in their materiality, but on their actions or effects on the human body. In the case of *laqvah*, this is manifested in the blockage of the facial nerve. The hakim's focus on the root cause of disease, i.e. what causes the excess of phlegm responsible for the blockage, is seen as the advantage of Unani vis-à-vis biomedicine, because Unani is said to look at the big picture and, in this way, to be capable of getting rid of the actual cause of disease, not only its manifestations. While a biomedical physician may not consider phlegm and, primarily, cold as the root cause of the disease, the hakim would address exactly those. In the case of Bell's palsy, excessive phlegm was seen as the product of excessive cold, and this is why dietary restrictions and avoidance of air conditioner at night were as important for the treatment as the oral expulsion of phlegm and the use of hot and dry medicines and foods. Hence, not the excess of phlegm, but the cold producing its excess was the root of the disease, affecting the physis and its response to different factors, whereas the excess of phlegm itself constituted the material cause, following the Aristotelian principle.

63 The text also mentions recipes for decoctions and other preparations containing drugs of different temperaments in order to counter the heat (and the possible constipation appearing as a consequence of it) caused as a side-effect of the hot and dry therapies (Kabīruddīn n.d. 198).

64 Compare with Langford's findings in the case of Ayurveda (2002: 39).

Hence, the principle of healing with the opposites through diet, lifestyle and drugs, as well as the use of mechanical techniques such as massage with an oil of hot and dry quality, all addressed the primary cause of the disease.

While hakims often employed the language of biomedicine—for example by using English names of diseases—, it would be misleading to assume that the use of this language automatically imposes biomedical nosologies. Harish Naraindas demonstrated how biomedical reasoning was given primacy by Ayurvedic practitioners who ruled out of conditions such as malfunctioning of the thyroid gland or worm infections first of all, whereby an Ayurvedic diagnosis, if used at all, was rather as 'a residual category' (2014b: 119). This may also be the case of institutionally trained Unani physicians working in government settings. As for the hakims whose practice I discussed above, the integration of 'biomedical' knowledge such as the functioning of the thyroid gland, hormone production or bacterial infections does not translate into a the biomedicalization of their practice because this knowledge is not conceived as biomedical, but as anatomical or pathological.

Writing on the overlapping of modern science and indigenous knowledge systems, STS scholars Helen Watson-Verran and David Turnbull suggested that these 'are polysemous, so that where one system leaves off and the other starts is a matter of strategic negotiation in the part of those involved in knowledge production enterprises' (1995: 131). For hakims, it is the way in which health and disease is approached that establishes the difference between Unani and other forms of medicine in clinical practice, whereas in terms of identity articulation the humoural paradigm is often recalled as Unani's essence. Differences drawn from the humoural theory of Unani alone are misleading because they assume that the 'essence' of Unani medicine resides also practically and not just narratively on concepts of bodily constitution rather than on understandings of how the body parts interact with each other and with the environment under the principle of Aristotelian causality (Attewell 2013; Savage-Smith 2013). This understanding appears to be the product of looping effects rooted in representations of Unani as humoural medicine discussed in the previous chapter, and of medical technologies as biomedical, as discussed above. However, it is not the presence or absence of substances, but rather the reasoning about how the causes operate and interact with the substances and other bodily parts that characterize the practice of hakims practising privately. In this way, epistemological gaps based on the opposition of humouralism with modern science dissolve in Unani clinical practices, because they transcend the boundaries of each of them.

5. Science and the Quest for Acceptance and Recognition

I visited the Central Research Institute of Unani Medicine (CRIUM) in Hyderabad for the first time in the summer of 2012. As I sat with the director of the institution at that time, Dr. M. Ataullah Shareef, and a few of his senior staff members in his large and comfortable office, he asked me first of all what I knew about the basics of Unani medicine. I said that I have read about them, but perhaps he could tell me a bit more. He nodded and began explaining that the humours and the elements constitute the basics of Unani medicine when, suddenly, he began telling me that the institute has a long experience with clinical research on diseases such as vitiligo, psoriasis, and sinusitis and that the treatments for these diseases have proven very effective so far. Intrigued by Dr. Shareef's preference to discuss the success of Unani treatments above its fundamental principles, I asked about the aim of this research, why is it actually conducted? His phone rang just at that moment. He excused himself and instructed Dr. Wahid, the then deputy-director who a year later would take over the direction of the institution, to answer my question. Obediently, Dr. Wahid turned to me as Dr. Shareef took the phone call, and calmly explained that research is conducted in order to translate the efficacy of Unani into the language of science, which will enable Unani to attain recognition from the WHO and the world. 'Now, with globalization, it is necessary' he added.

In the medical anthropological literature of Asian medicines, modern scientific research is commonly understood as pharmacological and clinical research based on a biomedical understanding of the body and its functioning. Scholars have used the term 'epistemic violence' coined by Gayatri Spivak (1988: 280) based on Foucault to describe the imposition of biomedical epistemologies on traditional medicine (Pordié 2014b: 50). However, from the perspective of researchers and scholars working on the validation of Unani medicine, modern scientific research is not considered to impose biomedical concepts. Quite the opposite: scientific research is considered a means by which the superiority—or at least the equality—of Unani medicine against biomedicine can be proven. To recall Dr. Wahid's words: 'We should see that today the ruling language is the language of science, and to attain recognition from the scientific fraternity research is needed.'

This chapter deals with the tensions involved in the use of modern scientific research in the quest for acceptance and recognition of Unani medicine. By exploring the history of modern research on Unani and the political economy behind it, and by examining how modern research has been integrated into Unani, I invite readers to rethink the idea that modern scientific research is necessarily incommensurable with Asian medicines, and to remember that while being political, 'what science becomes in any historical era depends upon what we make of it' (Harding 1991: 10).

Science as Means for Recognition

Unani research institutions such as the CCRUM are engaged in efforts to validate Unani medicine through modern science. The legitimation of Unani knowledge seems to be one of their highest priorities. The lack of scientific studies backing Unani medicine is often blamed for its subsidiary role in connection to biomedicine and Ayurveda in the Indian health-care system and in the global market of CAM. If the knowledge upon which Unani medicine was based could be recognized internationally and by the right authorities, Unani would have a more prominent role in global health care, so went a common claim. Most members of the Unani fraternity see modern scientific research as the only possible way for Unani to gain international (and, increasingly, also local) acceptance and recognition. The way to achieve this is described as a process of translation into the language of modern science, the expression used by Dr. Wahid and many other members of the fraternity.

Before the modernization of Unani through scientific research, it was the hakims themselves who strove for recognition of their own practice, a recognition that was granted by the patients—rulers included—when they were satisfied with the results of the therapies offered. This continues to be the case in private clinical settings (Schmidt Stiedenroth 2019a). The experimentation and the formulation of new treatments seems to have always been characteristic of Unani medical practice; a time-tested formula, for example, was described by hakims as *mujarrab*, meaning 'proved, tested, tried.' The testing of medicines for effectiveness was done in the *maṯabbs* by the hakims themselves with no record, except perhaps, for the own notes kept in the *bayāẓ*. In this way, Unani was 'Eminence-Based Medicine', i.e. it relied on the expertise of the hakim as professional authority. Some hakims boasted about the number of patients who came daily to their *maṯabbs* as a way to legitimate their practice and claim their good reputation and popularity.

The Urdu word *tajribah* (often pronounced *tajrubah*) refers to both 'experience' and 'experiment'. As argued in Chapter 2, experimentation refers to innovation in terms of treatment and is part of the art of Unani. Fabrizio Speziale pointed out that the experimentation and formulation of new medicines was characteristic of Graeco-Islamic medicine before institutionalization, and hakim families attained repute through own formulations prepared in the own *davāk̲h̲ānahs* that were inherited from generation to generation (2010b: 177f.). Experience allowed hakims to make proper judgments in terms of diagnosis, prognosis and treatment, something that was to be acquired through long-time practice and which included tacit knowledge, as in the case of pulse reading skills. This kind of knowledge embodied in the hakim constituted a sort of gnostic knowledge as defined by Bates, i.e. knowledge that is acquired through experience and learning and is centred in the knower (1995: 3).

The role of experience as a legitimate source of knowledge corresponds to a Greek legacy, although not only empiricism but also reasoning could lead to knowledge. Empiricists and Rationalists disagreed on which was the best epistemology: the first preferred experience (logos, *tajribah*) and lead medical investigations, the second favoured a specific method (Hankinson 1995; Pormann and Savage-Smith 2007: 9, 2007). Even today, Unani involves both experience and reasoning, as medicine is considered to be *fann* ('art' or 'craft') as well as *'ilm* ('science' or 'knowledge'). For the case of medieval Islam, art and science shall not be seen as opposed to each other, because the proper practice of science constitutes an art (Savage-Smith 2014: 158). This is the case of biomedicine too, which arguably combines scientific theory with clinical practice.

Manṭiq ('logic') and *falsafah* ('philosophy') continue to be part of the Unani curriculum, but many BUMS students fail to understand why these subjects are necessary. The head of the *Kulliyāt* Department (the subject dealing with the fundamental principles of Unani) in a prestigious Unani college explained that although these subjects constitute the basis for understanding Unani, students preferred to get closer to the chemistry and pharmacy departments of the college. They looked there for modern science, where the search for evidence has a priority over the discussion of epistemology. This appears a natural reaction, considering that most students enrolled in BUMS courses have trained in modern science at school, and is accentuated in the case of students coming from English medium schools, as teachers explained. Unlike classical Unani scholars, who addressed epistemological and ontological questions related to medicine (Savage-Smith 2014: 178f.), most contemporary practitioners of Unani hardly engaged in discussions about these topics, taking them for granted. This situation is not much different among Western scientific communities today (ibid.).

The confrontation with the fundamentals of Unani medicine such as the four elements and humours as basis for medical knowledge constitutes one of the major difficulties for many BUMS students. Among the Unani fraternity, it is resented but generally agreed that there are still no convincing scientific proofs—that is, proofs according to the modern scientific approach—of the existence of some of the fundamental principles, especially the four humours. Yet they are taken for granted and their importance is emphasized.

There have been numerous efforts to harmonize Unani with modern science. Through reasoning and experience, hakims and some Unani researchers agree that, for example, immaterial entities could be proved to exist through an observation of their physical effects, as discussed in the previous chapter. This form of reasoning is dismissed by modern science, for which the effect of the elements cannot be assessed objectively if their materiality cannot be verified. Pulse taking or the clinical falsification method practiced by hakims and discussed in Chapter 2 are not considered valid proofs according to this paradigm, which seeks truth outside of the human gaze in nature itself and favours reproducible results based on verifiable entities, an approach where some of the fundamental principles of Unani have, strictly speaking, hardly any possibility to be recognized as existent.

The close connection between experience and experiment that we find in Unani under the word *tajribah* was also acknowledged in Europe until the early eighteenth century (Scott 1991: 781). For a long time, seeing and knowing continued to be hand in hand in the European epistemological discourse: perception, observation and experience where all recognized as valid knowledge-producing practices (Kuriyama 2002 [1999]: 154). In Europe, as in the case of Unani, this was a Greek legacy. While modern science had already emerged by the mid-nineteenth century, it was not until then that experience was dismissed as scientific evidence and, instead, scientists began searching for knowledge independent from the knower (Daston and Galison 2010 [2007]: 17). Experience could no longer be reliable as scientific evidence because it was influenced by the observer: it became subjective (ibid.).

The current understanding of natural science as objective in the sense of obtaining truth independent from the knower extends to medicine. Valid evidence has to be reproducible and verifiable, as in the case pharmacological or clinical research generated to conform to what has been developed as Evidence Based Medicine (EBM) (Ecks 2008: 80; Lambert 2009: 16f.). And while this form of knowledge production seems to contradict important aspects of Unani medicine—including metaphysical entities and individualized approaches that may not be reproducible—, many of those involved in Unani considered its scientific validation a positive development constituting merely a translation process.

The view of validation through science as translation has to be understood from the backdrop of the development of modern science in India from the Colonial Period. Then, Western-trained Indians 'felt impelled to reinterpret classical texts and cast them in the language of Western discourse' producing 'the identification of a body of indigenous scientific traditions consistent with Western science' (Prakash 1999, 6). As Gyan Prakash argued, the British considered empirical sciences to be universal reason, and as such apt for the process of disenchanting natives from their superstitions (1999, 4). In the process, educated Indians appropriated science and its universality to construct a modern Indian nation (1999, 120), whereby science's authority was casted not as an imposition but as a translation in the sense of a 'realignment of power' and 'a renegotiation of the unequal rationality between Western and Indigenous languages' (1999, 49f.). While the translation process discussed by Prakash focuses on Hindu knowledge and the creation of a Hindu nation through it, the agenda pursued by Hakim Ajmal Khan suggests that also members of the Unani fraternity understood modern scientific research as a process of translation whose ultimate goal was to achieve the recognition of Unani by the colonial authorities by subscribing to its universality from the beginning.

The Beginnings of Modern Scientific Research on Unani

Hakim Ajmal Khan pioneered the introduction of new advances of chemistry in order to modernize Unani drugs and the art of *davāsāzī* ('compounding') (CCRUM 2009: 7; Ẓillurraḥmān 2004: 37). In 1926, he established the first department of the country conducting research on Unani using modern methods of chemistry and biochemistry (Bright 1998: 87; Ẓillurraḥmān 2004: 37f.). This was the response to his expressed concern about an apparent stagnation of Unani knowledge and the inadequacy of the classical books for teaching Unani in modern institutions (Habib and Raina 2005: 70).

Unani medicine was 'an expression of Muslim culture and a source of Muslim pride', and as Hakim Ajmal Khan was aware of the decline of Muslim culture, he considered the modernization of Unani the only viable way to preserve it (Metcalf 2004: 167). Aware of the need to convince colonial authorities about the value of Unani, he used arguments that implied his own recognition of modern science and even Western medicine as superior, at least in certain areas such as surgery (Metcalf 2004: 165). In order to secure both British and nationalist support, the secularization of traditional medicine and the emphasis on its scientific aspects increased during this period of revival. As a consequence, amulets and talismans lost their place in institutionalized settings such as colleges and medical conferences (Metcalf 2004: 167).

Hakim Ajmal Khan made medicine a politically relevant topic, whereby Unani was 'not a religious but a communal symbol of Muslim society' (Metcalf 2004: 154). For him, modernization was a means to preserve Unani and Muslim civilization, otherwise they would end 'in the hand of oblivion' (Metcalf 2004: 168). He saw modern science and medicine not as competition or antagonistic to Unani, but rather as means to achieving its further development (Habib and Raina 2005: 69). This aspect is crucial, as it still constitutes the dominant view among the Unani fraternity. Ajmal Khan's efforts to modernize Unani through modern science aimed not only at its recognition by the colonial authorities, but also at a renewal required to keep pace with the times.

The modernization of sciences in India arose in part from the perception of European economic and political advantage and the feeling of decline of the own sciences (ibid.). The modernization of Indian medicine was also part of a process of modernization of Indian sciences in general in the context of the nationalist struggle before Independence. Rather than signifying a submission to colonial—and hence Western—power, the acquisition and employment of modern scientific research to validate traditional knowledge systems such as medicine during the late Colonial Period can be read as a strategy for survival and competition. The introduction of scientific knowledge to modernize traditional thought was part of a 'culture of self-critique' which arose in the Colonial Period through a realization of differences between the Indian civilization and the West, whereby Western science was seen by some as the only way leading to progress and to avoid stagnation (Chakrabarti 2004: 13f.).

To accomplish the modernization of Unani through scientific research, Hakim Ajmal Khan sent Salimuzzaman Siddiqi, a young graduate of science, to Germany[65] in order to study chemistry and to later conduct modern research on Unani medicine (Ẓillurraḥmān 2004: 37). After Hakim Ajmal Khan passed away, the research department he opened became in 1930

65 Germany played an important role in the development of modern pharmacology from the 1880s through the generation of new methods to isolate active components and, from the mid-nineteenth century, to synthesize new drugs in 'fine chemical' industries (Whyte et al. 2002: 9).

an institute under the direction of Salimuzzaman Siddiqi, who pursued Hakim Ajmal Khan's research agenda using pharmacological parameters to validate Unani (ibid.). The isolation of the alkaloid Ajmaline from the plant Indian snakeroot (*rauwolfia serpentina*) is considered the milestone of modern scientific research on Unani and an example of its success. The alkaloid was named Ajmaline after Hakim Ajmal Khan (CCRUM 2009: 7; Habib and Raina 2005: 76). Later on, after World War II, a compound based on the Indian snakeroot plant was introduced as one of the first biomedical psychotropics under the name *Reserpine* (Reichmuth 2016). The medication was prescribed for schizophrenia and hypertension, but it is nowadays rarely prescribed because of its side-effects (ibid.). Medicines based on Ajmaline continue to be used in biomedicine for problems related to blood pressure (ibid.). Hence, from its earliest days, modern research of traditional forms of medicine was not only interesting for its supporters as a means for legitimation, but it was also attractive for Western scientists and pharmaceutical companies searching for new 'discoveries'.

The integration of modern scientific research into Unani was and continues to be contested. This debate is often articulated on the lines of a tradition (purist stance) and modernity (syncretic stance) dichotomy. The historiography of Unani in the late Colonial Period, for example, contrasts the divergent stances of the Sharifi lineage of physicians from Delhi—to which Hakim Ajmal Khan belonged—and the Azizi lineage from Lucknow. While the Sharifis advocated modernization, Hakim Abdul Aziz opposed the inclusion of modern subjects such as surgery into the Unani curriculum. In spite of the resistance of the Azizis to integrate modern research into their college, the very institutionalization of Unani training through the establishment of their *Takmil uṭ-ṭibb* College in Lucknow can be seen as the triumph of the modernizers, because of the adoption of the form of knowledge transmission used by modern medicine.

In the Postcolonial Period, Hakim Abdulhamid continued the support of Unani research through Jamia Hamdard—the educational institution which he incorporated as university in 1989—and its faculties of Medicine (dedicated until recently to Unani medicine only), Nursing, Pharmacy, as well as Science and History of Medicine and Medical Research (Bright 1998: 105). The Elementology project discussed in the previous chapter constitutes an example of the efforts pursued by Hakim Abdulhamid in order to gain recognition for Unani through its modernization. Unlike Hakim Ajmal Khan, Hakim Abdulhamid sought to validate not only Unani's pharmacology, but also the fundamental principles of Unani medicine. The correlation of Unani with modern science was one of his most important agendas. In his foreword to Altaf Ahmad Azmi's book *Basic Concepts of Unani Medicine–A Critical Study*, Hakim Abdulhamid wrote:

> Scholars of Unani Tibb cannot wholly agree with the approach of natural sciences in the study of human body and its ailments. To them medicine is a science as well as an art, as some of its aspects are demonstrable and some of them cannot be demonstrated on scientific parameters though proved on rational basis. [...] In due course they [other researchers] should bring out many more analytical research works on the subject and establish beyond doubt the truthfulness and validity of the basic principles of Unani medicine (Azmi 1995: viif.).

These statements are very important because they reveal not only the existence of concerns regarding the incommensurability of Unani medicine with modern science, but also the perceived need to make the theoretical basis of Unani acceptable in 'this modern scientific age.' This perception echoes today as the main reason behind conducting modern research on Unani medicine. It is necessary to remark that Hakim Abdulhamid was referring here to the fundamentals of Unani and not to Unani therapies as the objects of modern research. This distinction is extremely relevant in view of the literature on modern research of traditional therapies, which argues that proofs of efficacy in modern scientific terms will lead to the extinction of the underlying theories on which these forms of medicine are based (Banerjee 2004, 2008; Janes 1999).

Scholarly work on Unani medicine consisted for a long time of the compilation of medical texts and only recently shifted to a quest for validation based on science. Kristy Bright spoke of a 'shift from a text-based enterprise of translation of classical literature to a science-based industry of drug research and development,' particularly through the efforts of Hakim Ajmal Khan and Hakim Abdulhamid (Bright 1998: 78). Although the efforts of these entrepreneurs were crucial for the development of research in Unani medicine, they followed different aims. While Hakim Ajmal Khan focused on modern research as a means for survival of Unani and, with it, of Muslim culture, Hakim Abdulhamid further pursued a market-oriented revitalization of Unani, aimed also at competing in the growing (biomedical) pharmaceutical industry and to attain international recognition. For this, he organized conferences on Elementology with the support of the Indian government and the WHO, created a special Department of Elementology inside the Pharmacology Department at Hamdard University, and promoted research to validate the fundamentals as well as the development of new Unani drugs

(Bode 2008: 147). He conceived the validation of the fundamental principles as necessary for pharmacological research. Bridging epistemological gaps through translation, thus, seems to have been the means and not the goal of Elementology. To obtain the scientific validation of Unani medicine through modern scientific research was not considered, neither by Hakim Ajmal Khan nor by Hakim Abdulhamid, as the capitulation of Unani against modern science. On the contrary: through scientific validation, both hoped to obtain global acceptance, recognition, and respect towards Unani medical knowledge. Validation through modern science was for them not a question of modern science against ancient Unani principles, but rather a way to make Unani knowledge claims accepted in an environment which increasingly dismissed experience itself and the hakims' authority tied to it as epistemic virtues in Daston & Galiston's sense (2010 [2007]).

The Government's Agenda for Unani Research and Global Health Policy

Before and after independence, a number of committees were established in India to deal with policy regarding indigenous medicine (Wujastyk 2008: 44f.). Among those, the Bhore Committee Report of 1946 endorsed the support to biomedicine. Dominik Wujastyk argued that the ideological commitment to modern science led to the dismissal of experience as evidence of the effectiveness of indigenous forms of medicine, thus hindering a honest effort to seriously engage with traditional medicine. He further argued that this was based on what seemed like the plain ignorance about traditional medicine of the committee members, who were British-trained physicians (ibid.).

In post-independence India, the Chopra report was drafted. Like the Bhore report, it also subscribed to the idea of modern science—including medicine—as single and universal (Berger 2013: 163). The difference rested in the recognition of 'different aspects of and approaches to medical science' (ibid.), thus acknowledging possible contributions of indigenous medicine. However, it proposed the assimilation of traditional medicine into modern medicine, whereby modern science was to be used to validate the fundamental principles of traditional medicine or to conduct research on its materia medica (Wujastyk 2008: 65). The Chopra report was not implemented, and several reports followed, advocating for and against the inclusion of indigenous medicines in the health care system of post-independence India and recommending the establishment of different educational and research institutions in efforts to standardize indigenous forms of medicine (see ibid.). The government finally accepted the recommendations of the

Health Survey and Planning Committee Report of 1962, known as the Mudalier Committee Report. This report referred mostly to Ayurveda, but its recommendations affected policies pertaining to different recognized Indian Systems of Medicine, including Unani. A former member of the Bhore committee, Mudalier and his committee rejected the idea of medical pluralism through existing separate systems of medicine, advocating for the integration of useful aspects of traditional medicine into biomedicine instead, itself considered as the best system of medicine because of its syncretic nature (Government of India 1962: 457). Once again, it was suggested that research on indigenous medicine had to be conducted for the purpose of its integration into biomedicine. For this reason, the committee proposed that research should be carried out by persons having trained in both Ayurveda and biomedicine, and that they should also have 'familiarity with the methods of modern scientific research' (ibid.). The committee offered proposals for training of such professionals. It also recommended the training in Ayurveda and Unani medicine as post-graduate courses for biomedical graduates only, and the abolition of different, concurrent training in different systems of medicine (Government of India 1962: 456). In this way, the report explicitly advocated against medical pluralism as promoted in India today.

Not all the recommendations of the Mudalier committee report were adopted. Importantly, the synthesis of biomedicine with traditional medicine was never officially implemented in India. In spite of the goal to integrate traditional medicine into biomedicine, the systematization of indigenous forms of medicine was reinforced by recommendations of the Mudalier Report such as the following:

> One of the impediments to the progress of the indigenous systems and to a scientific evaluation of medical preparations under these systems is the absence of standards. [...] The task of developing appropriate standards for each preparation so that these standards can be enforced in a uniform basis throughout the country would appear therefore, to present formidable difficulties. However, some measure of uniformity can be attained and deliberate attempts at adulteration can be minimized if properly organized pharmacies can be established under State control and if the procedures for manufacture in respect of individual preparations are regulated in all State pharmacies [...] (Government of India 1962: 461f.).

The need for standardization was explained both through the necessity to facilitate research as well as to curb adulteration, facilitating the integration of traditional medicine with biomedicine. This integration was considered necessary in order to secure health funding from international organizations such as the WHO and the Rockefeller and Ford Foundations (Government of India 1962: 458). An important outcome following this suggestion was the amendment of the Drugs and Cosmetics Act 1940 in 1964 to include Ayurvedic (subsuming Siddha) and Unani drugs in an attempt to establish the basis for the standardization of these forms of medicine and facilitate their integration into biomedicine. The Drugs and Cosmetics Act of 1940, which previously regulated only biomedicine, was amended to provide the legal framework regarding purity, quality, and safety of single and compound Ayurvedic, Siddha and Unani drugs. These changes included the creation of pharmacopoeia committees of the different systems of medicine for the purpose of standardization of classical formulae. The first committee for the Unani Pharmacopoeia of India (UPI) focused on scientific research with the purpose to establish 'rigorous scientific testing and to lay down pharmacopoeial standards' in lines with the Drugs and Cosmetics Act of 1940 (CCRUM 2007b: iii). The standardization of drugs, which is a legacy from this report, continues to be a pillar of the research agenda for Unani nowadays.

The validation of traditional medicine through modern science worldwide was encouraged by the programme 'Health for All by the Year 2000' of the WHO (Pordié 2010: 59). The programme's objectives included to encourage the study and examination of traditional medicine and the promotion of the integration of traditional medical practices proved as efficacious through biomedical research (ibid.). Laurent Pordié argued that this approach focused on therapeutic evaluation as well as the integration of traditional practitioners into the health care system using biomedicine as a yardstick, and criticized that in spite of the critical literature on this approach, the WHO has done little to reorient its line of action (ibid.). The global quest for therapeutic efficacy was determined by the emergence of randomized control trials as dominating standard criterion for proving efficacy and by efforts to integrate traditional practitioners into health care delivery systems through biomedical training (Pordié 2010: 58). Twenty-five years later, the Executive Committee of the WHO recognized the need to integrate traditional medicine into health care policies, an approach which was consolidated in the Alma Ata declaration promulgated in 1978 (WHO 1978a). While the WHO provided lip-service to recognize experience as valid knowledge and a therapeutic scope that goes beyond the medicines themselves (WHO 1978b: 10), in practice the search for 'objective evidence' and the rejection of experience dominated WHO recommendations towards traditional medicine. Furthermore, following Pordié, the objectives of the programme to incorporate traditional healers into national health care systems encouraged the 'above all medical and not social' study of traditional medicine and herbal remedies (Pordié 2010: 59), in clear contrast to the recommendations of a meeting report from 1978 (WHO 1978b: 10).

In India, the state support towards traditional medicine preceded the Alma Ata declaration. The WHO report for the promotion and development of traditional medicine mentioned above argued that 'the integration of traditional medicine into the public health service is advancing satisfactorily' in India, describing the incorporation of traditional medicine in the Drugs and Cosmetics Act of 1940 as 'one major advance in the integration of traditional medicine' through the regulation of standards for practice and safety and control of drugs included in it (WHO 1978b: 12f.). Thus, standardization and safety were cemented as authoritative categories legitimizing indigenous medical knowledge for their inclusion in the public healthcare sector, whereby here 'integration' did not necessarily mean the absorption by biomedicine, as proposed by the Mudalier Report, but rather its inclusion in the biomedical-dominated health care system. This concept of integration influences the country's health policy towards indigenous medicines until our days as manifested, for example, in the integration of AYUSH practitioners in primary health care delivery through the National Rural Health Mission. However, the integration of Unani graduates in primary health care facilities is often cited as a critical example of the opportunistic approach of the Government of India, which employs practitioners of traditional medicine to overcome the shortage of qualified MBBS doctors (Priya 2013: 25).

After the institutionalization of Unani medicine as part of the public healthcare sector was consolidated with the Department of Indian Medicine (the precursor of today's Ministry of AYUSH), the next step was the setting up of autonomous bodies in charge of the research and development of traditional Indian medicine in order to align with the standards and safety recommended by the WHO. The Central Council for Research in Indian Medicine and Homeopathy (CCRIMH) was established in 1969. It was split into different research committees the same year when the Alma Ata declaration was promulgated, leading to the creation of the CCRUM in 1978 as an autonomous institution under the Ministry of Health and Family Welfare. The CCRUM started functioning independently on 10 January 1979 and, in this way, modern research continued hand in hand with the systematization of Unani. The CCRUM network extends all over India, having presence in 13 states (see Chapter 2). Its tasks include the development and coordination of scientific research on Unani as well as 'the formulation of aims and patterns of research on scientific lines in Unani Medicine' (CCRUM 2015b). In the years 2012 and 2013, the council spent 416,000,000 INR (ca. six million US dollars) in its activities (CCRUM 2015a). These can be divided into four areas: research on medicinal plants and Unani medicines and their efficacy, research on ancient Unani texts, the standardization of Unani medicines, and the propagation of Unani knowledge through the translation of classical texts, the reprinting of rare books, the publication of journals and other media, as well as the publication of original research conducted by the council. The CCRUM also organizes medical camps in low-income areas to deliver primary health care free of cost. These activities align the 'Health for All' programme with clinical research on experimental formulae as well as with Unani's core value of *k̲h̲idmat*.

In India, two main stakeholders carry out research on Unani medicine: the Unani colleges, particularly those offering research-oriented post-graduate degrees, and government research institutions, mainly those under the CCRUM's umbrella and the NIUM in Bangalore. Private Unani pharmaceutical companies did not have, to my knowledge, own notable research units and worked in cooperation with colleges and government research institutions. Hamdard Laboratories, for example, was linked with the university of the same name and worked closely with its Pharmacology Department—also in cooperation with the CCRUM—, while the Dawakhanah Tibbiya College Aligarh was linked with Aligarh Muslim University, in whose premises it produced Unani products sold all over the country. Other companies not related to any particular Unani college engaged MD students for research. An MD student at the Ayurveda & Unani Tibbia College in Delhi, for example, conducted clinical research on a proprietary formula produced by a private Unani pharmaceutical company. This is significant, because research at supposedly neutral institutions—i.e. state funded Unani colleges— was also market-oriented.

A speech by the former Indian Union Minister of Health and Family Welfare (at that time in charge of the former AYUSH department) expressed openly the interest of the Government of India in exploiting the global market of CAM and to become leaders in the training of traditional medicine in Asia:

> We are all aware of the increased interest worldwide in complementary, alternative and indigenous/traditional medicine. This is a reflection of the changing attitudes. The existing wellness market in India alone it is estimated to be of INR 110 billion [ca. EUR 1,67 billion] and is forecasted to grow at a rate of about 33%. [...] We are also training students from

> many neighboring countries and I am sure that India will continue to be the major hub for all systems of medical education, including alternative medicine, in Asia with its focus on excellence (Azad 2012).

This kind of development had certainly an impact on Unani and its research, as the government interests were expected to be reflected on new regulations and support. An important first move in this direction was the draft of a Memorandum of Understanding between the government of India and the SAARC (South Asian Association for Regional Cooperation) aimed at promoting co-operation in the field of 'traditional systems of medicines' in areas ranging from regulation of teaching and practice to mutual recognition of Unani pharmacopoeia (Alexander 2012). Another major step was the creation of a separate AYUSH Ministry in 2014, granting indigenous medicine autonomy from the Ministry of Health and Family Welfare. At the local level, the AYUSH Department (now Ministry) has funded 'centres of excellence' dedicated to specific diseases and therapies, although it is not very clear if these are aimed at targeting rural population with otherwise no access to health care or medical tourists from India and abroad. An example is the Centre for *'Ilāj bi-t tadbīr* (Regimental Therapy) in Puduvoyal, Tamil Nadu discussed in Chapter 6, which is supported by the AYUSH Ministry.

These developments reflect a serious commitment by the government to position India as a leading CAM destination. Not only global health policies have shaped this agenda. The global CAM market and the domestic demands for Unani pharmaceuticals have contributed to generate the need for modern research on Unani medicine.

A 'New Unani': The Unani Pharmaceutical Industry and the Global CAM Market

The idea of a 'New Unani' was often mentioned among practitioners. A Unani professor in Bangalore explained that patients want a new, modern Unani which integrates the advancements that were not available to Unani medicine before. According to him, people should understand that the 'New Unani' is totally different from the old one. He claimed that one of the reasons for the lack of popularity of Unani medicine was that people had in their minds the 'old' concept of Unani, which includes the prevailing idea of the hakim as a sex doctor, medicines consisting of bitter powders and characterized by poor hygienic standards in their production process, and the lack of regulations against quacks. This professor claimed that people nowadays do not trust the old Unani and, therefore, want a new, modern, and proven Unani medicine which integrates the latest advancements and provides a safe and natural alternative to biomedicine, which he addressed as noxious.

A medical officer at Majeedia Hospital in Delhi told me in 2012 that these are times of great changes for Unani medicine. According to him, Unani was becoming more and more prominent thanks to the growing interest in safer and side-effect free non-allopathic treatments, the world would be soon able to profit with the help of research in Unani medicines. He predicted that in ten to fifteen years a 'New Unani' proven efficacious by scientific standards and, as such, widely accepted by the population, will emerge. Even though Unani was associated with the Muslim community and Ayurveda with Hindus for historical reasons, the knowledge of Unani should be universal and not exclusive for Muslims, just like the Quran. He made an analogy referring to groups of people who opposed the translation of the Quran from Arabic into other languages and explained that the same happens to Unani: as a science, he argued, Unani should be universal knowledge available to anyone, regardless of faith or social class. If Unani medicine was to spread universally, it had to be proven as science, because science was universal.

The views of this practitioner echoed the opinions of others at the medical faculty of Jamia Hamdard and beyond. First of all, the optimistic perception of a growing global acceptance of Unani in the coming years. The perceived interest in alternatives to biomedicine was among the most commonly mentioned reasons backing the spread of Unani beyond South Asia. This was almost always linked to the idea that it could only happen through the process of translation into the language of science. The analogy with the translation of the Quran is striking: while this practitioner acknowledged that some groups exert resistance against the translation process, he used claims related to the universal character of the language of science as a legitimation to make Unani knowledge available to everyone in the world, beyond its cultural and historical context.

Although representations of Unani medicine as a CAM are rather rare among hakims, members of the fraternity are well aware of the potential of Unani medicine expanding internationally thanks to the growing CAM market. Manufacturers of Unani medicines, research and educational institutions but also Unani hospitals and individual practitioners often make claims contrasting Unani with biomedicine. They promote Unani as a side-effect free, natural, plant-based ancient tradition developed from the classical Greek humoral medicine.

The term CAM has been widely criticized in academia. The most common critique against the concept is that it subsumes everything that is not biomedicine, therefore including an extremely wide variety of therapeutic knowledge and practices under one category, which is defined only in opposition to biomedicine, thus implying (if not reinforcing) the dominance of the latter (Baer and Coulter 2008: 332). Here I do not use the term to refer to Unani as alternative or complementary to biomedicine, but to address the market of non-biomedical therapies in which Unani manufacturers and other members of the Unani fraternity seek to compete. While the term CAM is not part of the vocabulary of all the persons involved in the Unani field—the principal of a prestigious Unani college, for example, claimed in an interview that he had never heard about the term before—, the notion of a growing interest in Unani based on a decaying satisfaction with biomedicine and the search for side-effect free and natural medicines was mentioned by nearly everybody I met during fieldwork.

According to Banerjee, the global market of CAM has influenced the focus of the WHO support towards traditional medicine, leading to a shift towards herbal medicine (2002: 1143). This is significant because the category herbal medicine facilitates an integration of the therapies into biomedicine through their isolation from the form of medicine contributing to the pharmaceuticalization of traditional medicine (see ibid.). Interestingly, the term herbal medicine has also become very popular when referring to traditional medicine in India, including Unani, even though it is known that Unani materia medica also includes animal and mineral products. When I asked interlocutors why they refer to Unani as herbal medicine, they often said that Unani was '90 per cent' or even '99 per cent' herbal medicine, hence the label 'herbal medicine' was not considered problematic. Only a few practitioners and researchers reflected critically on the application of this term to Unani, arguing that it reduced its scope to pharamacotherapies only, neglecting diet and regimental therapies. After learning that I was conducting research on Unani, a physician said: 'You people talk only of Unani as herbal medicine!' Since she conducted clinical research on regimental therapies, she was wary of the dominance of drug research. However, most of the Unani fraternity seem not only to just accept but also to embrace the label herbal medicine, partly because it gives Unani a neutrality in terms of its Muslim identity. Through looping effects caused by demands of the market and WHO recommendations for regulation, Unani also became 'herbal medicine,' an enactment ubiquitous in its pharmaceutical industry. The rise of a pharmaceutical industry in India not only had an impact on the consumption patterns of drugs in India and the approach to health in general (Nichter 1996), but has also affected the quality of Unani medicine itself and even what we understand by it (Bode 2006, 2008; Bright 1998).

While the market of Unani medicine grows, new regulations are imposed and these are adopted, adapted or ignored, depending on the case. In the process, practices, institutions, and regulations create loopings that reinforce each other.

An example of this is how the brand Hamdard Laboratories became almost a synonym for Unani. Perhaps because of its massive presence, Hamdard was the focus of the few studies on Unani pharmaceuticals and the commoditization of Unani medicine (ibid.). Ask about Unani medicine in India and most lay people who have heard about it will mention 'Hamdard.' In conversations with members of the Unani fraternity, the shiny future of Unani and its increased global acceptance was often explained through the growing market of its pharmaceutical products, often mentioning Hamdard as an example. But while Hamdard was equated with Unani when it came to marketing success and monetary gains, the company has also been the target of criticism by hakims and other Unani companies, as discussed in Chapter 2. Notwithstanding these critiques, the success of Hamdard was undeniable. With a revenue of over 35 million USD in 1996 (Bright 1998: 180), it is by large the most successful producer of Unani medicines in the country. The reason for it may be in part explained through the early efforts to modernize the company through scientific research, as discussed in detail by Bright and Bode. The strong connection of Hamdard Laboratories with Jamia Hamdard and its close cooperation for research purposes with the departments of pharmacology and other modern sciences seem to have contributed to it. Perhaps more importantly, the marketing of Hamdard products as modern products to be consumed by the middle-class played a crucial role in its prosperity (ibid.). The company's advertisements could hardly be overseen from television to newspapers and on billboards alongside busy roads, they make Hamdard an important ambassador of Unani in India and abroad.

Although 80 percent of its products were sold over the counter and compete with similar Ayurvedic articles, fifty percent of its sales corresponded to four 'star products' (Bode 2008: 82). *Rooh Afzah*, the famous *sharbat* ('syrup') manufactured by the company, was not merely marketed as a product having health benefits, but it was also presented as a concurrent to Pepsi, as a 'cool' beverage encapsulating tradition, the family, and home in a modern context (Bright 1997). Through marketing strategies that addressed desires of becoming modern, Unani products manufactured by pharmaceutical companies became cultural commodities embodying local idioms of health reflecting the identities of Indian society in the postcolonial context (Bode 2006, 2008: 18f.; Bright 1998: 201f.). Thus, Hamdard embodies the 'New Unani' discussed above: scientific, modern, safe, convenient, and easily available (Bode 2001, 2006; Bright 1998; Nichter 1996).

While Hamdard was the first Unani manufacturer using industrialized production facilities, modern production units are widely available to producers seeking to satisfy consumers demanding the 'New Unani'. The appeal of Unani drugs in modern presentation packages was great, and only few hakims like Hakim Sadiq continued to prescribe almost exclusively Unani medicines produced conventionally in his dispensary. Hakims rely largely on branded Unani drugs (Bode 2008): they are easier to obtain and administer, they require no space for production (a matter of crucial importance in Mumbai, for example), and, most importantly, they do not require deep knowledge about the production processes or identification of medicinal plants and their effects. Last but not least, they are considered to be more attractive to their patients. Hakim Azim, for example, prepared only a very small part of the medicines he prescribed and relied mostly on branded products from the companies Dehlvi Remedies, Hamdard, and Dabur (a manufacturer of Ayurvedic medicines). The increased prescription of branded Unani drugs by hakims as well as the over the counter availability of Unani branded drugs in pharmacies and convenience stores is an important reason behind the perceived need for regulations ensuring quality and safety of Unani products.

The owner of a Unani pharmaceutical company explained that while the Indian market for Unani products is bigger, the international market is more lucrative and, hence, extremely important: although they sell less medicines abroad, the revenues are still greater. However, offering Unani products outside of India is connected to additional efforts because of the restrictions of the international pharmaceutical market through import regulations. These vary enormously from country to country. A producer explained that the US has the 'easiest' import policy as his company only needed to fill an online registration form for its products, which ranged from classical formulations to proprietary Unani drugs. A copy of that registration had to be included in every shipment, and that was enough. Europe, however, is a different story. He struggled to enter the European market and started with a country in Eastern Europe with more lax regulations: 'I need to send a copy of the laboratory tests with each shipment' he complained. By the time of writing, his products had also entered the European Union, albeit following a different strategy. His company sold single drugs marketed as Ayurvedic medicines through a television show in Germany, using a brand name different than the one used in India.

This producer was not the only one simplifying formulae in order to penetrate restrictive markets such as that of the EU. It is well documented that the import policies of countries have affected the way in which producers of traditional medicine define their marketing strategies and reformulate products (Pordié and Gaudillière 2014a, 2014b). The costs of safety controlling tests to prove the identity, purity, and quality of compound drugs is enormous (Schwabl 2009: 380), hence pharmaceutical companies producing traditional medicines have made the simplification of formulae a strategy to penetrate restrictive markets (ibid.). In the case of the EU, traditional medicine can enter the market either as herbal medicines or as food supplements. However, a regulation aiming at curbing abuse of the food supplement label in the EU has stipulated that claims of health benefits have to be backed by substantial scientific research (ibid.). As a consequence, pharmacological research and clinical trials have become necessary for the penetration of compound Unani drugs into the European Union.

The import regulations in the EU and other regions as well as the regulations for patent registration have led to the simplification of proprietary formulae through the combination of less ingredients (Pordié and Gaudillière 2014a, 2014b). The market, technologies, and institutions have changed the ways in which Ayurvedic pharmaceuticals are formulated and, thus, how medical knowledge is created (ibid.). However, the reformulation regime, as the authors call the phenomenon, should not be seen as a one-way development, as Ayurvedic companies make use of technologies and markets to create new medical knowledge 'building on strong continuities, both conceptual and material, with India's traditional medicines' (Pordié and Gaudillière 2014a: 7). In this way, while modern standards and approaches to research dominate and shape the ways in which traditional medicines are being produced, those are not simply absorbed but are instead dealt with in peculiar ways, much in line with the concept of originality valued in Unani medicine previously discussed in Chapter 2.

Validating Unani through Modern Science

Clinical Trials

The validation of traditional forms of medicine through modern scientific research has been discussed within the framework of colonialism, modernization, and globalization processes characterized by the dominance of Western paradigms of rationality and their influence on the global market economy, the pharmaceutical industry, global health policy as well as local health practices and institutions (Adams 2002a, 2002b; Adams et al. 2005;

Banerjee 2008; Bode 2009; Bode and Payyappallimana 2013; Kim 2007; Leslie 1992; Pordié 2010; Unschuld 1992). Evidence based medicine and randomized controlled trials have been condemned for being 'biomedically centered and therefore tied up with power relations' (Bode and Payyappallimana 2013: 1). Similarly, it has been argued that clinical trials are based on experimental science and biomedical understandings of the body, which 'share a significantly different notion of evidence than that of Indian medicine' because 'they address the body as biological entity rather than the body as a whole (i.e. physiological and cosmological) and, for that reason, claim universal validity and replicability' (Pordié 2010: 58). Other problems addressed by critics are related to establishing evidence or 'truths' and issues related to consent of participants, like for example awareness about the terms 'placebo' and 'randomized' (Adams 2002a; Adams et al. 2005). For Vincanne Adams, translating between disease categories constitutes an epistemological problem because they are based on unique approaches to the human body and its processes, which she deems untranslatable (2002b: 670). Further, she pointed out that 'it is assumed that disease *labels* may change but diseases themselves are universal' (2002b: 671), whereby it is the biomedical disease categories which are imposed in this kind of studies.

These critiques share the assumption that clinical trials impose biomedical categories and parameters into the study of traditional medicine, hence leading to epistemic violence. While I concur with the proposition that clinical trials are embedded in relationships of power that reinforce the hegemony of modern science as the only acceptable validating entity, I suggest that, in the case of Unani, their main problem does not rest on the imposition of biomedical concepts of disease causation and a possible incommensurability between Unani principles and those of biomedicine. Instead, they are problematic because they seek to assess the effectiveness of therapies in isolation, neglecting other aspects characteristic of the Unani therapeutic process. I suggest that this problem does not emanate mainly from divergent epistemologies between Unani and biomedicine, but rather from the characteristics of contemporary institutionalised Unani practice.

The CCRUM has been engaged in research of Unani treatment for *vajaʿ al-mafāṣil* ('rheumatoid arthritis' or 'joint pain')[66] since 1979. While it has focused mainly on drug formulations, clinical research has also included regimental therapies. In a brochure entitled *Unani Treatment for Waja-ul-Mafasil (Rheumatoid Arthritis): A Success Story*, the CCRUM justifies the relevance of research with WHO statistics about its prevalence—which is

66 See Pugh (2003) for concepts of 'arthritis' in Ayurveda and Unani.

higher in industrial countries— and describes the burdens to which patients are confronted with. It lists Unani literature on the disease, attributing the first compendium about it to Hippocrates, and mentions different causative factors which are prominently humoral based discussed by Unani authors (CCRUM n.d.). Regarding the therapies, it states: 'The principle of treatment aims at first correcting the imbalance of the Khilt (humor) through Emala (diversion) and Istafragh (evacuation) and then treating the patients with the drugs which were anti-inflammatory, analgesic, immunomodulatory and muscle relaxant in nature' (CCRUM n.d. 6).

Over the years, more than 40,000 patients have been treated for *vajaʿ al-mafāṣil* in different branch clinics all over the country, out of which 8,000 fulfilled the criteria for clinical studies (CCRUM n.d. 4). The diagnostic criteria initially followed 'the signs and symptoms as per Unani classification taking into consideration the involvement of different akhlat (humors) and the stage of disease etc.' until, in 1987, the ACR criteria[67] was also adopted 'to correlate the diagnosis with the modern parameters' (CCRUM n.d. 7). The CCRUM case sheet used for clinical research on rheumatoid arthritis included parameters such as temperament of the patient, the examination of pulse, and the physical examination of urine and stool, but these were not taken into consideration for the selection of patients. Only patients who fulfilled the ACR inclusion criteria for the study became part of it. The use of this criteria can be interpreted as a reaction to make the studies accepted by the scientific community in the first place, clearly reinforcing the hegemony of biomedical categories in validating what counts *scientifically* as evidence of efficacy.

Medical officers at one of the RRIUMs gave me a copy of the case sheet which was filled with data of the patients participating in the study. The officers said that the Unani parameters were important and therefore they were recorded, but none of them could specify their exact role in the research. Regarding the evaluation of the treatment outcome, a CCRUM brochure stated:

> Pathological investigations including complete hemogram [blood exam], E.S.R. [erythrocyte sedimentation rate], RA [rheumatoid arthritis] test and titre [a test used to measure the rheumatoid factor in blood] (in selected cases), urine analyses and C-reactive protein were done. Response to

67 The ACR criteria refers to the benchmarks stipulated by the American College of Rheumatology and which are commonly accepted as the standards for clinical research on rheumatology (American College of Rheumatology 2015).

> the therapy was assessed in terms and of subsidence in different signs and symptoms and normalization of laboratory findings. Subjective parameters such as pain, swelling, tenderness, etc. were assessed in terms of scores graded as mild, moderate and sever [sic.] whereas objective parameters such as grip strength, walking time and morning stiffness were assessed statistically by using various statistical tools to have an unbiased assessment (CCRUM n.d. 8f.).

As previously discussed, most members of the Unani fraternity considered disease categories as well as parameters obtained through modern technologies not as biomedical, but as universal and neutral concepts that cannot be ascribed to any form of medicine in particular and, thus, do not stand in opposition to Unani's epistemology. The perceived neutrality of science makes the use of modern research for validating purposes acceptable for the fraternity in the first place. This becomes clear in the CCRUM brochure: the aetiologies of the disease (and therefore the treatments) are explained in humoural terms, whereas the selection criteria and the final assessment of the therapy efficacy included clinical as well as pathological parameters based on blood tests and X-rays, for example. The discussion of the role of diet was also significant:

> Unani physicians laid emphasis on Ilaj bil Ghiza (dieto-therapy) at first line of treatment in the management of Wajaul Mafasil. According to them all cold and phlegm producing food articles are harmful in this disease. Clinical experiences of the Council's researchers show that frequent use of such article [sic.] not only delays the response but also aggravates the symptoms (CCRUM n.d. 19f.).

Diet was not assessed in this clinical trial. The patients were treated with experimental drugs developed from classic recipes, sometimes combined with cupping therapy. While the treatments being tested do fit the fundamental framework of Unani medicine, an important point needs to be noted. Unlike in the private practice of hakims, who adapt the course of therapies to the responses of the patients in the process of 'clinical falsification' (Obeyesekere 1992), the course of treatment in the trials is followed during the whole process even with those patients who show no response to the therapies. This aspect is significant, because the success of Unani treatment is not just based on the therapies themselves, but on finding out the best therapy for a specific patient and in a specific environment. In this sense, the therapies require a (skilled) hakim in order to work optimally, and effectiveness cannot be separated from the physician and his clinical practice. This distinction may be interpreted as the imposition of a different epistemology, i.e. a different approach towards health and disease. But we need to be careful with such an assumption that focuses on the fundamental principles of Unani, namely the humoural paradigm. Even though the principles of Unani medicine are not entirely forsaken in clinical research design such as in the present example, the clinical procedure characteristic of Unani medicine is completely neglected as integral to the therapy. This aspect, however, is not only a problem characteristic of clinical trials but seems to affect institutionalized practices in general. Thus, the problem of scientific validation through clinical research on Unani formulations does not rest mainly on the imposition of biomedical understandings of diseases and their causation—which is certainly present and determines the selection of participants in the first place—, but rather on the neglect of Unani clinical practice procedures and the role of a physician's experience as crucial parts of the therapeutic process itself. Consequently, the problem of scientific validation is not so much a problem of divergent epistemologies, but mainly of divergent understandings of the therapeutic process and their influence on the therapeutic outcome. In other words: not the science (*ʿilm*) part of Unani is neglected, but the art (*fann*) part. To a certain extent, that could be said to apply for trials testing biomedical drugs, too.

It is from this backdrop that I should point towards the institutional context where clinical trials take place as part of the problems involved in them. It is important to remember that epistemological choices are made within the social context of those involved in the research process, thus being influenced by the training, institutional affiliation, value system, and socio-geographical location of the researchers (Sujatha 2011: 196). Also, the asymmetries characterizing power relations between traditional forms of medicines and biomedicine when it comes to research need to be acknowledged (Naraindas et al. 2014). It would be naive to deny the hegemony of biomedicine and the threat of rationalization in biomedical terms when it comes to clinical studies. In institutionalized settings, Unani medicine is practiced in ways which are very different from that found in private clinical settings of more traditional hakims. Unani college hospitals and the OPDs of the CCRIUM branch offices employ medical officers or MD students who have been educated in an environment where many aspects related to the *asbāb-i sittah ẓarūriyah* and traditional diagnostic methods have been neglected, or even substituted, through biomedical training. Many of these practitioners are admittedly not in a position to understand the complexities involved in the healing process from a Unani perspective.

This has consequences for research, too, as the fundamental principles are sometimes acknowledged rhetorically only, and some researchers may not understand their actual meaning.

Clinical research on traditional medicine is not only imposed externally, but it is also produced locally within the social context of researchers (Sujatha 2011: 196). This involves their own cognitive universes and the political economy that frames clinical research (ibid.). The cognitive universes of most BUMS graduates are biomedicalized to a great extent, and the social context as well as the political economy in which Unani medicine is framed makes critical reflection on the process of research itself rather scarce. Through this looping, the need for clinical trials to prove the validity of Unani has been naturalised. In this way, modern research is not perceived as a threat to Unani by most members of the fraternity, but rather as a chance to prove its validity, and as such it is largely supported and contested only by very few members of the fraternity.

'The Method Has Changed but Not the Principles'

After I visited the Nizamia Tibbia College and Hospital in Hyderabad for the first time, I was walking out of the building when a student who had seen me inside the college approached me. Someone had told her that I was working on my PhD thesis about Unani. 'I am about to finish my BUMS course and I would like to do a postgraduate course in Europe. How can I get a PhD in Unani from Germany, what are the requirements?' she asked politely. I explained that I was not doing my PhD *in* Unani but *on* Unani, as I was actually pursuing a degree in social anthropology. For that, I told her, usually a master's degree in social sciences is required. She looked puzzled. 'But you are writing about Unani, so it is a Unani degree, right?' I had to disappoint her. The spark in her eyes, which was the only part of her face I could see as the rest was concealed under her dark blue niqab, was gone. This brief encounter helped me understand one of the puzzles I was struggling with during fieldwork: that of disciplinary boundaries in Unani medicine.

The seats for postgraduate (PG) courses in Unani in India are very limited. As of 1 April 2014, a total of 8 Unani colleges all over India shared a total admission capacity of 100 seats for post-graduate courses in Unani (Ministry of AYUSH 2014). In the past years, this number fluctuated because the former AYUSH department, through the CCIM, did not allow admission for PG-courses in all colleges for not meeting minimum requirements, such as the number of faculty members or beds in the college hospital. This situation made each seat very sought-after, as BUMS graduates hoped for better job opportunities—particularly those in the government service—through MD degrees. At the time of fieldwork, the government of India recognized two post-graduate academic grades: *Māhir-i ṭibb* ('Doctor of Medicine'), which included subjects such as *'Ilm al-adviyah*, *'Ilm aṣ-ṣaidlah*, *Mu'ālijāt*, and *'Ilm al-amrāẓ* ('pathology'), and those granting the *Māhir-i jarrāḥiyat* ('Master of Surgery') degree, including subjects like *tashrīḥ al-badan* ('anatomy'), *jarrāḥiyat* ('surgery'), and *'ilm al-qabālat o amrāẓ-i nisvān* ('obstetrics and gynaecology'). The curriculum for each of these subjects is regulated by the CCIM. The post-graduate course in *'Ilāj bi-t tadbīr* ('Regimental Therapy') was introduced recently given the demands I explore in the next chapter. A look into its syllabus, which was finalized in April 2015, reveals the complexities of establishing boundaries in terms of disciplines (CCIM 2015c).

During the first year of the postgraduate course on Regimental Therapy, students are expected to learn the fundamentals of research methodology according to modern scientific standards, including clinical research and clinical trials, experimental research, placebo control, and randomization. They are trained in different guidelines for research given by the WHO, the Indian Council for Medical Research (ICMR) and the Committee for the Purpose of Control and Supervision of Experiments on Animals (CPCSEA). Following this, they are taught research ethics following the Declaration of Helsinki (the ethical principles developed by the World Medical Association, WMA), including the constitution of ethical committees and the informed consent of the patients. Also, postgraduate students are expected to learn and apply biostatistics, i.e. to measure their research according to methods and procedures accepted in the natural sciences. Apart from the methodologies of modern research, the contents of the course include Applied Anatomy and Physiology, General and Specific Regimental, Principles of Diagnosis and Treatment (based on traditional Unani methods and biomedical sources), 'Biomechanics' (based on biomedical sources) as well as the Application of Therapeutic Regimens in Systemic Disease (based on Unani classical sources and biomedical ones) (CCIM 2015c: 3f.).

The case of *'Ilm aṣ-ṣaidlah* ('Pharmacy') is very similar. According to it, students should learn research methodology and biostatistics, methods of drug analysis and quality assurance of single and compound drugs, pharmacognosy and plant nomenclature following modern standards and not classical Unani classification schemes, as well as general and experimental pharmacology. The only methods corresponding to the classical Unani tradition were subsumed under the topic 'Specific Unani Pharmaceutical Procedures' and included methods of preparation of Unani formulations, but also newly introduced procedures such as Good Manufacturing Practices

(GMP) and shelf life (CCIM 2015b). In these postgraduate courses, modern research is the central component, being clearly oriented towards the standardization of Unani medicine. As a result, students write their theses using modern research methods in order to provide comparable results, whereby Unani is reduced to the object of study. This led me to ask what defines the discipline: is it the object of study or the methods? I kept asking myself this question in the course of fieldwork because it seemed that all the methods and also the underlying epistemologies of modern scientific research had been borrowed, and the fundamental principles of Unani played only—if any—a marginal role in the postgraduate degree courses. This implied that postgraduate Unani degrees were less about a qualification in knowledge about Unani medicine, but more about modern science research engaged in the study of Unani medicine with the aim to prove its validity.

A great number of employees in research institutions such as the CCRUM were not BUMS graduates, but had degrees in subjects like biology, chemistry, pharmacology, toxicology and botany instead. The RRIUM in Srinagar, for example, collaborated with the University of Kashmir. Students pursuing postgraduate degrees in pharmacology or botany worked in research projects at the institute and obtained the degrees in their disciplines from the University of Kashmir. Much of the research conducted in Unani medicine was pharmacological research and clinical studies aiming at standardizing medicines and proving the efficacy of Unani classical single and compound drugs, including the testing of proprietary formulations. The first was often carried out in the numerous departments of *'Ilm al-adviyah* across the country. During visits to these departments in different Unani colleges, students and faculty members often proudly told me that they followed the latest standards for pharmacological research, that they have state of the art equipment and that they hoped to publish the results in international journals.

Pharmacological research on Unani drugs was commonly conducted by BUMS graduates pursuing an MD degree in *'Ilm al-adviyah*. Although a BUMS degree was required for admission in these MD courses, most students used the methods of modern pharmacology. From the perspective of Unani practitioners, teachers, and students, researchers had the right to borrow methods from modern science. According to Prof. M.A. Jafri, who was director of the National Institute for Unani Medicine (NIUM) in Bangalore when we met in 2012, Unani needs modern science to make correlations. When asked about the role of the fundamental principles in these correlations, he explained that they do not change at all, they remain stable across time. 'The use of other disciplines is necessary for Unani, their integration is essential in order to correlate the knowledge and gain acceptance', he firmly added. Upon the question if these disciplines could be considered to be a part of Unani or if they should be separated, he vehemently denied the first. Prof. Jafri argued that the sciences are related to Unani medicine and this is why it is pertinent to study them together, especially at the postgraduate level, since they are all required to establish correlations.

Similarly, Prof. M.A. Siddiqi, who at the time of our meeting was the head of the Department of *Muʿālijāt* (Medicine) at the NIUM and later succeeded Prof. Jafri as the NIUM director, expressed that nothing happens to the fundamental principles of Unani when research on it is combined with the methods of other disciplines. He claimed that the same Unani principles that were accepted as the result of observation were those used today in experimentation. Just like an old hakim would diagnose by looking at the urine through the glass, basic principles like *arkān*—whose translation as elements, he argued, is misleading—and *ak̲h̲lāt* ('humours') have not changed, it is just the way of assessment that has changed. 'The old hakim knew which *arkān* are there through observation only, the method has changed but not the principles.' In his example, Prof. Siddiqi referred to the use of modern diagnostic methods.

Unani medicine is mostly understood by members of the fraternity as knowledge itself—produced, accumulated, adjusted—, whereas science is understood as means of knowledge production and validation. The prevailing view among the fraternity echoes Hakim Ajmal Khan's understanding of science as a way of obtaining knowledge, in contrast to Hakim Abdullatif's view of science as a 'form of knowledge' (Liebeskind 2002: 64). Hakim Abdullatif's understanding of medicine as science did not prevail. However, drawing a strict line of divide between medicine and methods would be misleading. In Urdu, the Arabic term *ʿilm* is used to denote both science and knowledge, they are not explicitly separated. *ʿIlm,* thus, encompasses the processes of production and validation of knowledge as well as knowledge itself, the method *and* the object of study. And since modern science is considered to be the method of choice at the moment, it is integrated into the framework of Unani medicine or science (*ʿIlm-i ṭibb*).

The understanding of modern science as methodology constitutes an important clue to understand why the fraternity generally accepted it as means to prove the validity of Unani medicine. Neither Prof. Jafri nor Prof. Siddiqi saw an epistemological gap between Unani and other disciplines using what is often considered to be biomedical-based research criteria. Members of the Unani fraternity tended to see modern scientific research as a means to achieve acceptance and recognition, not as an end in itself. Just as in the case of modern diagnostic methods discussed in the previous chapter, modern science including its technologies and advances were not regarded as different forms of knowledge, but as different sources of knowledge instead. And as such, applying a modern scientific method was not considered the same as applying a different epistemological basis. As a method, modern research was regarded as a part of science, which itself was seen as a universal and neutral domain to which all forms of medicine are subordinated to, including biomedicine. This understanding of modern science as neutral remains, however, problematic, even if limited to methodology only. I will return to discuss this problem below.

Is Translation Possible?

From the late 1970s, different publications touched upon the topic of the reconciliation of Unani's fundamental principles with modern science, which was considered the key for Unani's further development. In 1979 Hakim Muhammad Said, Hakim Abdulhamid's brother who migrated to Pakistan after partition and established Hamdard in Karachi, published a book entitled *Traditional Greco-Arabic Medicine and Modern Western Medicine: Conflict or Symbiosis*. Using different sources ranging from classical Unani treatises to modern scientific books as well as works of history, philosophy and even poetry, Hakim Muhammad Said attempted to reconcile the basic tenets of Unani with modern science. In a similar effort, Azmi's book *Basic Concepts of Unani Medicine–A Critical Study* (1995) is perhaps the most important publication aiming at translating the fundamentals of Unani into the language of modern science as part of the Elementology project previously discussed.

While the project pursued by Hamdard focused on the validation of the four elements, the CCRUM engaged in a different project entitled 'Fundamental Research' which strived to validate the humoral theory through research on the four temperaments. Alokananda Chakraborty, one of the officers involved in this project at the CRIUM in Hyderabad, has worked on the correlation of the four temperaments with modern scientific parameters for more than twenty years. She spoke about her work in terms of a translation of the basic principles of Unani medicine into modern science. This was to be achieved through establishing correlations of the temperaments of patients with physiological, pathological and biochemical parameters. At the time of my visit in 2012, the fourth phase of the project was just getting started. This phase was concerned with establishing the genetic bases of the four temperaments. A biochemist, Ms. Chakraborty had no training in Unani medicine. When I asked what happens to the fundamentals of Unani medicine once they are translated, she and her colleagues stated that the fundamentals always remain and that the scientific parameters constitute merely an addition to them. I was told that the outcome of the previous research has been positive so far, thus upholding the concept of the temperaments through modern science.[68]

The CCRUM was, to my knowledge, the only institution with a permanent research agenda aiming at scientifically proving the fundamental principles of Unani. Although recognized as important, research of this kind has been marginal compared to pharmacological and clinical studies aiming at testing standards, efficacy, and safety following state and market requirements. Fundamental research seems to have failed in its purpose. Referring to the four humours, a CCRUM officer put it like this 'Until now, it is not scientifically proven that they exist.' Sighing, he added: 'You cannot prove everything.'

Proving the existence of the humours through modern science was arguably far more challenging than proving the efficacy of Unani treatments in clinical studies. In spite of this, the fundamentals continued to be acknowledged as the very basics of Unani medicine. Those who still truly acknowledged their existence based their conviction on the classical scientific methods of logic and reasoning. Regarding the elements, we may recall Hakim Zillurrahman's arguments focusing on the action of the elements rather than their materiality discussed in the previous chapter. He also spoke about *rūḥ* ('pneuma' or 'soul'), explaining that 'it is the delicate part of the humours, it is connected to them' and arguing that they are 'something non-material'. According to him, *rūḥ* is like *quvvā'e* ('powers' or 'faculties'): we cannot see them, but we can see their action. As an example, he mentioned hearing: we cannot see what is heard, but that does not mean that is not there. Hearing takes place through the hearing power (*quvvāt-i sāmʿa*), he explained, and it cannot be seen or tested in the laboratory.[69] The same happens with *rūḥ*: 'If *rūḥ* is over, then one's life is also over. A human is not empty matter like a machine is. In allopathy, a human is understood as matter, but it is not like that. A

68 I was not able to verify this information. A study conducted at Jamia Hamdard seeking to correlate the four temperaments with blood groups provided a vague conclusion: 'a possible correlation between temperaments and blood group certainly do [sic.] exist' (Ali et al. 2007).

69 Audiometry is used in biomedicine, but involves the subjective assessment of the test-subject. The point that Hakim Zillurrahman is making here is that what a person hears cannot be assessed objectively, i.e. independently from the test-subject.

machine has no *rūḥ*. A human is no empty matter, he is made out of the mixture of body and *rūḥ*.' The connection of *rūḥ* to actions takes place through the faculties (*quvvā'e*), and these are connected to the organs (*aʿẓā'*) which, in turn, are connected to the actions (*afʿāl*). While *rūḥ* and *quvvā'e*, being part of the metaphysical level, are dismissed by modern scientific paradigms, *aʿẓā'* and *afʿāl* can be and indeed are the object of modern scientific inquiry. Considering this seemingly enormous gap between modern science and the metaphysical concepts of the cosmology underlying Unani medicine, why do those engaged in Unani not see a problem of incommensurability between the acceptance of Unani's basic principles and the use of modern scientific research for the legitimation of Unani knowledge?

In the area of medicine, Ibn Sina was very clear regarding the role of the physician when it came to the fundamental principles upon which medical knowledge is based. According to him, practitioners should be concerned with practical knowledge about health and disease, but they should not engage in questioning the theories upon which this knowledge is based (Ibn Sīnā 1993: 4f.). A physician, thus, has to accept the fundamental principles underlying his medical knowledge and practice, as the questioning of such a basis is considered to be the task of different disciplines, namely philosophy and physics (ibid.).[70] The influence of this idea is reflected in the statement 'the fundamentals remain' uttered by many informants, as seen above. This differentiation between disciplines—and the difference between medicine as knowledge itself and modern scientific research as method discussed above—is crucial for an understanding of how modern science is used to obtain validation without creating sentiments of epistemic violence among most members of the fraternity. The distinction between method and knowledge allows to see modern science as separate from biomedicine, which, as medicine, constituted a form of knowledge in the same way that Unani does. In this way, the use of modern pharmacology corresponds to an integration of modern scientific methods without rejecting Unani medical knowledge: drugs continued to be classified according to the degrees of quality and potency, while phytochemistry parameters—seen as modern advances, and not as biomedical concepts—were added to this classification. As a method, its main purpose is seen not as the generation of new knowledge about Unani medicine or as questioning its fundamental principles, but as

70 However, even the fundamentals cannot be assumed to be static, as their interpretations have been discussed in the literature and continue to be discussed today (King 2013; Speziale 2014a; 2014b; 2018).

translating existing Unani knowledge into the globally accepted language of modern science in order to generate acceptance and recognition.

Modern science privileges observation and reproducible evidence. Hakims acknowledge the empirical character of modern science while they simultaneously accept the existence of fundamental principles based on metaphysics, whose existence, according to them, can and has been proven through logic and reasoning. This corresponds to an Islamic cosmological view that does not separate between the natural and the supernatural as having different verification systems and where 'knowledge claims were joined in a single epistemology' (Liebeskind 2002: 66), whereby Greek concepts—especially Ptolemaic and Aristotelian—were integrated into it (Good and DelVecchio Good 1992: 260). Unani researchers and hakims with a sound understanding of *kulliyāt* do not consider the Graeco-Islamic cosmology upon which Unani medicine is based to be incommensurable with modern science, mainly because the origin of modern science and biomedicine is considered to be located within the same cosmological and epistemic framework of Unani, sharing a common origin.

After explaining how pharmacological research of Unani drugs is conducted taking into consideration metaphysical aspects, Prof. Amin from the *'Ilm al-adviyah* ('Pharmacology') Department in the Ajmal Khan Tibbia College of Aligarh Muslim University concluded: 'This is the sophistication of Unani medicine, that it is able to get an initial indication and holism, holistic comparison by the *mizāj* a priori method, and then it confirms it by clinical or empirical method, just as Western medicine does. So, in fact, it is wider than Western medicine.' Following his understanding of pharmacological research in Unani, Prof. Amin did not consider the integration of metaphysics to be incommensurable with modern pharmacological research. Instead, the integration was seen as an addition to modern science which does not interfere with the basic principles of Unani medicine.

For Hacking, styles of reasoning[71] arise in historical contexts and determine which data and methods are eligible to present proofs of truth and falsehood, or, in his words, 'what brings in the possibility of truth and falsehood' (2002: 167). Taking Hacking's idea as point of departure, I propose that talking about 'translating Unani in the language of science,' as Dr. Wahid and many others did, does not present a problem of incommensurability because translation is not reduced to the level of language only: it always

71 Hacking took the word style from A.C. Crombie's (1994) *Styles of Scientific Thinking in the European Tradition* (Hacking 2002: 161). See also Ludwig Fleck's *Entstehung und Entwicklung einer wissenschaftlichen Tatsache. Einführung in die Lehre vom Denkstil und Denkkollektiv* (2019 [1935]).

involves reasoning (Hacking 2002: 171). From the perspective of the Unani fraternity, using modern science as method means arguing using the style of reasoning preferred by the scientific community. In order to obtain acceptance, claims of validation have to be made in the dominant language of modern science.

Hakim Abdullatif's view of Unani and Western medicine as corresponding to different styles of reasoning—just like the purist conception of Unani pursued by the Azizis in general—did not prevail. The views of most hakims and researchers nowadays represent a continuation of those of Hakim Ajmal Khan and Hakim Kabiruddin during the late Colonial Period. The legacy of these two hakims continues to be very influential in contemporary Unani medicine. They claimed that the legitimation of Unani knowledge was only achievable through an approach that framed Unani and Western medicine within a common, neutral realm of science. This understanding did not constitute a break with the own tradition because, through the history that connects the distinct trajectories of Unani and Western medicine, modern science was seen as part of the same knowledge tradition as Unani. While practitioners of Western medicine in South Asia did distinguish between them and practitioners of indigenous medicine, the common ancestry between Unani and Western medicine 'was not finally rejected in the West until the nineteenth century' (Liebeskind 2002: 59). Although the loopings of the systematization process discussed in Chapter 1 contributed to promote and accentuate the division between Unani and biomedicine in postcolonial India, this division did not extend to the conceptualization of scientific research. Modern research corresponds to the methods used to present proofs of efficacy of Unani and biomedicine, while Unani and biomedicine are understood as distinct systems of medicine, meaning as separate bodies of knowledge and epistemologies that provide the basis for medical practice, not research. For most Unani practitioners, Unani has always been scientific. The language of science is considered to have evolved in the West in a different way, leading eventually to the language of modern science using pharmacological research and clinical trials to provide proofs of efficacy. However, this development is not considered to create a chasm or a complete rupture. Rather, it is conceptualized as a different form of expression which can and should be translated. This idea corresponds to the pragmatic approach pursued by Hakim Ajmal Khan, for whom the theory underlying the causation of a specific disease was not relevant as long as the actual treatment was effective (Liebeskind 2002: 65).

Those pursuing modern research on Unani agree that the language of modern science is currently the dominant one, as they could not escape its powerful grip from the laboratory to the market. Its dominance emerged from and is being reinforced by the political economy. As the global scientific community, the WHO, the CAM market and even the Government of India accepts only modern science as the lingua franca for the validation of medicine, proofs of efficacy and safety of Unani medicine have to be framed using its language. However, from the perspective of most members of the Unani fraternity, its dominance does not necessarily make modern science in any sense superior or even different from Unani forms of expression, neither does its use result in the biomedicalization of Unani. Conceptualized as neutral and universal, science and its modern scientific method are considered by the fraternity apt instruments to achieve recognition without presenting a problem of incommensurability. This, from an outside perspective, reinforces the hegemony of modern scientific research over indigenous forms of knowledge production. From the emic perspective, however, it demonstrates the superiority of Unani, which is said to have a broader scope than Western medicine. What these different versions of what scientific research reveal, is not that science and its objects are neutral or universal. Quite the opposite: they confirm what scholars of science and technology studies have long stated: that science and its objects are 'inextricably *symbolically* and *politically construed*' (Knorr Cetina 1995: 143). Using Mol's practice ontology approach once again, it could be argued that Unani research scholars enact their own version of modern scientific research, a version which does not conflict with Unani's fundamental principles or metaphysics but which, for the fraternity, reframes modern science as a language necessary to obtain recognition, a language that constitutes an addition, but not a substitution, to Unani knowledge and its producing practices.

In his study on the current pharmaceutical industry of Ayurveda, Laurent Pordié criticized the idea of epistemic violence for 'freezing unequal relations of power over time,' pointing out to the need to acknowledge rearrangements in power relations and asymmetries, particularly addressing the leading role of China and India in the CAM market by addressing 'the contemporary reordering of global asymmetries' as 'a transformative agent in healthcare' (2014b: 50). Another limitation of epistemic violence in this context is the assumption that modern research imposes a different epistemology into Unani. While the process of institutionalization has certainly contributed to the biomedicalization of Unani practice to a great extent, this dominance is by no means absolute. On the contrary: through claims of scientificity that enact an own version of modern science as universal and neutral, the Unani fraternity appropriates modern scientific research as means to achieve recognition. At the same time, it allows it to claim superiority based on an enhanced reality, rendering Unani 'amenable to biopolitical structures' in a way similar to how Ayurveda transformed its therapeutics through modern technologies (Mukharji 2016), without necessarily rejecting the epistemic framework in which it was based. If any violence is involved in the process, it does not emanate from the episteme itself, but rather from political economies that establish the hierarchies by which a specific enactment of modern science 'wins' instead.

6. Unani Medicine and Muslims in India

The struggle for legitimation of traditional forms of medicine is often loaded with the sentiments of the communities with which they are associated. The anthropological and historical study of Asian medicine has recognized the importance of nationalistic and religious interests when analysing historical developments such as the revival of medical practices or medical systems (Alter 2005a; Hardiman 2009; Langford 2002). There is consensus that cultural and religious plurality, which is characteristic of India, has played a central part in shaping different forms of medicine (Bode 2002, 2008; Smith and Wujastyk 2008; Weiss 2009). Medicine, thus, is a platform where social, political as well as religious interests and identities are articulated. To understand the multiple enactments of Unani medicine and their looping effects, one has to consider also the connection of Unani with Muslim communities.

Unani medicine has been closely related to Muslim societies through its history. This link has played a relevant role in its development in spite of past efforts pursued by the Government of India to de-Islamize Unani's identity (Speziale 2005, 2010a: 321ff). After the de-Islamization process described by Speziale (ibid.), which was pushed forward in the Postcolonial Period mainly by the Indian government, we find now a resurgence of the identification of Unani with its Muslim past, especially among some Unani private practitioners and, more recently, even by the government of India (Schmidt Stiedenroth 2019b). Neshat Quaiser identified this trend, which he described as an 'essentialization of Unani' (2013) and as 'medical communalism' (2012a).

This chapter addresses the historical and political connections between Unani medicine and Muslims in India and their role in contemporary enactments of Unani. The focus rests on Muslims in general and not on sectarian differentiations among them. Although sectarian differences among the fraternity played a role in some conflicting representations, the differentiation of Unani as Muslim medicine (subsuming all sectarian groups) vis-à-vis other religious or social groups in India emerged as a prominent topic. Consequently, I examine how members of the fraternity use Unani to position themselves vis-à-vis other religious communities in India, and how Unani is enacted as Islamic medicine. In other words, I attend to how the Unani fraternity articulates its Muslim identity through Unani, and how this identity stands in relation to political economy and the global CAM market.

Unani Medicine and Muslim Culture

Historical Background

The role of Unani as a factor of cultural identification for Muslims in India has been studied mostly from historical perspectives (Alavi 2007; Attewell 2007; Quaiser 2001, 2012a). Unani medicine arguably constitutes 'an integral part of the Indian Islamic culture' (Pordié 2011) and most of its practitioners today are Muslims. In South Asia, Unani medicine was strongly connected to Muslim rulers. Official representations tend to portray the Mughal period as the 'golden era' of Unani medicine (CCRUM 2009: 3). The courts of Mughal rulers became intellectual centres which attracted Muslim scholars from other regions in Asia, hence the production of medical works flourished at that time (Speziale 2010a: 306, 2018), contributing to the 'making of Mughal political culture', as health topics were engaged with kingship and sovereignty through proper rules of conduct and etiquette (Alavi 2007: 30).

Apart from the support of court physicians, the establishment of hospitals also belongs to the contributions of Muslim culture to India. During the Mughal rule, hospitals in India were tied to Graeco-Islamic medicine before they became instruments for the spreading of Western medicine under the British (Speziale 2012a: 1f.). Although some clinics or hospitals in nineteenth century India were located in premises belonging to *dargāhs* (Sufi shrines), they were not necessarily religious institutions (Speziale 2012a: 3). However, Islam, and particularly Sufism, were instrumental in the development of the Graeco-Islamic textual tradition in South Asia, facilitating the introduction and adaptation of Galenic knowledge (Speziale 2010b). The link between medicine, science, and Islam, thus, was a tight one. Hence, we cannot conceive science as separated from religion in the case of Unani (ibid.).

The history of Unani medicine in South Asia continued to go hand in hand with the history of Muslim communities during the Colonial Period. The production and transfer of medical knowledge took place mainly in Arabic, Persian, and later Urdu, the languages associated with Islam and Muslim communities. However, the decline of the Muslim rulers affected the practice of hakims negatively, and Unani received state patronage almost exclusively in Muslim princely states (Preckel 2012; Speziale 2010b: 65ff).

Religious schools such as the *Dar al-Ulum* in Deoband included medicine in their curriculum, but their medical content was not much profound, as these institutions were not aimed at training medical practitioners (Speziale 2010b). They integrated medical knowledge as part of general knowledge (ibid.). Although Graeco-Islamic medicine was a popular subject in the *Dar al-Ulum*, its inclusion in the curriculum was contested and did only happen by the end of the nineteenth century (Metcalf 1982: 103). The increased influence of Islamic reformist movements that opposed Sufi thought and the institutionalization of medical education which was initiated during the Colonial Period gave Unani a new, secular identity which contributed to the decline of its authority (Speziale 2010b: 76).

Notwithstanding this new secular identity, which became dominant in government representations, Unani continued to be strongly connected with Muslim milieus. For example, the most prominent families of elite physicians in India were Muslim families. The identification of Unani as a primarily Muslim system of knowledge in contrast to Ayurveda—considered to be a Hindu knowledge tradition—was reinforced during the Colonial Period and persisted among the public and even in the historiography. For instance, some scholars continued to distinguish between Unani and Ayurveda as Islamic and Hindu medicine, respectively (Liebeskind 2002: 59; Sheehan and Hussain 2002: 124).

This representation of Unani as Muslim was—until very recently—not found in official discourses of Unani after independence (Schmidt Stiedenroth 2019b). Following modernizing efforts striving to separate strictly between science and religion (Latour 1993), efforts of standardization removed religious aspects and focused on the legitimation of Unani as a secular and scientific system of medicine (Speziale 2010a: 322). The choice of 'Unani' as the official name was a strategic attempt to develop Unani as a modern system of medicine, exalting its Greek origin and—thus—historical connection with modern science and medicine, while at the same time undermining its connections to Islam (Speziale 2005, 2010a: 324f.). Notwithstanding the active efforts of the government to enact Unani as secular and modern—i.e. as scientific and separate from religion—, it continues to be strongly associated with Muslims in the country. To understand this, it is useful to explore the relationship of Muslims with Urdu language in India.

Unani, Muslims, and Urdu

Even though neither government institutions nor certain well-known companies like Hamdard focus on Islam or Muslim culture in their representations of Unani (Bode 2008: 208), most people in India continue to associate Unani primarily with Muslims. Most Unani practitioners in India nowadays are Muslims, and the most common reason I was given for this is the official use of Urdu as the medium of instruction in the institutions imparting BUMS training. Prospect Unani students shall know Urdu in order to obtain entrance into a BUMS course. Hence, they have been ideally trained in Urdu-medium schools or madrasas.

Urdu is required for Unani training because most textbooks included in the BUMS curriculum have not been translated into English yet. Some practitioners and lecturers argued that Urdu had to be used because not all terms can be translated easily into English, and because translations into the language associated with biomedicine may be confusing for students lacking a profound knowledge of Unani medicine.[72]

Urdu-medium schools were avoided by non-Muslims, and even most Muslims I spoke to about it preferred to send their children, if they could afford it, to English-medium schools. This had consequences for pursuing training in Unani, as a conversation in a *maṭabb* in Mumbai revealed. A friend of the hakim who ran the clinic came to visit him and the three of us had a jovial conversation. While sipping chai, the hakim told me that his friend held a BUMS degree but did not practice Unani at all. I asked the friend if this was true, he said yes and told me that his wife also had a BUMS degree, but she practiced allopathic medicine. Apologetically, he added that his son was pursuing an MBBS degree. 'It is because he went to an English-medium school, so he does not know Urdu.'

English-medium education opens opportunities for Muslims into more prestigious careers while at the same time closing the door for formal Unani training. In the competitive Indian context, parents think about future job opportunities for their children when deciding about their language education (Oesterheld 2002: 131). The director of a Unani research institution explained:

> Now, since independence, the Hindu majority has imposed the displacement of Urdu as a national language. So, the problem today is that many people don't know Urdu. Even I attended only up to the eight grade in an Urdu-medium school, and my children are being educated in English-medium schools only. It is necessary if the children are to attain good positions in their careers. This is why so many do not know Urdu. However, in every batch there are some three seats occupied by non-Muslims, and three seats are reserved for foreigners.

Educated Muslims take the chance of sending their children to English-medium schools in order to secure access to the best possible education

72 While Hindi is also an official language in India, the possibility of translating Unani textbooks into Hindi was not discussed among the fraternity.

at their reach. Unani education is less appealing not only because its practitioners are paid less than their MBBS colleagues, but also because it requires the command of Urdu at a level that, nowadays, can only be acquired through schooling in an Urdu-medium school or madrasa, both educational institutions which were not favoured by the Muslim middle-class.

Urdu was not considered an exclusively 'Muslim' language until the Colonial Period, even though it emerged through the influence of Muslim rulers and its literature flourished under their patronage (Matthews et al. 2003: 26). While Urdu never had the sacrosanct status that Arabic has in Islam, in South Asia it became associated with Muslims and Islam through its usage by several religious groups when reformist movements such as *Ahl-i Ḥadīs̱*, *Barelvī*, and *De'obandī* used it to spread their message among the masses (Metcalf 1982: 102f.; Rahman 2006).

Although Urdu is still officially recognized in India, it has completely lost the elite status it once had. Even though in India it is regarded primarily as a literary language (especially of poetry), this does not make it attractive to young people (Oesterheld 2002: 131f.). Many native Urdu speakers migrated to Pakistan after partition. Hindi, along with English, were chosen as the two official languages of India. Urdu was recognized as the state language of Jammu and Kashmir because of its comparatively high Muslim population, even though Kashmiri and Dogri are the most spoken languages in that state. Urdu was still used in Kashmir as a language of learning by Muslims and Hindus some decades back, as I was told by the principal of a private Unani college in the Kashmir Valley in a mix of Urdu and English:

> Basically, Urdu is needed for Unani, a bit of Arabic and Persian knowledge is required, it is very necessary. This is why a lot of kids of Muslim families come [to attend the Unani college in Srinagar], who know Urdu and so on. [...] When I did my BUMS here in Kashmir, those days several, a lot, fifty percent of the population was Hindu. But now, today's scenario is that, they [students] come from all over Kashmir [...]. When I went for my MD, we went three from the Kashmir Valley those days, one was Hindu and the other was Muslim. Both spoke better Urdu than me. He [the Hindu student] could also write Arabic, and he wrote very good Urdu. But today's scenario is totally different.

Most pandits left the Kashmir Valley in the 1990s due to persecution by Islamist groups, and now it is mostly Muslims who learn the language in the region. This is the case of the rest of the country, too, as madrasas and Urdu-medium schools are attended, mostly, by low- and middle-class

Muslims (Farouqui 1995: 165; Government of India 2006: 17). The neglect of Urdu, it has been argued, 'stems from a public perception that it is a language of the Muslims and separatist Muslims at that' (Engineer 2012: 118), as 'it was equated with a language that divided up the country' (Farouqui 1995: 158). The comparatively few Urdu-medium schools remaining are characterized by a low quality of teaching, vacancies of teachers for years and the recruitment of Hindu teachers to fill these gaps (Government of India 1962: 18).

The state of neglect of Urdu in India also affects Unani education, as even those having a certificate in Urdu are weak in reading and writing in the language (Qadīr 2004b: 452). The increased number of biomedical subjects, whose textbooks have not been translated into Urdu and are taught in English, has further contributed to the problem (ibid.). As a consequence, not only Muslims, but also Unani education in general has suffered from the decline of Urdu language and Urdu education in India. This situation exacerbated a general feeling of neglect among Muslims in the country, manifested in the medical realm by 'medical communalism' (Quaiser 2012a).

Medical Communalism

The status of Muslims in India suffered with the decline of their ruling power. Today, Muslims are not only a religious minority, but they also constitute a marginalized and neglected section of Indian society. The partition of the country and the subsequent tensions with Pakistan have been held responsible for the existential fear of the Muslim population in India, as well as general suspicion and disdain towards Muslims by other religious groups, especially Hindus (Gayer and Jaffrelot 2012; Jeffrey and Sen 2014). After independence, communal tensions lead to communal motivated violence which continues to erupt to date and contributed further to foster negative sentiments against Muslims, having consequences in different areas (Shaban 2012b).

Although the Indian constitution ensures equal opportunities and rights to all of its citizens, the Sachar Committee Report revealed that this was not necessarily the case in practice (Government of India 2006). Muslims reported feelings of discrimination not only by certain sectors of society but also by government and public institutions (Government of India 2006: 11f.). Also, the media was perceived as perpetuating these stereotypes (ibid.). These sentiments resonate with their underrepresentation in different areas of public life. For example, Muslims are not proportionally represented in government services (Shaban 2012a: 11) and are marginalized in the private labour market, where urban Muslims constitute only eight per cent against the 21 per cent national average in the formal sector, while the literacy rate of male Muslims 'was only one percent above that of Dalit men' (Gayer and Jaffrelot 2012: 3f.). Apart from that, Indian Muslims have been increasingly segregated into Muslim neighbourhoods in a process that has been called 'ghettoisation' by some authors (Gayer and Jaffrelot 2012: 21f.; Shaban 2012a: 1). These 'ghettos', where Muslims prefer to live due to security fears (Government of India 2006: 14), contribute further to the marginalization of Muslim communities through an imagined de-nationalization implied in the common reference to them as 'mini-Pakistan' by non-Muslims (ibid.). Further, the deficient infrastructure that often characterizes these areas also contributes to the marginalization of their population (Shaban 2012a: 9f.). The discrimination of Muslims in India is further manifested in the partisan pro-Hindu stance of police officers during communal riots (Punwani 2012), in aspects of everyday life like those related to employment and education (Fazal 2014; Jeffery et al. 2007), and in poverty, which is considered the main cause for the low educational levels (Government of India 2006: 15). I could often sense this feeling of neglect pouring through conversations with Unani practitioners, manufacturers, as well as with students—all of them Muslims—, who often blamed the 'Hindu government' for the lack of support towards Unani medicine.

In India, most Unani practitioners are Muslims, and professional demands to the Government of India were often articulated in communalist terms, even though the government supports Unani as well as other forms of indigenous medicine following a secular approach. Neshat Quaiser identified this phenomenon and named it 'post-colonial medical communalism' (2012a). He focused on how Unani has been instrumental in the creation of an 'eastern collective self' that served maintaining 'a distinct Muslim/Islamic identity' (Quaiser 2001: 318). This 'eastern collective self,' which during the Colonial Period might have established alliances with representatives of Ayurveda, now embodies Muslim minorities against the majority Hindu state, represented by the dominant Ayurveda. As a result, many secular aspects related to health and health policy acquired a communal note (Quaiser 2012a: 131f.).

The term communalism, as used by Quaiser, echoes Pandey's definition of its common Indian usage, referring to 'a condition of suspicion, fear and hostility between members of different religious communities,' but also its academic usage applied to 'organized political movements based on the proclaimed interests of a religious community [...] that make sectional demands on state policy for a given share in jobs, education and legislative positions [...]' (Pandey 2012: 6). The Unani fraternity can be considered such an interest group. When discussing the challenges that Unani medicine has to face, fraternity members often mentioned government support as a central issue. A hakim and I were talking about the Unani fraternity when we came across the topic of government support. He complained that the government was not giving enough support to Unani, but it gave a lot of support to Ayurveda instead. He said that Ayurveda was closer to 'theirs' (meaning the religion of those in power, i.e. Hinduism): 'This is why the government is not supporting Unani' he concluded. This criticism towards the government echoed conversations with other members of the Unani fraternity who complained about the lack of support towards Unani by the 'Hindu' government. To prove such claims, I was often asked to compare the total number of dispensaries and other Ayurvedic facilities supported by the government with those for Unani. As a matter of fact, there are many more Ayurvedic colleges (163 Ayurvedic colleges approved for 2014) than Unani ones (42) in India (CCIM 2015a, 2015d), and the same applies to the dispensaries and hospitals, which for Ayurveda accounted to 15,353 and 2,458 respectively against to only 1,146 and 269 for Unani in 2010 (Department of AYUSH 2010).

The government of India, through the then AYUSH department (now AYUSH Ministry), guaranteed the support to each of the recognized medical systems without officially differentiating on the basis of religion. The budget allocation proposals for AYUSH were made at the state and not the central level. An official explained that the state directories tend to focus on the demands of patients in the process. Consequently, Unani received a smaller budget allocation because the state directories considered the religion of their population when making the proposal, and assumed that Hindus would prefer Ayurvedic and Muslims Unani facilities. As a reflection of this, we do find greater government support towards Unani in states with more numerous Muslim populations, such as Jammu and Kashmir and Andhra Pradesh,[73] whereas some states with a scarce Muslim population, like Chandigarh or Arunachal Pradesh, have no Unani facilities at all (Department of AYUSH 2010). Hence, even the secular commitment from the central government could not prevent the communalization of health at state levels.

Medical communalism also influenced the way in which certain policies affecting drug production were interpreted by members of the fraternity. A Unani practitioner who manufactured medicines on a small scale explained the problems related to musk as an ingredient. According to him,

73 The state of Andhra Pradesh was split into Andhra Pradesh and Telangana in 2014. Being the data from 1 April 2010, I am referring to both territories here.

the production of musk had been hampered since the BJP (Bharatiya Janata Party) was on the government because the BJP does not want the animals to be killed. However, as discussed in Chapter 1, the production of musk in India was banned by the Wildlife Protection Act of 1972. This act was passed during the ruling period of the Indian National Congress party with Indira Gandhi as prime minister. However, the BJP government was accused by this practitioner who attributed the ban to Hindu nationalist values such as vegetarianism rather than to environmentalist agendas enforced upon international pressure. Claims such as this reflect sentiments of discrimination and lack of support by what is called the 'Hindu government' against Unani medicine and Unani professionals on the basis of religion, accounting for deep resentments among the Unani fraternity against the ruling political parties.[74]

Following this line, informants often argued that Ayurveda was well known and spreading in the West thanks to government support, whereas Unani remained almost unknown in Europe and the United States due to its neglect. However, evidence suggests that the spread of Ayurveda to the Western world was not only the result of conscious efforts made by the Government of India, but it was initiated as the consequence of a combination of various developments, notoriously the New-Age movement of the 1980s (Diem and Lewis 1992; Smith and Wujastyk 2008). Hence, it is valid to ask why those involved in Unani medicine blame the government for the disadvantaged position of Unani, especially vis-à-vis Ayurveda. Quaiser analysed this development from the Colonial Period to our days, arguing that the communalization of health was increased after independence, when Muslims were accused of dividing 'Mother India' (2012a). He argued that Ayurveda and Unani 'were projected as markers of Hindu and Muslim interests and identity respectively' and that Muslims were seen as responsible for safeguarding the interests of Unani medicine (Quaiser 2001: 318, 2012a: 133). Protecting and developing Unani medicine, thus, was also protecting and developing Muslim identity. Ayurveda became 'the principal antagonistic other and constant comparison between the two emerged as critical strategy of complaint' (Quaiser 2012a: 141ff.). Complaints against the government for giving Ayurveda a preferential treatment have accompanied the development of Unani throughout the Postcolonial Period.

74 It was only after my fieldwork research that Narendra Modi (BJP) was elected Indian prime minister (in office since May 2014) and established a separate Ministry of AYUSH in November 2014. The reactions toward this important health policy change among the Unani fraternity have not been included in this study.

These concerns have been addressed in electoral campaigns and have been used to articulate a Muslim identity, whereby Ayurveda represents the 'other' (Quaiser 2012a: 151f.).

A prominent hakim spoke about an 'inferiority complex' among Unani practitioners. According to him, Unani practitioners felt treated as inferior in comparison to Ayurvedic practitioners, and as practitioners of traditional medicine they felt like second class citizens vis-à-vis biomedical doctors. This, he argued, caused them to act only for money purposes, indulging in what he considered questionable practices like prescribing allopathic medicines, for example. Although the wording 'inferiority complex' seems harsh, it was evident in conversations that a sentiment of marginalization of Unani medicine was present among the fraternity: as a professional community of Muslims, they felt discriminated at the state and national health policy levels, and as professionals of traditional medicine, they felt marginalized among the medical and scientific communities.

It is necessary to stress that this sense of marginality was neither universal nor unique. The link between Unani and Muslim cultures was regarded very positively when it came to job opportunities in the Persian Gulf states, for example. In this scenario, the interest on Unani therapies considered to be part of Islamic medicine was seen as a great opportunity to achieve professional success, especially with a clientele of Muslim patients in India, in rich Muslim countries like the United Arab Emirates or Saudi Arabia, or in countries with a notorious South Asian Muslim diaspora, like the United Kingdom. Thus, an analysis taking into consideration medical communalism shall not only focus on the demands and sense of neglect expressed by Unani practitioners as members of the Muslim minority in India, but it should also attend to the sentiment of attachment to the ummah bringing together Muslims around the world. While the ties of Unani with Islam as a religion are mainly downplayed by the government of India and, often, by practitioners and manufacturers as well, there are also plenty of situations where exactly these ties are stressed while enacting Unani.

Islamic Medicine?

Unani and *Ṭibb-i Nabavī*

After I had spent a couple of months with Hakim Ahmad and before I left for Hyderabad in April 2013, I asked him for an interview, which he was happy to give. When I finally set the recorder on, my first question was:

'What is Unani for you?' He told me about the Greek origins of Unani, but he stressed that Unani is actually Islamic medicine. The sound of the *azān* ('call for prayer') coming from the mosque nearby filled the small *maṭabb* and Hakim Ahmad asked me to stop the recording. We stopped talking until the *azān* was over. Later on, when we resumed the interview, I asked him explicitly about the relationship between Unani and Islam. He explained:

> Look, actually, Unani medicine is Islamic medicine. To be practiced in India it had to be called Unani medicine because here there are people of other religions also. Because if it was named Islamic medicine, if that had been done, then people of other religions would worry about using it, like 'it is Islamic medicine, I don't know what is it, what they use…' So, the hakims then, the Unani hakims gave it that name, because it is from Greece, so that name would do. But its principles are quasi Islamic. […] A lot of its formulations, a lot of… prescriptions, a lot of discoveries of herbal medicines were done in the times of Jesus (peace be upon him), Jesus (peace be upon him) who was a prophet and who also gave birth to Islam. Afterwards Moses (peace be upon him) came,[75] and after him Muhammad (peace be upon him) came, so Muhammad (peace be upon him) is the one in whose times there was also *ṭibb,* there was that, and a lot of treatments he… apart from that he discovered 850 medicinal plants and told people about the benefits of 850 medicinal plants, he told people like, 'brothers, they heal', and told about different forms of treatments among which cupping is a celebrated one […]. That's it, this way [of treatment] is Islamic, from that I understand that Unani medicine is the same as Islamic medicine. And there is so much literature and so on there in Arabic and Persian, because most hakims were from Arab countries, and Islam… they were Muslims. This is why in my understanding there is not much difference between Unani medicine and Islamic medicine.

The meaning of 'Islamic medicine' as medicine based on ancient Greek medicine is to be distinguished from the popular or religious Islamic medicine, which 'covers also hygienic, dietetic or healing instructions that they attribute to the Prophet and the Imams' (Ebrahimnejad 2005: 127), meaning also *ṭibb-i nabavī*, or prophetic medicine. While the historiography tends to differentiate between two kinds of Islamic medicine—scholarly and popular traditions—Hakim Ahmad, like many other Unani practitioners,

75 Like in Christianity, in Islam Moses lived before Jesus.

mingled the history of Graeco-Islamic with prophetic medicine, allowing Unani medicine to emerge as one and the same.

Ṭibb-i nabavī, or prophetic medicine, as its name suggests, is a common term used for the recommendations and practices related to health preservation and healing, as described in numerous Hadiths or sayings about the prophet Muhammad, custom (Sunna) and the Quran (Pormann and Savage-Smith 2007: 72). Hadiths have been described as 'a corpus of traditions upon which the life of the Muslim community is largely based and its institutions rationalized' (Rahman 1987: 22), thus constituting a central aspect not only of religious practice, but of everyday life of Muslims around the world. The actions and deeds of the prophet Muhammad are considered as exemplary for all human beings and constitute the traditional portion of Muslim law called Sunna, Arabic for 'tradition', 'path' (Elgood 1962: 36). The Sunna is considered authoritative for the leading of life in Islam, especially among Sunni Muslims.

Prophetic medicine constitutes a genre in Islamic literature based on compilations of Hadiths, Sunna and the Quran. These texts are related to practices regarding health in general or giving concrete advice and even recipes of remedies or procedures to treat specific ailments (Pormann and Savage-Smith 2007: 71; Rahman 1987: 41ff.). Works on prophetic medicine were authored mainly by religious scholars and not by physicians (Pormann and Savage-Smith 2007: 71). A renowned example of this kind of work is represented by Al-Jauzyah's *Aṯ-ṯibb an-nabavī,* a compilation of Hadiths related to health maintenance and recovery and a common source of reference for prophetic medicine (ibid.).

There are several theories about the creation of the prophetic medicine genre. Manfred Ullmann suggested that it was established to challenge the authority of Greek medicine, which for orthodox Muslims was 'suspect as being a science of heathen origin' (Ullmann 1997 [1978]: 5). Similarly, Pormann and Savage-Smith proposed an anti-philosophical tradition opposing earlier Greek thinkers as possible reason (2007: 72). Fazlur Rahman criticized Ullmann's position, arguing that prophetic medicine combines elements of Greek medicine in it and does not oppose, but complements the Graeco-Islamic medical tradition instead, suggesting that the main reason behind its creation was probably the aim of spiritualizing medicine (1987: 42).

Prophetic medicine had no comprehensive underlying theory from the medical point of view, combining 'elements of Greek medical learning (in Arabic dress) and religious elements specific to Islam with pre-Islamic Arabian practices' (Pormann and Savage-Smith 2007: 74). The recommendations of certain practices by the prophet were initially not considered important by the medical milieu until they were later collected and interpreted through concepts of Greek medicine (Ullmann 1997 [1978]: 5). In like manner, Thomas Bauer downplayed the popularity of prophetic medicine, arguing that patients probably expected from physicians' treatments with drugs and venesection following 'solid humoral-pathological standards' instead of honey-recipes (2011: 194). As a matter of fact, Unani and prophetic medicine overlap in some therapies. Among them, the most prominent example may be *ḥijāmah* ('cupping therapy').

Unani Medicine and Islam

Some hakims integrated Islamic elements in clinical practices. After a *ḥijāmah* session, Hakim Ahmad told one of his patients, who was Muslim, to go to the nearby mosque for prayers. When asked if that was part of the treatment, the hakim seemed to weigh what would be a good answer. After a few seconds, he said that god is happy with everyone who prays. 'God is the one who cures, it is better if one prays', he concluded. While he did not explicitly connect Unani to Islam here, Hakim Ahmad agreed that pleasing god contributes positively to the therapeutic process. His explanation resonates with the conviction among hakims that god is the ultimate healer, being the health of patients ultimately in god's hands.

The idea of adhering to the Sunna in order to avoid disease seemed to be wide spread. This found expression inside some *maṭabbs* and even in the practice of Hakim Sadiq, who commonly separated strictly between Unani and prophetic medicine:

> A patient told the hakim that he prays a lot and reads the Quran even though he works a lot. Hakim Sadiq asked him what does he do in the day of Eid,[76] and the patient said that one should not work on Eid. Hakim Sadiq then talked about food and the Quran, telling the patients about the timings for eating and sleeping. He said 'it is Sunna' and explained that it is written in the books (meaning in compilation of Hadiths) and in the Quran that one has to eat systematically (*niẓām ke sāth*). Hakim Sadiq pointed out that whoever follows the Sunna does not get sick.

Hakim Sadiq occasionally used the Sunna as a means to legitimate his claim that keeping specific timings for waking up and sleeping as well as for eating were necessary in order to convince certain patients to follow his advice.

76 A Muslim religious holiday.

He did so with patients who were visibly pious Muslims: those wearing a shalwar *qamīẓ* and topi not only on Fridays, and those women being very particular about purdah. This suggests that, more than issuing a disclaimer attributing full responsibility to the patients' behaviour for the cause of sickness, the hakim invoked the prophetic tradition in order to appeal to the conscience of pious patients to stick to the regimen of treatment. While healing is ultimately in god's hands, own efforts were necessary for health recovery.[77] Hakim Sadiq once said to a patient 'Diseases come from the lord Allah, every affliction comes from Allah. It is Sunna to treat [or be treated] and to keep the regimen.' While it is god who is responsible for causing the diseases, Hakim Sadiq claimed that in Sunna, the responsibility of getting treatment and applying a regimen to recover health rests on the patient. Muslim hakims agreed that it is Allah, and not the physician, the one who cures patients. Patients are reminded about the limitations of the hakim's power in front of god through the following Quran verse, which is displayed in many *maṭabbs*: 'And when I am ill, it is He who cures me' (26: 80).[78]

Many members of the Unani fraternity included *ṭibb-i nabavī* in the realm of Unani or explained that Unani was also 'Islamic medicine.' These assertions, however, were not shared by everyone. When discussing government support, Hakim Zillurrahman claimed that Unani received much less support than Ayurveda because of the association of medicine with religion, something that—he plainly stated—made him sick. While arguing that religion should not be mixed up with medicine, he complained that it still had a huge influence on the government, being a communal issue. Like Hakim Zillurrahman, other members of the Unani fraternity also considered the association of Unani with Muslims problematic. A BUMS graduate practicing allopathic medicine explained:

> The problem of people thinking of Unani as Islamic medicine is that they are dismissive with it. People would not like to use Unani, they think it is related to Islam because 99 per cent of the people trained in Unani are Muslims. But that has nothing to do with Unani being a Muslim medicine,

77 On the link between sickness and un-Islamic behaviour see Parkin, who for the case of Zanzibar stated: 'Sometimes people say that Islamic morality is the necessary condition of any form of well-being, and that an unpolluted natural environment only provides good health if that condition is met. But this is tantamount to saying that Muslim virtue is a necessary but not always sufficient condition of well-being [...]. This further amounts to a claim that God's omnipotence is the *sine qua non* of well-being but that humans can only achieve this well-being through their own efforts at keeping the environment clean' (2007: 202).

78 *'Vāiẓā mariẓat u fahuva yashfīn'* (Quran 26: 80).

> it is only because Urdu is required. And almost no Hindus know Urdu, because they say that it is a Muslim language. But Urdu is not a Muslim language, it is a young language, some 400 years old, but it is an Indian language and not a Muslim language.

This opinion, apart from resonating with Hakim Ahmad's notion that the term Unani was chosen in order to make Unani more attractive to patients with religious affiliations other than Islam, reflects the resentments that I encountered during fieldwork. The idea that the general public would avoid using Unani medicine if it was represented as Islamic medicine is a plausible one. Maarten Bode has cautioned against concluding that costumers of Unani (in his example, consumers of Hamdard products) were mainly Muslim since, according to his observations, most of the patients at the Majeedia Hospital in Delhi were Hindus (2008: 110). In the private clinics I observed, however, most patients were actually Muslims. This can be explained not mainly through a preference by Muslims for Unani over other forms of medicine, but because the clinics were commonly located in Muslim areas, thus being conveniently accessible to Muslims (Quaiser 2012a: 159f.).

Most patients seemed to choose their practitioners pragmatically. Hindu patients consulting Unani physicians did mainly so based on recommendations from family members and neighbours. Some Muslim patients I spoke to in the waiting room of the clinics thought that the hakim they were consulting practiced Ayurveda. Another patient, who consulted one hakim regularly, told me once that she was now taking ayurvedic medicines because the allopathic drugs did not help her. When I asked her if she meant Unani medicines, she said that ayurvedic and Unani are the same. Further research focusing on the patients' perspectives is required to prove these impressions.

The separation of Unani from everything religious followed the modernization of Unani medicine as medical science, which allowed no space for any religious connection with medicine (Speziale 2010a). This process was initiated during the Colonial Period (Metcalf 2004: 167). Making Unani appealing to the whole population was a requirement for it in order to survive in India after partition, a time when its representation as indigenous medicine was, strategically speaking, by far more adequate than a representation as Islamic medicine. Although Unani continues to be associated with Muslims in spite of government efforts to stress its secular character, it seems that it was not until recently that Unani medicine began being explicitly defined as Islamic medicine by some hakims and even patients. This phenomenon is clearly manifested in the revival of prophetic medicine in the private Unani sector and its influence on official representations (Schmidt Stiedenroth 2019b).

Producers selling Unani medicine to non-Muslims make use of ambiguous representations of it as *desi* ('local', 'Indian') in India or as herbal medicine abroad. While these vague labels help manufacturers sell their products to different audiences, they also hinder the spread of Unani medicine as a cultural commodity attached to the Muslim communities it is closely connected to. Likewise, representations of Unani medicine or some of its therapies as Islamic or even prophetic medicine target a specific Muslim audience and are not necessarily connected to Unani. In other words, the logic of the market, driven in great part by consumer demands, generates a vicious circle where the labelling of Unani medicines and practices as Unani are often avoided because of its association with Muslim communities.

The use of different denominations for health products related to Unani medicine hampers the establishment of Unani as a global name in the CAM market, in contrast to Ayurveda, Tibetan or Chinese medicine. This is also because Unani is known under different names in Muslim countries: in Iran it is *Ṭibb-i Sunnatī* while in Pakistan it is Eastern Medicine. This hinders the internationalization of a single name, which Ayurveda has successfully achieved. The different names used for Unani medicine, its products, and practices in different contexts account for the multiplicity of Unani, whereby marketing strategies and identity politics determine which version of Unani is enacted in a specific context.

Although Unani products already circulate in the global CAM market, its reach is by far smaller than that of other forms of Asian Medicine such as Ayurveda, Chinese or Tibetan medicine. As a matter of fact, Unani medicine remains largely unknown in Europe except, perhaps, among migrant populations with South Asian background. The Unani fraternity regards the success of what they consider to be the export of Ayurveda to the West with ambivalence. On the one hand, it is considered as a model to follow, giving hope for the expansion of Unani both as a form of medicine and as a cultural commodity. On the other hand, the growth of Ayurveda in North America and Europe is seen by some as the outcome of a greater government support towards Ayurveda as against Unani, as previously discussed.

In view of the increasing knowledge about and acceptance of Ayurveda and Tibetan Medicine in Germany, for example, the lack of awareness about Unani seems paradoxical: being the form of Asian medicine more closely connected to biomedicine for historical reasons, it does not attract Western patients in the way that other forms of Asian medicine do. Apart from the labelling problem discussed above, a possible reason for this lack of popularity outside of South Asian or Muslim contexts could be that, precisely because of its historical connections to biomedicine, Unani is not exotic enough for a Western audience which may seek for spirituality and otherness in traditional Asian medicines (Smith and Wujastyk 2008; Zysk 2001).

When Unani is linked to spirituality, then it is to a Muslim spirituality, a trend which was increasing in the private sector where Unani was often presented as 'Islamic medicine'. However, producers marketing Unani products abroad preferred the labels 'herbal medicine' or even 'Ayurveda,' whereas the local Muslim segment may be targeted through the labels 'Islamic medicine', 'Unani' or even 'prophetic medicine', depending on the case. The associations of Unani medicine with Muslims and Ayurveda with Hindus have a deep impact on the marketing strategies and labelling of medicines. This is, in India, linked to assumptions such as that Unani uses lizards in their preparations, while Ayurvedic drugs use cow's urine, thus making both forms of medicine mutually non-usable for orthodox Hindus and Muslims due to food taboos. It goes almost without saying that this typologization of Unani and Ayurveda as Muslim and Hindu respectively is, at its best, simplistic, but it was mentioned way too often to be ignored.[79] In a similar vein, a hakim once explained to a patient that homeopathic medicines are manufactured using alcohol and hence 'are not allowed in Islam,' even though some practitioners of homeopathy were Muslims.

During an informal meeting with Unani government officials and the owner of a Unani pharmaceutical company in Delhi, one of the first stated: 'We have to pose the question why has been Ayurveda able to spread so much whereas Unani has not, and we have to find an answer for this question.' He remarked the need to adopt the latest standards for Unani and commented that members of the Unani fraternity keep comparing Unani and Ayurveda and resent less support given to the former by the government instead of taking the issue in their own hands, adopting the same standards as the 'Ayurvedic people' did. The manufacturer who was present expressed that, as a businessman, he was aware of the associations of Unani with Muslims, hence he had to be very careful when introducing a new product that he would like to market beyond the Muslim milieu. Because of this, he commonly labelled a product as 'Unani' only after it has been already

79 Contrary to common assumptions, classical Ayurvedic texts have not only allowed but even recommended the consumption of meat and blood, for example (Zimmermann 2011 [1982]). Further, Dominik Wujastyk suggested that the origins of Ayurveda, culturally speaking, do not seem to be found in the Vedic religious literature as it is often claimed, and pointed out to a Buddhist origin, as suggested by Kenneth Zysk (Wujastyk 2003: xxixf.).

accepted in the market. The same applied to a new magazine he wanted to bring out through his company: they would first publish it in English in order to target a wider audience, and after the publication had been accepted by the public, they would launch an Urdu version of it.

These statements reveal that the need for consumer acceptance draws producers to avoid the label 'Unani' associated with Muslims in India. Unlike Ayurveda, Unani can hardly offer the appealing 'full package' of spirituality and herbal medicine to non-Muslim consumers, and manufacturers were faced with the need to decide which consumer group to target through marketing strategies. Consequently, we find Unani manufacturers selling their products outside of India under the label 'Ayurveda,' a strategy criticized among the fraternity but which one of the producers justified as the only possible way to penetrate foreign markets and make a start in the spread of Unani worldwide because 'No one knows what Unani is in Europe'. Often, I had to disappoint those who asked me if Unani was popular in Germany. The dismay of my interlocutors was even greater when, after being asked, I would tell them that nowadays many people in Germany do know Ayurveda. Even in India, manufacturers of Unani products sometimes preferred to sell Unani single drugs labelled as Ayurvedic, natural, herbal or desi medicine instead of as Unani, because those labels were said to sell better (Bode 2008: 75). Unlike Ayurveda, which has been arguably represented and marketed outside and inside of India—in simple terms—as a single Indian, ancient, natural, spiritual and gentle medical tradition (Bode 2008; Hardiman 2009; Langford 2002; Reddy 2002; Smith and Wujastyk 2008; Zysk 2001), Unani was offered using audience-dependent—sometimes overlapping and sometimes mutually exclusive—labels such as Islamic medicine and herbal medicine when addressing national and international audiences. In this way, the consumers and the companies adapted representations, thus enacting different realities of Unani medicine.

Attending to labelling strategies reveals how Unani's multiplicity unfolds in practice, and also how enactments are situated and context dependent, involving economic as well identitarian recognition interests. These conflicting interests make coordination work difficult. As a result, Unani medicine has failed to establish itself in the CAM market as a cultural commodity in the way Ayurveda has, its ontologies remaining largely distributed between "herbal medicine" and "Islamic medicine". Some members of the fraternity, especially those involved in the pharmaceutical sector, considered that multiple labels helped propagate Unani in the long term. This practice, however, remains highly contested among the Unani fraternity. It is said to betray Unani's core identity and the possibility of recognition as a unified system of medicine for the sake of profit. As such, it goes against *k̲h̲idmat*, accounting for a problematic moral economy.

Secular or Islamic? Unani and Prophetic Medicine

Ḥijāmah in the Context of Unani

Discussed in medical books as part of regimental therapies (*ʿilāj bi-t tadbīr*) or surgery (*jarrāḥiyat*), *ḥijāmah* has been a therapy in Unani medicine since its origins, but its practice seems to have been neglected by elite hakims in South Asia. Pharmaceutical preparations or dietary advice appear to have been preferred in the therapeutic practice of most hakims during the Colonial Period, as suggested by some influential Unani books (Kabīruddīn 1934; K̲h̲ān 2010).[80] Fabrizio Speziale argued that all Unani medical aspects that did not match modern scientific criteria, like Unani surgery and pathology, were gradually excluded from Unani medicine during the modernization period (2012a: 9). As cupping disappeared from the practice of Western medicine in its process of becoming biomedicine, it is possible that *ḥijāmah* became associated with a medical practice of the pre-modern period and begun to be seen as archaic, losing its appeal during the institutionalization of Unani training and practice, and through the growing interest on validation through modern scientific criteria analysed in the previous chapter. Policies supporting modern research targeting pharmaceutical products have led to the neglect of non-pharmaceutical knowledge and practice (Speziale 2010a: 327). Another possible explanation for the apparent disuse of *ḥijāmah* in Unani until recently is that it may not have been practiced by elite hakims at all, but only by barber surgeons (called *ḥijām*) or street healers instead (Hardiman and Mukharji 2012: 27). This was the case of cupping in fifteenth century Europe. In Germany, for example, cupping was among the tasks of the *Bader* (the person in charge of the bath house), who would not only shave, cut hair, and massage those attending public baths, but also treat them with cupping (Martin 1906: 70).[81] As for medieval Islam, cuppers were not learned physicians and were regarded as having a low social status instead (Pormann and Savage-Smith 2007: 121). If *ḥijāmah* was also in India practiced by non-elite practitioners, then most probably

80 Further research is required to establish if *ḥijāmah* was widely practiced before the 20th century, and, if yes, why did its practice decline.
81 I thank Claudia Preckel for pointing this out to me.

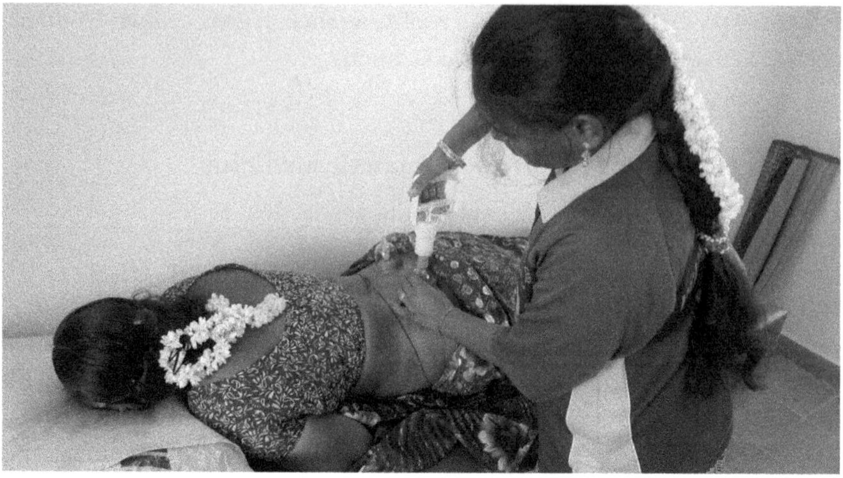

5. A patient receives cupping treatment at the 'Centre for Ilaj bit Tadbeer (Regimental Therapy)' funded by the former AYUSH Department in Puduvoyal, Tamil Nadu (2012).

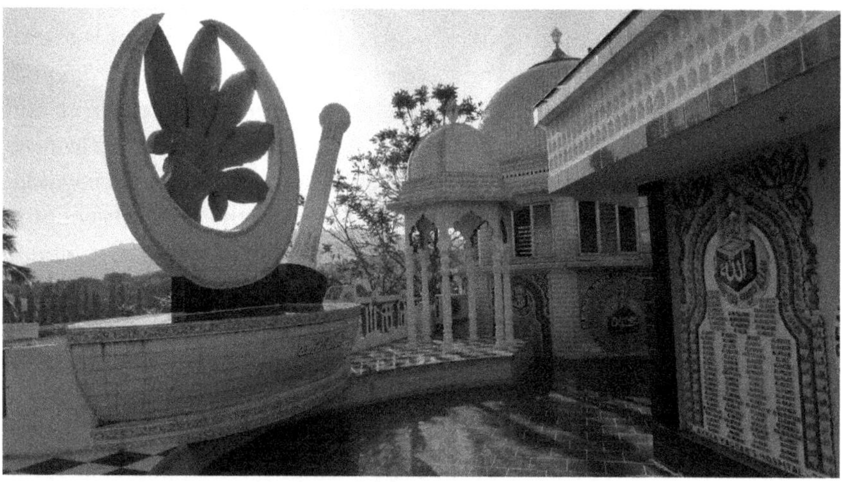

6. Hakim Akbar Kausar's symbol: a mortar and pestle with the crescent and the *kasni* plant. The walls display the 99 names of Allah (2012).

the elite physicians involved in the creation of Unani training institutions lacked practical knowledge about it and could, consequently, not transmit it in institutionalized settings. In postcolonial India, Unani medical colleges did, and some continue to, teach about cupping, but according to BUMS students and graduates this was done only in theory and not in practice, even though most Unani colleges had a section of *ʿIlāj bi-t tadbīr*—often as part of the *Muʿālijāt* (medicine) department (Schmidt Stiedenroth 2019b: 187).

This situation of neglect has been changing rapidly since the time of my fieldwork. The government of India, through the Ministry of AYUSH (former AYUSH department) has been promoting the practice of *ḥijāmah* and other regimental therapies in a development influenced by the boom of Ayurvedic panchakarma therapies both as wellness therapeutic and relaxation practices. Authorities in Unani departments of state institutions have taken an example from the success of Ayurveda in this sense, seeing there a chance for Unani to target a broader audience too, through the promotion of medical tourism for regimental therapies. The revival efforts pursued by the government, thus, aim at a promotion of Unani through an emulation of the panchkarma therapies which have flourished notably in the state of Kerala and in the west, albeit in a simplified manner that focuses on gentle therapies such as massage, and avoids more violent ones such as vomiting (Zimmerman 1992). These versions of panchakarma, which focus on catharsis, evacuation, and purification (ibid.), are similar to Unani's regimental therapies in which the latter also aim at evacuating superfluous matters that cannot be eliminated through digestion only (Ibn Sīnā 1993: 264ff.; Pormann and Savage-Smith 2007: 43f.). Government officials regarded panchakarma therapies as an example to be followed by Unani given their role in the popularization of Ayurveda not only among medical tourists coming to India, but also worldwide (Schmidt Stiedenroth 2019b: 188)

Due to its growing popularity and its potential as an export product, the CCIUM recently approved a new postgraduate programme on regimental therapies, the syllabus for which was published in April 2015 (CCIM 2015c). Before that, it was not possible to pursue a post-graduate degree in *ʿilāj bi-t tadbīr*, as opposed to the MD course in *ʿilm al adviyah*, which has a comparatively long tradition in India.[82] Apart from the regimental therapies sections present in some Unani government hospitals, the former AYUSH department recently started the support of a few projects related to *ʿilāj bi-t tadbīr* at the time of my fieldwork research, two of which were located in Tamil Nadu and which I had the chance to visit in 2012. The first was the construction of a hammam in cooperation with Hakim Akbar Kausar in Vaniyambadi, and the second was a centre of excellence in *ʿilāj bi-t tadbīr* in Puduvoyal in cooperation with Hakim Syed Khalifatullah and his sons. The latter institution is particularly interesting because, although its focus rested on the regimental therapies, it was also intended to provide primary health care to the rural population of the area where it was located. At the

82 The *ʿIlm al-Adviyah* department at Aligarh Muslim University, for example, was established in 1972 (Aligarh Muslim University 2014a).

same time, the centre was supposed to attract medical tourists from other parts of India and abroad.

The Centre of Excellence in *ʿIlāj bi-t Tadbīr* opened in 2011 with the financial support of a government scheme funded by the former AYUSH department in the form of a public-private partnership for non-profit organizations. The scheme covered the costs of construction as well as the staff's salary for the first five years, after which the centre should become self-sufficient and must run for another 25 years.[83] According to Dr. Syed M.A. Iqbal, administrator of the centre in Puduvoyal and son of Hakim Khalifatullah, the condition for receiving financial support was that, for an extended yet limited period of time, fifty percent of the patients treated in the centre should be persons below the poverty line (which they can demonstrate through a card); these patients should be treated for free. Located in a village, the centre for regimental therapies followed two aims: to provide health care to the village population, as well as becoming a place of attraction for medical tourists from India and abroad. The strategy, Dr. Iqbal explained, was to first attract the local rural population and, after five years, to address people from all over the country and abroad. Dr. Iqbal held a PhD in medical tourism and had come all the way from Brunei, where he had been living for the past 21 years, to support the centre administratively. The centre also organized medical camps targeting the local population in order to spread awareness on public health related issues.

Although it was a centre for regimental therapies, the OPD was open for general consultations and also provided pharmacological treatment. There was also a kitchen serving meals to the IPD patients according to dietary recommendations. The persons in charge of the centre explained that the government wanted to build it in a rural area without a primary health care centre nearby. However, the centre did not work as a proper primary health care centre, as it did not conduct vaccinations or treated acute cases because, they insisted, it should provide Unani services only. This exclusivity was remarked when I asked if the son of a Unani practitioner working at the centre, who was pursuing an MBBS degree at the time of my visit, would join as a staff member after obtaining his degree. I was told that this would not be possible because the centre is 'only for Unani.' The emphasis on Unani as a closed system, thus, was reinforced through this institution.

The premises, which had been recently constructed for the purpose of the centre, consisted of various therapy rooms offering diverse forms of

83 Other Unani institutions recently opened through this scheme included a Centre for Paralysis in Hyderabad and a Centre of Excellence for the treatment of arthritis in Deoband.

regimental treatment: one was a small gym featuring exercise machines, another one had a whirlpool for herbal baths, other ones were equipped for massages or infrared therapy. The centre had also a meditation room: with images of the Kaaba, green lightening and praying carpets on the floor, it looked like a Muslim prayer room. Medicinal plants abounded in the green areas of the centre, where *ḥijāmah* and leeching therapies were offered, too. In this clinical institution, *ḥijāmah* was just one among the several other regimental therapies offered in the luminous and spacious cottages.

Although *ḥijāmah* is also linked to *ṭibb-i nabavī*, institutions like the one in Puduvoyal stressed its secular character, making it also attractive to Hindu patients. Until very recently, official representations of cupping never linked it with prophetic medicine. An AYUSH publication on Unani medicine had an image of Galen performing *ḥijāmah* in it, and, just as with other topics, no link between Unani and Islam was explicitly made as the text merely described the therapy and its effects (Department of AYUSH 2013b).

The Revival of Prophetic Medicine in the Context of Unani

Enactments of Unani medicine as Islamic medicine seemed to depend much on the targeted audience. Some hakims often referred to Islam when treating Muslim patients, but not when talking with patients of other religious affiliations. Dressing as a Muslim, for example by wearing a shalwar *qamīẓ* and topi, was also considered by some hakims, especially young ones, to be important in order to inspire trust in their patients. However, the relevance of the dress may be more important as means to project the image of an experienced hakim than as a symbol of Muslim religiosity. Some Unani manufacturing companies were increasingly addressing Muslim patients as Muslims, as did private practitioners who claimed to practice prophetic medicine. This development can be observed through the revival of *ḥijāmah* (Schmidt Stiedenroth 2019b), as well as through the introduction of brands selling prophetic medicine. One of those brands was Sunnah Remedies.

Sunna Remedies was launched in 2014 by Mohsin Delhvi, the owner of Delhvi Naturals (a Unani pharmaceutical company), on the occasion of a conference on Urdu language. Under the slogan 'The Prophetic Testimony – *Sanad Nabavī*', Sunnah Remedies advertised different products under their Arabic name with the respective Hadiths mentioning them in its website. It also promoted *ḥijāmah* and sold *misvāk*, a stick used to clean the teeth which is claimed to have been used by the prophet Muhammad. Most of the other products were common spices, part of the stock of any South Asian kitchen. These spices are also considered to be single drugs in

Unani medicine. They are marketed as prophetic medicine in convenient modern packages that can be purchased as gift-packs also. With this, Delhvi Naturals clearly targeted a more specific consumer segment from that of Unani medicine. It is worth noting that, while the website of Delhvi Naturals offering the Unani products was in English only and it includes a section on *ṭibb-i nabavī* in it (Dehlvi Naturals 2015), the website of Sunnah Remedies was in no way linked to Unani and it offered information both in English and Urdu. Moreover, the website of Dehlvi Naturals (former Dehlvi Remedies) often referred to Unani as herbalism, hence targeting an even wider audience than that seeking Unani treatments only.

Social media discussions among hakims about this brand and other companies selling prophetic medicine products revealed divided opinions about the marketing of prophetic medicine. While some condemn the profit-oriented marketing of common spices in the name of Islam, others comment very positively about it and praise any efforts to promote *ṭibb-i nabavī* and, hence, Islam.

The case of *ḥijāmah*, a therapy at the intersections between Unani and prophetic medicine, constitutes perhaps the most striking example of how Unani is being re-Islamized through its revival (Schmidt Stiedenroth 2019b). Increasingly promoted as a 'forgotten Sunna', the practice of *ḥijāmah* was growing in Muslim urban areas at the time of my fieldwork. Not all practitioners offering *ḥijāmah* were registered Unani practitioners, while at the same time not all hakims practiced *ḥijāmah*.

Hakim Ahmad was among the BUMS graduates who offered this therapy. He came to know about *ḥijāmah* being prophetic medicine and decided to train and practice it as to emulate the positive example of the prophet Muhammad (Schmidt Stiedenroth 2019b: 189ff.). While he had learned about *ḥijāmah* in theory during his studies, it was not until he participated in training workshops that he learned how to actually practice it (ibid.). Because *ḥijāmah* was relatively expensive, his patients spent considerable time weighing the advantages and disadvantages of this therapy. Their concerns were mostly about the efficacy, the safety, and the price. When offering this treatment option to patients, Hakim Ahmad legitimated the practice both on the base of Hadiths that mention it as well as using his own credentials as a certified Unani physician. Sometimes patients came to his clinic asking explicitly for *ḥijāmah* treatment, as they had heard or read about it from the growing number of advertisements and articles published in newspapers such as the Urdu Times of Mumbai (ibid.). While *ḥijāmah* was promoted as part of spiritual healing in non-Unani contexts (Sax 2013), Hakim Ahmad practiced it in the context of Unani medicine, explaining its action in accordance with the fundamental principles of Unani. However, *ḥijāmah* was also used as a therapeutic method to treat psychological problems, as the following consultation exemplifies:

> On one occasion, a woman wearing a black niqab and her sister came to Hakim Ahmad's clinic because of her foot, which was swollen and full of patches that seemed to cover numerous wounds. She explained that she was taking antibiotics and that with painkillers the pain goes away for two hours, only to come back again. [...] She said that she was hoping to get *ḥijāmah* treatment today. The hakim said: 'the thing is, this will be a bit difficult for *ḥijāmah*.' After feeling the patient's pulse, the hakim wrapped the sphygmomanometer around her arm and checked her blood pressure. He said 'For this you will have to take medicines from outside' (meaning biomedical drugs). The hakim diagnosed a liver disease. The patient asked about her allergy, and the hakim said that it is related to the blood: 'These things come from the blood, they remain in the body and the liver throws them in the blood.'
>
> The patient said that she wanted to be treated with *ḥijāmah* today and asked if this treatment would be suitable for her condition. 'It will work, but I will also give you medicines', replied the hakim. They discussed the price of the therapy, and the patient asked for a discount. Hakim Ahmad agreed to charge Rs. 450,- today instead of the Rs. 1000.- he normally charged for a cupping session. 'What about the coming sessions?' asked the patient. 'We will see', said the hakim.
>
> [...] She then asked about other doctors practising *ḥijāmah*, to which he replied: 'I am very knowledgeable about medicines and I have been practising *ḥijāmah* for two years'. The patient turned to her sister saying 'May Allah make this treatment work' and her sister repeated the same words. After discussing her menstruations and stool with the hakim, the patient explained that she had been feeling very depressed since she suffered from an accident. She said that she is fine, but the other person involved passed away. 'She has a lot of depression, doctor',[84] said her sister. The patient explained that she was taking medicines for that, but she stopped taking them. 'May Allah give you peace of mind', said the hakim. The sister explained the details of the accident to the hakim. The patient explained that she could not sleep for a whole week.

84 During this whole consultation, which took place in Urdu, the term 'depression' was always mentioned in English by the hakim, the patient, and her sister.

Patient: In the name of Allah, I read the Quran a lot, mahshallah!
Hakim Ahmad: The devil keeps doing his work. You will keep doing yours. There is one medicine, *k̲h̲amīrah muqavvī dimāg̲h̲* ('brain strengthening *k̲h̲amīrah*'), this will do good for you and so will *ḥijāmah.*
Patient: The mind says one thing but the heart says another.
The hakim talked to the patient in a gentle and reassuring manner.
Patient: And, do I have any other problem?
Hakim Ahmad: No, it's a depression. Dr. Sajjid does *ḥijāmah* with me.

This consultation exemplifies how some patients consulted Hakim Ahmad asking explicitly for *ḥijāmah*, and also how the therapy was combined with Unani as well as biomedical medicines. It also reflects how Hakim Ahmad positioned his medical authority vis-à-vis other practitioners offering *ḥijāmah* through his deep knowledge on drugs (he held a post-graduate degree in Unani pharmacology) as well as his—at that time—comparatively long experience practicing *ḥijāmah*.

Hakim Ahmad legitimated the practice of *ḥijāmah* in front of his patients both on the basis of its being prophetic medicine and of its being Unani. While performing *ḥijāmah* on the female patient introduced above, the hakim explained to the patient's sister, who was present during the cupping session, that 'the dirty blood from the belly is collected and expelled.' He said that he had tested this kind of dirty blood in the laboratory and explained that 'if there is no dirty blood, then nothing will come out'. He added: 'Allah's prophet said this, but I have confirmed it.' Hence, Hakim Ahmad claimed that the effectiveness of *ḥijāmah* was not only based on religious, but also on scientific principles.

Unani is facing an unprecedented opportunity to gain acceptance as Islamic medicine in the global CAM market. As the practice of *ḥijāmah* grows in popularity among Muslims worldwide, the fraternity held great hopes to make the most of Unani's position as an institutionalized system of medicine. Claiming *ḥijāmah* expertise on the basis of its long tradition as part of Unani's regimental therapies, while simultaneously stressing the overlap of Unani with prophetic medicine, the Unani fraternity was aware of Unani's unique position to make claims of recognition in Muslim countries where the demand for prophetic medicine is growing. The Government of India, following its agenda to make India the leading CAM destination, has recognized this potential, too. After decades reinforcing the secular character of Unani, an official brochure for an AYUSH conference and exhibition taking place in Dubai in 2017 described Unani as Islamic (and also as herbal) medicine for what was perhaps the first time (Schmidt Stiedenroth 2019b: 184).

While I have examined this recent and important development in detail elsewhere (ibid.), it is important to note here that Unani remains fluid, subjected to the historical conditions in which its ontologies emerge: Unani (and *ḥijāmah*) can be a secular form of complementary and alternative medicine and at the same time (a part of) prophetic medicine. As the example of *ḥijāmah* reveals, Unani's reality multiplies (Mol 2002: 4f.) as different enactments of it emerge. Because some enactments are simultaneous, a hierarchy is established, depending on the case (Mol 2002: 63). These divergent—yet not always mutually exclusive—versions of Unani medicine require coordination and distribution which, as the examples above have shown, hakims play a very active role in. Further, coordination and distribution are also influenced by professional interests, economic agendas, and political contexts, the difference of which makes the coordination efforts at times more difficult. They also produce looping effects: hakims mentioning that *ḥijāmah* is Sunna in newspaper articles and advertisements, newspaper articles attracting patients to pursue *ḥijāmah* as Islamic medicine, the increase in demand for *ḥijāmah* by Muslim patients, the government's decision to establish Unani postgraduate programmes on regimental therapies, and the support towards institutions promoting them as part of an AYUSH scheme are examples of how Unani is being increasingly enacted as Islamic medicine by emphasizing practices connected to prophetic medicine.

The case of *ḥijāmah* epitomizes the malleability of Unani practices, the historical trajectories of therapies, and Unani's inherent multiplicity. This is done in a way that is not necessarily fragmentary, on the contrary: as the practice of hakims attest, the multiplicity of Unani appears to be coherent with the idea of Unani as a system of medicine. Unani was officially enacted by emphasizing its scientific and, hence, secular character, following modernizing aims that separated strictly between religion and science. The complex dynamics involved in local and global politics and markets contribute to a reconfiguration of enactments that emphasize its character as Islamic medicine. In this context, we may talk about a re-Islamization of Unani medicine (Schmidt Stiedenroth 2019b). This re-Islamization, however, does not correspond to a restoration of all magico-religious elements that were de-attached from Unani through the process of standardization in efforts to validate it as scientific (Speziale 2010a). Rather, it is characterized by the revival of remedies and therapies considered also to be prophetic medicine as means to claim professional authority over other practitioners of Islamic medicine and to specifically target Muslims as potential patients and consumers. It remains to be seen, however, if the Unani fraternity succeeds in the process.

Summary and Reflexions for Future Engagement

Almost six years after my fieldwork, as I write these words from my desk in Germany, *ḥijāmah* therapy is only a phone call away. Websites advertising this practice in German language have proliferated in the past few years, but instead of targeting the 'wellness' or 'New Age' sector, as the advertisements of Ayurvedic therapies in magazines about organic farming and natural living in Germany often do, these websites are oriented towards a Muslim audience looking for prophetic medicine. In contrast to *ḥijāmah*, Unani as a system of medicine has not yet managed the international breakthrough that the fraternity was hoping for at the time of fieldwork. This development reflects that therapeutic practices are not bound to the medical systems they are often attached to, and that they can proliferate on their own under particular circumstances. *Ḥijāmah* owes its international success among Muslim communities to its unambiguous connection to Hadiths and the Sunna, coupled with it being an easy to learn, relatively safe, and cheap procedure, but also to the popularization of cupping as a form of alternative and complementary medicine.

It may seem strange that in today's highly scientized and technicized field of medicine, specific therapeutic practices linked to religion and spirituality such as *ḥijāmah* are thriving, whereas Unani as a system of medicine has been less successful in spreading itself through validation using modern scientific terms. This not only speaks for asymmetries regarding authorities of scientific recognition, but it also confirms that it is not necessarily the modern scientific paradigm what determines the destiny of particular therapeutic practices. Also the global therapeutic market where they can thrive, including commercial interests, the possibility of specific therapies to be commoditized against others, as well as the potential of specific practices to articulate identities, religious or otherwise, play a crucial role.

This book has discussed the making of Unani medicine through an examination of its generative practices in contemporary India. I addressed the question of what Unani is based on several issues emanating from the existing literature on traditional Asian medicines. Each chapter analysed a different problem: the acceptance of Unani as a single system of medicine in spite of its multiplicity, the conflict between efforts of systematization and the inherent heterogeneous nature of Unani practice, the essentialization of Unani as humoural medicine, the apparent incommensurability of

Unani with biomedicine and with modern science, and the association of Unani with Muslims and Islam notwithstanding efforts of de-Islamization pursued by the government since independence. The study of Unani practices and representations through a combination of Mol's ontology of practice and Hacking's historical ontology allowed me to trace the multiplicity of Unani medicine in the making and to explain how certain enactments of it are naturalized to the extent of influencing academic scholarship. Consequently, the findings of this book allow me to re-examine some of the current literature on traditional Asian medicines. Perhaps one of the most important claims of this study is that the modernization of traditional forms of medicine does not invariably lead to their biomedicalization by threatening to erode the fundamental principles underlying their practice.

Taking up on the critique addressing the idea of Unani as a system of medicine, I investigated how regardless of its apparent multiple practices and representations there was still a consensus among the Unani fraternity about it being a system of medicine. Like other officially recognized forms of medicine in India, Unani underwent a process of systematization. This was backed mainly by the post-independence Indian state but emerged already in the Colonial Period. The consequent reduction of state support and patronage lead to a re-organization of the profession and the emulation of institutional structures of Western medicine through the establishment of Unani colleges and the introduction of a degree requirement for practice (Alavi 2007; Attewell 2007).

In independent India, the Unani sector is characterized by competition with other forms of medicine for funding and support based on a differentiation of Unani as a distinct system of medicine, as established through its official recognition. Consequently, different budget allocations, institutions and facilities such as research units, colleges and dispensaries have contributed to cement the separation of Unani as a system. This was coupled with the identification of forms of medicine with unique textual traditions, the codification of materia medica in separate pharmacopoeias, and the role of eminent hakims considered to embody the knowledge and values associated with Unani medicine, leading to looping effects reifying the understanding of Unani as a clear-cut and unified system of medicine. Having a systematized Unani one can get hold on at any time makes it possible to have an inclusive category to stick to and secure support, even though in practice what is subsumed under this category may be anything but structured and homogeneous.

The official status granted to Unani medicine in the postcolonial context has brought to light the tensions between efforts of state regulation and the inherent multiplicity of Unani. Chapter 2 dealt with the problem of imposing standards on Unani medicine, since the reputation of hakims has traditionally been based on innovation and originality. I contrasted traditional forms of knowledge transmission with institutional training, concluding that college education fails to provide an adequate framework for the transmission of practical knowledge—the art aspect of Unani medicine—because of the compact syllabus, the lack of extensive exposure to Unani clinical practice, and the missing intimacy required for the transmission of exclusive knowledge. The latter constitutes an important part of Unani medicine and is not delivered through books. Further, because original or exclusive knowledge is still considered to be a necessity for Unani physicians in order to establish a reputation as a good hakim, the government recognition of practitioners through degrees has failed to establish itself as the main source of legitimation and authority. Using Pordié & Blaikie's concept of taskscapes (2014), I proposed that, similarly to the case of Tibetan Medicine, the qualification of Unani graduates does not apply to all the taskscapes. For instance, young graduates who are interested in becoming hakims seek traineeships with established physicians in order to gain more exposure to Unani practice, hoping to obtain exclusive knowledge as well. Because the Unani fraternity and patients not only accept, but moreover require physicians to innovate in order to produce original knowledge, hakims defy standardization efforts in practice, giving shape to the intrinsic multiplicity that characterizes Unani medicine and which is currently threatened in strict institutional settings. Variations and multiplicity, it can be argued, constitute an important aspect of medicine in general and of Unani medicine in particular.

The analysis of clinical practices of hakims and the theories underlying them lead me to conclude that representations of Unani as humoural medicine are misleading. The examination of the fundamental principles of Unani and their role in clinical practices reveal that humoural imbalance is not considered to be the primordial cause of disease, since this is located mainly in the six essential factors closely connected to lifestyle. Taking into consideration recent research questioning the role of the humours in so-called humoural forms of medicine (Attewell 2013; Horden 2013; Savage-Smith 2013), I argue that enactments of Unani as humoural medicine are the product of looping effects and dynamic nominalism (Hacking 2002). The modes of diagnosis and treatment suggest that the qualities (mainly heating and cooling) are even more important than the humours in clinical practice, much in line with Emilie Savage-Smith's argument on medieval Graeco-Islamic medicine (2013).

In view of these findings, I examined the supposed incompatibility of Unani medicine with scientific advances, including the use of diagnostic technologies and the adoption of modern medical concepts. The views of members of the Unani fraternity suggest that modern advances are not regarded as imposing a biomedical epistemological framework upon Unani medicine. Rather, they are seen by the fraternity as the product of a neutral and universal realm of science which encompasses all forms of medicine, including biomedicine. The use of modern diagnostic methods in the context of Unani should be regarded as an appropriation of technologies rather than a mere integration. This is because instead of exporting an understanding of the human body and its functioning, modern diagnostic methods are utilized as neutral tools adjustable to the needs of hakims' medical practice. These needs vary from diagnostic aids to proof of therapeutic success. Further, the acceptance of the biochemical parameters provided by modern diagnostic methods does not necessarily conflict with the fundamental principles of Unani medicine as applied by hakims. Instead, hakims regarded them as an addition. This is because the technologies do not provide explanations about disease causation (Sieler 2015: 187), the aspect considered most central in the differentiation hakims make between Unani and biomedicine. Similarly, the use of (biomedical) anatomical knowledge and various re-interpretations of the concept of elements in line with modern scientific knowledge does not oppose theories of disease causation used by hakims and produces no epistemological collision between Unani and biomedicine. This allows hakims to make claims of superiority vis-à-vis biomedicine, arguing that their understanding of disease causation goes deeper than the biomedical one. In this way, also hakims are involved in the power struggles inherent to the production of what is medical and, thus, scientific, and in assertions of authority in these fields.

I acknowledge that the institutionalization of Unani training and practice has led to a narrowed approach towards patients and their treatment. Brief observations and conversations suggested that practitioners in institutionalized settings focus more on symptomatic treatment instead of addressing the root cause of disease. However, the term biomedicalization seems inadequate to describe this phenomenon, as these changes in Unani medical practice were not merely triggered by the influence of biomedical knowledge. Rather, institutionalized training and its limitations as well as the healthcare system itself with its arrangements for consultations, focus on drug therapies, and a limited number of drugs available as well as the restricted time frame given to consultations may better explain this shift. The very use of the term biomedicalization in the literature to address the use of medical technologies, scientific research, institutionalization, and the influence of biomedical knowledge reminds us of the necessity for a more differentiated approach towards biomedicine and even medicine as a category, as proposed for example by Alter (2005b: 20) and Sieler (2015: 159). Long term participant observation in institutional settings will be required to provide sustained claims regarding the role of the fundamentals of Unani and the influence of biomedical knowledge in those contexts.

Chapter 5 dealt with the role of modern science in the search for acceptance and recognition of Unani ever since the loss of its previous hegemony against Western medicine. The search for legitimation has been shaped by the changing political, economic, and social environments that surround Unani medicine. With a focus on the best possible evidence, biomedicine has increasingly relied on modern scientific research and statistical data as against the clinical experience of the physician when it comes to setting standards (Adams 2016; Ecks 2008). Because biomedicine is favoured by international organizations and governments around the world, the standards applying to it have been imposed on traditional forms of medicine worldwide in order to comply with regulations and acquire legitimacy. The adoption of standards as means for legitimation mirror national and international health policies (Pordié 2010: 57). Critics have pointed out the negative implications of standards applied to the pharmaceutical industry and research aiming at the validation of traditional forms of medicine. They have focused mostly on the decontextualization of therapies, the alienation from the fundamental principles underlying traditional medicine and the subsequent loss of traditional medicine through a rationalization process which underplays its epistemological tenets. It has been commonly criticized that modern scientific research reinforces the hegemony of biomedicine through imposing its own rationale as a yardstick to prove the efficacy of traditional medicines. While this is indeed often the case, the majority of the Unani fraternity does not see a problem with what they consider to be merely a translation process. In spite of the justified scepticism of scholars of Asian medicines, most Unani researchers and practitioners continue to perceive standardization and modern research positively as means to attain acceptance and recognition, and not as a threat against Unani.

One of the greatest puzzles of the present work was the question of reconciliation between modern science and the fundamental principles of Unani medicine. Part of the problem was solved through the examination of clinical practices and the rhetoric towards modern advances: Unani medicine cannot be reduced to a humoural form of medicine, and modern science is not considered to impose biomedical understandings but is regarded by most hakims as neutral instead. This dissolves possible epistemological gaps in clinical practices. However, the question still had to be addressed: how does the fraternity reconcile Unani's scientific approach—which includes metaphysical elements—with modern science, which arguably rejects them? I attempted to explain this through a very brief examination of the history of science and the common trajectories—until a certain point in history—of Unani (Graeco-Islamic) medicine and European thought: while the development of positivism in Europe lead to a break with metaphysics and the dismissal of experience as proof of evidence, in Unani science continued to conceive both the material and immaterial as parts of reality in the same way that experience continued to be accepted as evidence. Both are grasped by the Unani fraternity as a single style of reasoning in Hacking's sense (2002: 169). Hence, from the point of view of the fraternity, Unani and modern science are not incommensurable.

While hakims condemn biomedicine for its reductionist view of the human body, critics against traditional forms of medicine often point out that they have not been able to prove their fundamental principles scientifically. This criticism has been discussed as a form of epistemic violence. However, I argued that this violence does not emanate from the episteme itself, but from the political economy that backs its dominance instead. Without underplaying the asymmetrical relationships in which Unani scientific research is framed, as the discussion on the political economy determining the quest for acceptance and recognition evinced, it is important to understand that the Unani fraternity appropriates modern science to claim a position within the scientific community for itself. Unlike other forms of Asian traditional medicine, the history of Unani is rooted in the same intellectual tradition that gave birth to modern science. From the perspective of the fraternity, a 'translation into the language of science' is actually possible. However, the acceptance of this translation remains subjected to power relations determined by health and import policies, the WHO, and the market of CAM, among others.

As for the relationship of Unani medicine with Muslim identity in India, language politics have done their part for Unani college education to be accessed almost exclusively by Muslims, thus perpetuating the stereotype that a hakim is necessarily a Muslim. As history shows, this was not always the case: neither were all classical authors Muslims during the medieval Islamic period (Savage-Smith 2014: 171), nor all hakims in pre- and postcolonial South Asia. It has been noted that there were (and there still are, although very few) Hindu Unani physicians and Muslim Ayurvedic scholars, and that Unani medicine was also patronized by Hindu aristocrats in the past (Leslie 1974: 89f.). Also important, the exchange of masters and pupils between the

Ayurvedic and Unani traditions that was common until the Colonial Period disappeared later through the institutionalization of training that reinforced the difference between both traditions as separate systems of medicine (Speziale 2018: 133). Unani medicine was re-defined as a scientific form of medicine in modern terms during the Postcolonial Period by de-attaching religious elements and transforming Unani into a secular 'Greek' medicine (Speziale 2005). However, its identification as Islamic medicine seems to be growing among a number of practitioners. Presently, we find multiple but not necessarily mutually exclusive representations of Unani, for example as secular, scientific or Islamic. When looking back at the history of Unani, the looping effects of these enactments become apparent, as historical and political developments have impacted and continue to influence the way in which Unani has been represented in connection to religion and how Indian Muslims, particularly those involved in Unani medicine, articulated their identity through it. Through enactments of Unani as Islamic medicine, Unani is used by Muslims to express identification with their religion, be it for themselves, on a personal level, or for others.

As a minority since independence, Muslims in India have been subjected to increased marginalization in different spheres, from education and employment to actual 'ghettoisation' in urban settings. In this scenario, Unani may offer unique opportunities to Muslims to access much sought-after government jobs in different institutions related to it. As Islamic medicine, it also makes it possible for hakims and patients to pursue medical treatments according to the Sunna and, hence, more in line with their moral local worlds, i.e. the 'moral accounts [which] are the commitments of social participants in a local world about what is at stake in everyday experience' (Kleinman 1995: 45). While the government of India and its related institutions focus on a portrayal of Unani as a secular and scientific medical practice which shares a common history with biomedicine and which can offer successful treatments not only for the local population, but also for the rest of the world, some private practitioners like Hakim Ahmad preferred to focus on the sentiments and interests of their Muslim patients when the case required. While not all patients opting for Unani are Muslims, the majority certainly is, although not necessarily for ideological reasons, often simply because many Unani clinics are located in Muslim areas, making them conveniently accessible for the Muslim population living there.[85] It is likely that Unani will continue to be associated with Muslims in India in spite

85 However, my observations in the *maṭabbs* revealed that not few patients come from far away areas, some indeed from very far away, covering distances over 300kms, a few times even more.

of government efforts to stress its secular character, an effort that has also been changing recently (Schmidt Stiedenroth 2019b). Future engagements with Unani medicine in India should examine the role of rising Hindu nationalism in its representations and practices.

The revival of prophetic medicine is emblematic in terms of how a medical practice has been re-invented through secular globalization processes and re-Islamization. Cupping therapy has received increasing government support as a regimental therapy, following an agenda aiming to establish India as a global health care destination inspired by the success of 'global Ayurveda' (Smith and Wujastyk 2008). Cupping therapy appears to have been re-introduced into Islamic countries as TCM. It appears that efforts of legitimation as well as marketing strategies lead to the re-discovery of *ḥijāmah* as a 'forgotten Sunna', as it is currently promoted among private practitioners in India (Schmidt Stiedenroth 2019b). Hacking's concept of looping effects is useful to understand this phenomenon, as denominations and categories influence what we understand by Unani while, simultaneously, practices, institutions and ideas related to them naturalize them (Naraindas et al. 2014: 5). Unani, thus, is naturally enacted as Islamic medicine by Hakim Ahmad, for example, given his personal commitment towards leading a life following the example of the Prophet, a view that is shared by his religious community and by many of his patients. Both Muslim patients as well as Muslim practitioners articulate their Muslim identity through enactments of Unani as Islamic medicine. Hakim Sadiq, on the other hand, also emphasizes the importance of Sunna when talking to patients, even though for him *ḥijāmah* is simply not a part of Unani and, thus, he does not consider integrating it into his practice. Another crucial point emanating from the case of prophetic medicine is that the categories scientific and religious/Islamic as well as Unani and prophetic medicine are not necessarily mutually exclusive (Schmidt Stiedenroth 2019b). Muslim physicians and patients, thus, co-constitute Unani medicine in ways that best suit their own purposes, enacting their own and multiple versions of it. Herein lie Unani's multiple ontologies, which emerge from the political and moral economies in which Unani's generative practices are embedded. Through a constant making of different Unanis—from Greek to Islamic—and their looping effects, the multiplicity of Unani and its contingent nature remain characteristics of it.

The context in which Unani medicine is practiced today is not fully subjected neither to biomedical understandings of the body and its diseases, nor to paradigms of knowledge production dominant in Western societies and in certain spheres of the Indian one. While the interest to translate Asian medicines into the language of science is often interpreted in the literature as a subjugation to dominant scientific models, scholars engaged in their study should not forget to look at practices that either appropriate these models for the sake of an own, distinct narrative, or reject them as reductionist and simplistic, articulating not only superiority but also, clearly, the necessity of broader paradigms more congruent to the own worldview. Indigenous knowledge systems are 'no more innocent than contemporary scientific knowledge, yet they are a useful counterweight because, as subjugated knowledges, they are less likely to deny the critical and interpretative core of all knowledge' (Watson-Verran and Turnbull 1995: 131). In this sense, the Unani fraternity engages in its own power practices of science.

The present book attended to some of the processes involved in braiding science, a science constituted by a myriad of spools already composed by heterogenous threads (Mukharji 2016). One of the tasks of scholars of Asian medicine is to disentangle the braids, identify their constitution and origin, and to answer the question why a particular thread or spool has become part of the braiding at a particular time and place. Often, the answers lie beyond the medical realm. Thus, scholars need to keep questioning this category as point of departure for our engagement with medical practices (Alter 2005: 20, Deb Roy and Attewell 2018). It is also useful to recall that the study of biomedicine from an anthropological perspective emerged from the necessity to examine it as another form of culturally produced knowledge (Lock and Nguyen 2018: 53). The practices of Unani medicine in India discussed in this book demonstrate that understandings of the body and therapeutic approaches are not being universalized through the hegemony of biomedicine, even as hakims make use of modern diagnostic methods such as urine examinations or blood tests. On the contrary: they reflect processes of contestations and appropriations that further question the dominance of biomedical science.

Challenging the hegemony of the biomedical paradigm has important consequences. It allows us to question its relevance, advantages, and disadvantages. In today's Anthropocene, at the verge of ecological catastrophes of global scale brought about by capitalist production, anthropologists and scholars of Asian medicine also have the important task to keep questioning the status quo. We need to think about our role in presenting and discussing existing modes of knowledge production and practices that may help societies find sustainable alternatives. Without romanticizing our subjects and objects of study, nor isolating them from the political and moral economies in which they are embedded, we may take a closer look at what we can learn from the multiple ontologies we encounter in our work, and to think seriously about how to bring them into conversations beyond our fields, also into the public sphere. This invitation is certainly not an easy task, as the biomedical scientific community is often wary about engaging in conversations with para-sciences, to use Mukherji's term (2016). More than assuming and advocating role, I suggest that anthropologists and scholars of Asian medicine could maintain a critical one. As put by Watson-Verran & Turnbull, 'the strength of social studies of science is its claim to show that what we accept as science and technology could be better than it is; its great weakness is the general failure to grasp the political nature of the enterprise and to work toward change' (1995: 138). While the study of Asian medicines has gone a long way to identify and problematize the social, political and economic dimensions of medical practices, we still have a long way to go towards change. Recognizing that differences go beyond epistemologies and are importantly rooted in political economy is, however, the first step.

Bibliography

Adams, Vincanne. 2002a. 'Establishing Proof: Translating "Science" and the State in Tibetan Medicine'. In Mark Nichter & Margaret Lock (eds.), *New Horizons in Medical Anthropology: Essays in Honour of Charles Leslie*, 200–220. London: Routledge.

Adams, Vincanne. 2002b. 'Randomized Controlled Crime: Postcolonial Sciences in Alternative Medicine Research'. *Social Studies of Science* 32(5/6). 659–690.

Adams, Vincanne (ed.). 2016. *Metrics: What Counts in Global Health*. Durham: Duke University Press.

Adams, Vincanne & Fei-Fei Li. 2008. 'Integration or Erasure? Modernizing Medicine at Lhasa's Mentsikhang'. In Laurent Pordié (ed.), *Tibetan Medicine in the Contemporary World: Global Politics of Medical Knowledge and Practice*, 105–131. London: Routledge.

Adams, Vincanne, Suellen Miller, Sienna Craig, Nyima, Sonam, Droyoung, Lhakpen & Michael Varner. 2005. 'The Challenge of Cross-Cultural Clinical Trials Research: Case Report from the Tibetan Autonomous Region, People's Republic of China'. *Medical Anthropology Quarterly* 19(3). 267–289.

afʿāl al-adviyah. n.d. In *Ferozson's Urdu-English Dictionary: (Revised Edition)*, 62. Lahore: Ferozsons.

Ahmed, Sayed Ishtiaq. 2009 [1980]. *Introduction to Al-Umur Al-Tabi'yah: (Principles of Human Physiology in Tibb)*. New Delhi: Central Council for Research in Unani Medicine.

Āl Īnḍyā Yūnānī Ṭibbī Kānfrans. 1984 [1951]. *Qarābādīn-i Majīdī*. Dihlī: Āl Īnḍyā Yūnānī Ṭibbī Kānfrans.

Alavi, Seema. 2007. *Islam and Healing: Loss and Recovery of an Indo-Muslim Medical Tradition, 1600 – 1900*. New York: Palgrave Macmillan.

Alavi, Seema. 2008. 'Medical Culture in Transition: Mughal Gentleman Physician and the Native Doctor in Early Colonial India'. *Modern Asian Studies* 42(5). 853–897.

Alexander, J. 2012. 'India Takes Lead to Forge Ties Between SAARC Nations to Promote Traditional Medicines'. *Pharmabiz.com*. 2012. http://pharmabiz.com/NewsDetails.aspx?aid=67148&sid=1 (accessed 8 December 2015).

Ali, Syed Mahtab, Rashid Ul-Islam & Mahe Alam. 2007. 'A Scientific Correlation between Blood Groups and Temperaments in Unani Medicine'. *Indian Journal of Traditional Knowledge* 6(2). 319–323.

Aligarh Muslim University. 2014a. Department of Ilmul Advia. http://amu.ac.in/departmentpage.jsp?did=89 (accessed 6 December 2014).

Aligarh Muslim University. 2014b. Department of Kulliyat. http://amu.ac.in/departmentpage.jsp?did=91 (accessed 27 August 2018).

Alter, Joseph S. (ed.). 2005a. *Asian Medicine and Globalization*. Philadelphia: University of Pennsylvania Press.

Alter, Joseph S. 2005b. 'Introduction: The Politics of Culture and Medicine'. In Joseph S. Alter (ed.), *Asian Medicine and Globalization*, 1–20. Philadelphia: University of Pennsylvania Press.

American College of Rheumatology. 2015. ACR-endorsed Criteria for Rheumatic Diseases. http://www.rheumatology.org/Practice-Quality/Clinical-Support/Criteria/ACR-Endorsed-Criteria (accessed 29 July 2015).

Andersen, Tavs Folmer & Gavin Mooney. 1990. 'Medical Practice Variations: Where Are We?' In Tavs Folmer Andersen & Gavin Mooney (eds.), *The Challenges of Medical Practice Variations*, 1–15. London: Macmillan Press.

Appadurai, Arjun. 1996. *Modernity at Large: Cultural Dimensions of Globalization*. Minneapolis: University of Minnesota Press.

Appadurai, Arjun (ed.). 2013 [1986]. *The Social Life of Things: Commodities in Cultural Perspective*. Cambridge: Cambridge University Press.

Arnold, David. 1993. *Colonizing the Body: State Medicine and Epidemic Disease in Nineteenth-Century India*. Berkeley: University of California Press.

Arnold, David. 2013. *Everyday Technology: Machines and the Making of India's Modernity*. Chicago: University of Chicago Press.

Attewell, Guy. 2005. 'The End of the Line? The Fracturing of Authoritative Tibbi Knowledge in Twentieth-Century India'. *Asian Medicine* 1(2). 387–419.

Attewell, Guy. 2007. *Refiguring Unani Tibb: Plural Healing in Late Colonial India*. New Delhi: Orient Longman.

Attewell, Guy. 2013. 'Yunani Tibb and Foundationalism in Early Twentieth-Century India: Humoral Paradigms between Critique and Concordance'. In Peregrine Horden & Elisabeth Hsu (eds.), *The Body in Balance: Humoral Medicines in Practice*, 129–148. New York: Berghahn.

Attewell, Guy. 2016. 'Alignments? X-ray Diversions, Haptics, Credibility—With a "Bone-Setting" Clinic in Hyderabad City'. *Medical Anthropology* 35(1). 5–16.

Aʿvān, M.Ḥ. n.d. *Kitāb al-Mufradāt: Al-maʿrūf bah ḵẖāṣ al-ādviyah biṭ arz jadīd*. Lāhor: Shaiḵẖ G̱ẖulām ʿAlī and Sanz.

AYUSH. 2015. Welcome to AYUSH. http://indianmedicine.nic.in (accessed 29 September 2015).

Azad, Ghulam Nabi. 2012. *Sh Azad Calls Upon Overseas Indian Medical Professionals to Partner with Institutions in India*. http://pib.nic.in/newsite/erelease.aspx?relid=79409 (accessed 23 April 2020).

Azmi, Altaf Ahmad. 1995. *Basic Principles of Unani Medicine: A Critical Study*. New Delhi: Department of History of Medicine Jamia Hamdard.

Azmi, Altaf Ahmad. 2004. *History of Unani Medicine in India*. New Delhi: Centre for History of Medicine and Science Jamia Hamdard.

Baer, Hans A. & Ian Coulter. 2008. 'Taking Stock of Integrative Medicine: Broadening Biomedicine or Co-option of Complementary and Alternative Medicine?' *Health Sociology Review* 17(4). 331–341.

Baer, Hans A., Merrill Singer & Ida Susser. 1997. *Medical Anthropology and the World System: A Critical Perspective*. Westport: Bergin & Garvey.

Banerjee, Madhulika. 2002. 'Public Policy and Ayurveda: Modernising a Great Tradition'. *Economic & Political Weekly* 37(12). 1136–1146.

Banerjee, Madhulika. 2004. 'Local Knowledge for World Market: Globalising Ayurveda'. *Economic & Political Weekly* 39(1). 89–93.

Banerjee, Madhulika. 2008. 'Ayurveda in Modern India: Standardization and Pharmaceuticalization'. In Dagmar Wujastyk & Frederick M. Smith (eds.), *Modern and Global Ayurveda: Pluralism and Paradigms*, 201–214. Albany: State University of New York Press.

Bates, Don. 1995. 'Scholarly Ways of Knowing: An Introduction'. In Don Bates (ed.), *Knowledge and the Scholarly Medical Traditions*, 1–22. Cambridge: Cambridge University Press.

Bauer, Thomas. 2011. *Die Kultur der Ambiguität: Eine andere Geschichte des Islams*. Berlin: Verlag der Weltreligionen.

Beckerleg, Susan. 1994. 'Medical Pluralism and Islam in Swahili Communities in Kenya'. *Medical Anthropology Quarterly* 8(3). 299–313.

Belo, Catarina. 2018. 'Elements'. In Kate Fleet, Gudrun Krämer, Denis Matringe, John Nawas & Everett Rowson (eds.), *Encyclopaedia of Islam, Three*: Brill. http://dx.doi.org.ubproxy.ub.uni-heidelberg.de/10.1163/1573-3912_ei3_COM_26149 (accessed 27 August 2018).

Berg, Marc & Annemarie Mol (eds.). 1998. *Differences in Medicine: Unraveling Practices, Techniques, and Bodies*. Durham: Duke University Press.

Berger, Rachel. 2013. *Ayurveda Made Modern: Political Histories of Indigenous Medicine in North India, 1900 – 1955*. Basingstoke: Palgrave Macmillan.

Besch, Florian. 2006. 'Tibetan Medicine Off the Roads: Modernizing the Work of the Amchi in Spiti'. PhD thesis, Heidelberg University. http://www.ub.uni-heidelberg.de/archiv/7893 (accessed 27 August 2018).

Bode, Maarten. 2001. 'Indigenous Pharmaceuticals: The Articulation of Modernity and Tradition in India'. In Bidare V. Subbarayappa (ed.), *Medicine and Life Sciences in India*, 549–573. Delhi: Project of History of Indian Science Philosophy and Culture, Centre of Studies in Civilizations.

Bode, Maarten. 2002. 'Indian Indigenous Pharmaceuticals: Tradition, Modernity and Nature'. In Waltraud Ernst (ed.), *Plural Medicine, Tradition and Modernity, 1800-2000*, 184–203. London: Routledge.

Bode, Maarten. 2006. 'Taking Traditional Knowledge to the Market: The Commoditization of Indian Medicine'. *Anthropology & Medicine* 13(3). 225–236.

Bode, Maarten. 2008. *Taking Traditional Knowledge to the Market: The Modern Image of the Ayurvedic and Unani Industry, 1980 – 2000*. Hyderabad: Orient Longman.

Bode, Maarten. 2009. 'On the Effectiveness of Ayurvedic Medical Treatments: Humoral Pharmacology, Positivistic Science, and Soteriology'. *eJournal of Indian Medicine* 2. 1–20 (accessed 20 January 2018).

Bode, Maarten. 2012. 'Ayurveda in the Twenty-First Century: Logic, Practice and Ethics'. In Venkatesh Sujatha & Leena Abraham (eds.), *Medical Pluralism in Contemporary India*, 59–76. New Delhi: Orient Blackswan.

Bode, Maarten. 2015. 'Assembling Cyavanaprāsh, Ayurveda's Best-selling Medicine'. *Anthropology & Medicine* 22(1). 23.

Bode, Maarten & G. Hariramamurthi. 2013. 'Integrating Folk Healers in India's Public Health: Acceprance, Legitimacy and Emancipation'. *eJournal of Indian Medicine* 7. 1–20. https://ugp.rug.nl/eJIM/article/view/24752 (accessed 20 January 2018).

Bode, Maarten & Unnikrishnan Payyappallimana. 2013. 'Evidence Based Traditional Medicine: For Whom and to What End?' *eJournal of Indian Medicine* 6. 1–20. https://ugp.rug.nl/eJIM/article/download/24746/22196 (accessed 19 January 2018).

Bright, Kristy. 1997. 'Cool, Cool Beverage'. *Seminar* (433). 33–37.

Bright, Kristy. 1998. 'The Traveling Tonic: Tradition, Commodity, and the Body in Unani (Graeco-Arab) Medicine in India'. PhD Thesis, University of California.

Bürgel, Johann Christoph. 1976. 'Secular and Religious Features of Medieval Arabic Medicine'. In Charles Leslie (ed.), *Asian Medical Systems: A Comparative Study*, 44–62. Berkeley: University of California Press.

Büttner, J. 1991. 'Urina ut signum: Zur historischen Entwicklung der Urin-Untersuchung'. In Walter G. Guder & Hermann Lang (eds.), *Pathobiochemie und Funktionsdiagnostik der Niere: Deutsche Gesellschaft für Klinische Chemie Merck-Symposium 1989*, 1–21. Berlin: Springer.

CCIM. n.d. Niṣāb-i Taʿlīm barā'e Kāmil-i Ṭibb o Jarrāḥat. Na'ī Dihlī: Sinṭral Kaunsil āf Īnḍī'an Meḍīsin.

CCIM. 2004. 'Notification No-8-5/2002 – Ay. (MM)'. New Delhi: Central Council of Indian Medicine.

CCIM. 2015a. 'Introduction to Central Council of Indian Medicine'. http://www.ccimindia.org/introduction.php (accessed 20 August 2015).

CCIM. 2015b. 'Syllabus of Doctor of Medicine (MD-Unani) (Pharmacy): 3 Years Degree Course'. http://www.ccimindia.org/pdf/PG%20syllabus%20of%20Ilmul%20Saidla.pdf (accessed 24 July 2015).

CCIM. 2015c. 'Syllabus of Doctor of Medicine (MD-Unani) (Regimental Therapy): 3 Years Degree Course'. http://www.ccimindia.org/pdf/pg-Syllabus-Ilaj-Bit-Tadbeer.pdf (accessed 24 July 2015).

CCIM. 2015d. 'Unani Colleges'. http://www.ccimindia.org/unani-colleges.php (accessed 27 August 2018).

CCRAS. 2013. 'CCRAS News Bulletin 27 (2): Central Council for Research in Ayurvedic Sciences'. http://ccras.nic.in/bulletin/News%20letter%20English%20Vol%2027%20No.2.pdf (accessed 5 June 2014).

CCRUM. n.d. 'Unani Treatment for Waja-ul-Mafasil (Rheumatoid Arthritis): A Success Story'. New Delhi: Central Council for Research in Unani Medicine.

CCRUM. 2001 [1979]. *Ṭibb-i yūnānī maiṉ gharelo adviyah aur 'ām mu'ālijāh kī kitāb*. Na'ī Dihlī: Sinṭral kaunsil fār rīsarc in yūnānī meḍīsin.

CCRUM. 2006 [1981]. *National Formulary of Unani Medicine*. New Delhi: Central Council for Research in Unani Medicine.

CCRUM. 2007a. *National Formulary of Unani Medicine*. New Delhi: Central Council for Research in Unani Medicine.

CCRUM. 2007b. *Unani Pharmacopoeia of India*. New Delhi: Central Council for Research in Unani Medicine.

CCRUM. 2009. *Unani Medicine in India*. New Delhi: Central Council for Research in Unani Medicine.

CCRUM. 2010. *Unani Pharmacopoeia of India*. New Delhi: Central Council for Research in Unani Medicine.

CCRUM. 2012. *Standard Unani Medical Terminology*. New Delhi: Central Council for Research in Unani Medicine.

CCRUM. 2015a. 'Budget Allocation 2012-2013'. http://www.ccrum.net/wp-content/uploads/2012/08/Plan-Non-Plan-Budget-Allocation-headwise-2012-13.pdf (accessed 13 February 2015).

CCRUM. 2015b. 'Establishment of CCRUM'. http://www.ccrum.net/ccrum/establishment-of-ccrum/ (accessed 23 February 2015).

Central Council of Indian Medicine Notification. 2013. 'No. I t-76120t l-UG Regl'. In *The Gazette of India*. http://www.ccimindia.org/downloads/UG%20REGULATIONS.pdf (accessed 23 April 2020).

Chakrabarti, Bhupati. 2007. 'Fifty Years of the Metric System in India and its Adoption in our Daily Life'. *Current Science* 92(3). 390–391.

Chakrabarti, Pratik. 2004. *Western Science in Modern India: Metropolitan Methods, Colonial Practices*. Delhi: Permanent Black.

Chatterjee, Partha. 1993. *The Nation and its Fragments: Colonial and Postcolonial Histories*. Princeton: Princeton University Press.

Chipman, Leigh. 2018 [2012]. 'Botany'. In Kate Fleet, Gudrun Krämer, Matringe, Denis, John Nawas & Everett Rowson (eds.), *Encyclopaedia of Islam, THREE*. http://dx.doi.org.ubproxy.ub.uni-heidelberg.de/10.1163/1573-3912_ei3_COM_23874 (accessed 3 February 2018).

Chipman, Leigh. 2018 [2014]. 'Dioscorides'. In Kate Fleet, Gudrun Krämer, Matringe, Denis, John Nawas & Everett Rowson (eds.), *Encyclopaedia of Islam, THREE*. http://dx.doi.org.ubproxy.ub.uni-heidelberg.de/10.1163/1573-3912_ei3_COM_26047 (accessed 3 February 2018).

Craig, Sienna R. 2012. *Healing Elements: Efficacy and the Social Ecologies of Tibetan Medicine*. Berkeley: University of California Press.

Daston, Lorraine & Peter Galison. 2010 [2007]. *Objectivity*. New York: Zone Books.

Deb Roy, Rohan; Attewell, Guy N.A. 2018. 'Introduction. Locating the Medical'. In Rohan Deb Roy und Guy N.A. Attewell (eds.): *Locating the Medical. Explorations of South Asian History*, 1-20. New Delhi: Oxford University Press.

Dehlvi Naturals. 2015. 'Herbal Tibb-e Nabavi Products List'. http://www.dehlvi.com/product-listing.php?pid=0 (accessed 14 December 2015).

Delhi Government. 2015. 'Ayurvedic and Unani Tibbia College'. http://www.delhi.gov.in/wps/wcm/connect/doit_health/Health/Home/Ayurvedic+and+Unani+Tibbia+Collage/ (accessed 25 October 2015).

Department of AYUSH. 2010. 'Summary of Infrastructure Facilities under AYUSH'. http://indianmedicine.nic.in/showfile.asp?lid=44 (accessed 26 January 2015).

Department of AYUSH. 2013a. 'Essential Drug List: Unani Medicine'. http://ayush.gov.in/sites/default/files/1378112724-Essential%20Unani%20Medicines%20LR%20%204.pdf (accessed 29 August 2019).

Department of AYUSH. 2013b. 'Unani System of Medicine. The Science of Health and Healing'. New Delhi: Ministry of Health and Family Welfare.

Diem, Andrea Grace & James R. Lewis. 1992. 'Imagining India: The Influence of Hinduism in the New Age Movement'. In James R. Lewis & J. Gordon Melton (eds.), *Perspectives on the New Age*, 48–58. Albany: State University of New York Press.

Dutta, Sumi Sukanya. 26 Mach 2018. 'Doctors Threaten Indefinite Strike from April 2 if Government Doesn't Amend National Medical Commission Bill'. *The New Indian Express*. 26 Mach 2018. http://www.newindianexpress.com/nation/2018/mar/26/doctors-threaten-indefinite-strike-from-april-2-if-government-doesnt-ammend-national-medical-commis-1792442.html (accessed 27 August 2018).

Ebrahimnejad, Hormoz. 2005. 'The Development of Galeno-Islamic Medicine: Assimilation of Greek Sciences to Islam'. *Disquisitions on the Past and Present* 13. 127–140.

Ebrahimnejad, Hormoz. 2009a. 'Introduction: For a History of Modern Medicine in Non-Western Countries'. In Hormoz Ebrahimnejad (ed.), *The Development of Modern Medicine in Non-Western Countries: Historical Perspectives*, 1–22. London: Routledge.

Ebrahimnejad, Hormoz (ed.). 2009b. *The Development of Modern Medicine in Non-Western Countries: Historical Perspectives*. London: Routledge.

Ecks, Stefan. 2008. 'Three Propositions for an Evidence-Based Medical Anthropology'. *The Journal of the Royal Anthropological Institute* 14(s1). S77-S92.

Elgood, Cyril. 1962. 'Tibb-ul-Nabbi or Medicine of the Prophet'. *Osiris* 14. 33–192.

Engineer, Irfan. 2012. 'Indian Muslims: Political Leadership, Mobilisation, and Violence'. In Abdul Shaban (ed.), *The Lives of Muslims in India: Politics, Exclusion and Violence*, 107–130. New Delhi: Routledge India.

Fangerau, Heiner & M. Martin. 2012. *From Quality to Quantity: On the History and Conceptual Embedding of Urine Tests*. Paper presented at the conference History, Culture and Science: Asian and European Perspectives on Complementary and Alternative Medicine, Ruhr-University Bochum.

Farage, Samar. 2008. 'The Ethics of s Physician in the Galeno-Islamic Tradition'. In Jonathan E. Brockopp & Thomas Eich (eds.), *Muslim Medical Ethics: From Theory to Practice*, 21–37. Columbia: University of South Carolina Press.

Farouqui, Ather. 1995. 'The Problem of Urdu in India: Political or Existential? (An Interview with S. R. Faruqi)'. *The Annual of Urdu Studies* 10. 157–167.

Fārūqī, 'Abd-ul Nāṣir. 1995. *Aṯibbā' ke ḥairat angez kārnāme*. Na'ī Dihlī: Ai'jāz pablishing haū's.

Fārūqī, Rahbar. 1999 [1937]. *Islāmī Ṭibb: (Shāhānah sarparastyon̲ main̲)*. Ḥaidarābād: Maktabah-i 'Ain al-'ulūm.

Fazal, Tanveer. 2014. '"Being Muslim" in Contemporary India: Nation, Identity, and Rights'. In Robin Jeffrey & Ronojoy Sen (eds.), *Being Muslim in South Asia: Diversity and Daily Life*, 201–223. New Delhi: Oxford University Press.

Fleck, Ludwig. 2019 [1935]. *Etnstehung und Entwicklung einer wissenschaftlichen Tatsache: Einführung in die Lehre vom Denkstil und Denkkollektiv*. Mit einer Einleitung herausgegeben von Lothar Schäfer und Thomas Schnelle. Frankfurt am Main: Suhrkamp.

Foucault, Michel. 2005 [1963]. *Die Geburt der Klinik: Eine Archäologie des ärztlichen Blicks*. Frankfurt am Main: Fischer-Taschenbuch-Verlag.

Ganguly, Ritika. 2014. 'Sense and Evidence: Ayurvedic Experiments and the Politics of an "Open-minded" Science'. *Asian Medicine* 9(1-2). 102–140.

Gaudillière, Jean-Paul. 2014a. 'An Indian Path to Biocapital? The Traditional Knowledge Digital Library, Drug Patents, and the Reformulation Regime of Contemporary Ayurveda'. *East Asian Science, Technology and Society: An International Journal* 8(4). 391–415.

Gaudillière, Jean-Paul. 2014b. 'Herbalized Ayurveda? Reformulation, Plant Management and the "Pharmaceuticalization" of Indian "Traditional" Medicine'. *Asian Medicine* (9). 171–205.

Gayer, Laurent & Christophe Jaffrelot. 2012. 'Introduction: Muslims of the Indian City: From Centrality to Marginality'. In Laurent Gayer & Christophe Jaffrelot (eds.), *Muslims in Indian Cities: Trajectories of Marginalisation*, 1–22. London: Hurst.

Good, Byron J. & Mary-Jo DelVecchio Good. 1992. 'The Comparative Study of Greco-Islamic Medicine: The Integration of Medical Knowledge into Symbolic Contexts'. In Charles Leslie & Allan Young (eds.), *Paths to Asian Medical Knowledge*, 257–271. Berkeley: University of California Press.

Government of India. 1962. 'Report of the Health Survey and Planning Committee (August 1959-October 1961)', vol. 1,. http://www.nhp.gov.in/sites/default/files/pdf/Mudalier_Vol.pdf (accessed 23 February 2015).

Government of India. 2006. 'Social, Economic, and Educational Status of the Muslim Community in India. A Report'. New Delhi: Ministry of Minority Affairs. http://www.minorityaffairs.gov.in/sites/upload_files/moma/files/pdfs/sacharcomm.pdf (accessed 23 January 2015).

Green, Nile. 2008. 'Breathing in India, c. 1890'. *Modern Asian Studies* 42(2-3). 283–315.

Gutas, Dimitri. 2011 [1987]. AVICENNA ii. 'Biography'. In *Encyclopaedia Iranica*, 67–70. http://www.iranicaonline.org/articles/avicenna-ii (accessed 3 February 2018).

Habib, S. Irfan & Dhruv Raina. 2005. 'Reinventing Traditional Medicine: Method, Institutional Change, and the Manufacture of Drugs and Medication in Late Colonial India'. In Joseph S. Alter (ed.), *Asian Medicine and Globalization*, 67–77. Philadelphia: University of Pennsylvania Press.

Ḥabīburraḥmān, Ḥ.S. 2000 [1988]. *Hindūstān ke mashhūr aṭibbā'*. Na'ī Dihlī: Taraqqī Urdū Byūro.

Hacking, Ian. 1995. *Rewriting the Soul: Multiple Personality and the Sciences of Memory*. Princeton: Princeton University Press.

Hacking, Ian. 1999. *The Social Construction of What?* Cambridge: Harvard University Press.

Hacking, Ian. 2002. *Historical Ontology*. Cambridge: Harvard University Press.

Hacking, Ian. 2002 [1995]. 'The Looping Effects of Human Kinds'. In Dan Sperber, David Premack & Ann James Premack (eds.), *Causal Cognition: A Multidisciplinary Debate*, 351–394. Oxford: Clarendon Press.

Hadolt, Bernard, Viola Horbst & Babette Muller-Rockstroh. 2012. 'Biomedical Techniques in Context: On the Appropriation of Biomedical Procedures and Artifacts'. *Medical Anthropology* 31(3). 179–195.

Hamdānī, S.K.H. 2011 [1998]. *Uṣūl-i Ṭibb*. Na'ī Dihlī: Taraqqī Urdū Byūro.

Hameed, Abdul. 1993. 'Preface. In *Al-Qānūn Fi'l-Ṭibb* (*English translation of the critical Arabic text*), xiii–xvi. New Delhi: Jamia Hamdard.

Hankinson, Robert James. 1995. 'The Growth of Medical Empiricism'. In Don Bates (ed.), *Knowledge and the Scholarly Medical Traditions*, 60–83. Cambridge: Cambridge University Press.

Hardiman, David. 2009. 'Indian Medical Indigeneity: From Nationalist Assertion to the Global Market'. *Social History* 34(3). 263–283.

Hardiman, David & Projit Bihari Mukharji. 2012. 'Introduction'. In David Hardiman & Projit Bihari Mukharji (eds.), *Medical Marginality in South Asia: Situating Subaltern Therapeutics*, 6–35. Abingdon: Routledge.

Harding, Sandra. 1991. *Whose Science? Whose Knowledge? Thinking from Women's Lives*. Ithaca: Cornell University Press.

Hildebrand, Vanessa M. 2012. 'Scissors as Symbols: Disputed Ownership of the Tools of Biomedical Obstetrics in Rural Indonesia'. *Culture, Medicine, and Psychiatry* 36(3). 557–570.

Hinojosa, Servando Z. 2004. 'Bonesetting and Radiography in the Southern Maya Highlands'. *Medical Anthropology* 23(4). 263–293.

Horden, Peregrine. 2013. 'Introduction'. In Peregrine Horden & Elisabeth Hsu (eds.), *The Body in Balance: Humoral Medicines in Practice*, 1–21. New York: Berghahn.

Horden, Peregrine & Elisabeth Hsu (eds.). 2013. *The Body in Balance: Humoral Medicines in Practice*. New York: Berghahn.

Ḥussain, I. 2003. *Ajmal-i Aʿẓ am*. Lāhor: Sang-i Mīl Pablīkeshanz.

Ibn Sīnā. 1993. *Al-Qānūn Fi'l-Ṭibb: (English translation of the critical Arabic text)*. New Delhi: Jamia Hamdard.

Idrīsī, Ḥussain ʿAlī. n.d. *Nabẓ Baul-o Barāz*. Mukẖtaṣir Noṭs. Lakhna'ū: Irām yūnānī meḍīkal kālaj.

Iftekhar, J. S. 2012. 'Unani Hospital Sans Medicines: Government Nizamia General Hopsital Allocated Shoe-string Budget'. *The Hindu*. 20 January. http://www.thehindu.com/todays-paper/tp-national/tp-andhrapradesh/unani-hospital-sans-medicines/article2816343.ece (accessed 27 August 2018).

Iṣlāḥī, M. M. 1987. *Aṭ ibbā' aur un kī massīḥā'ī*. Bomba'ī: Iṣlāḥī yūnānī ṭ ibbī rīsarc insṭīṭyūṭ.

Jaggi, Om Prakash. 1977. *Medicine in Medieval India*. New Delhi: Atma Ram & Sons.

Janes, Craig R. 1999. 'The Health Transition, Global Modernity and the Crisis of Traditional Medicine: The Tibetan Case'. *Social Science & Medicine* 48(12). 1803–1820.

Janes, Craig R. 2002. 'Buddhism, Science, and Market: The Globalisation of Tibetan Medicine'. *Anthropology & Medicine* 9(3). 267–289.

Jefferey, Roger. 1982. 'Policies Towards Indigenous Healers in Independent India'. *Social Science & Medicine* 16(21). 1835–1841.

Jeffery, Patriticia, Roger Jeffery & C. Jeffrey. 2007. 'Investing in the Future. Education in the Social and Cultural Reproduction of Muslims in UP'. In Mushirul Hasan (ed.), *Living with Secularism: The Destiny of India's Muslims*, 63–89. New Delhi: Manohar.

Jeffery, Roger. 1988. *The Politics of Health in India*. Berkeley: University of California Press.

Jeffrey, Robin & Ronojoy Sen. 2014. 'Introduction: Diversity and Daily Life'. In Robin Jeffrey & Ronojoy Sen (eds.), *Being Muslim in South Asia: Diversity and daily life*, xvi–xxx. New Delhi: Oxford University Press.

Kabīruddīn, Muḥammad. n.d. *Aksīr-i Aʿẓam: Jadīd Munaqqaḥ Shakl*. Lāhor: Maktabah Dānyāl.

Kabīruddīn, Muḥammad. 1934. *Kulliyāt-i Nafīsī: (ʿAlāmah Burhānuddin Nafīs kī Mashhūr Kitāb Nafīsī kī Tarjumah-o Shuruḥ)*. Lāhor: Idārah Maṭ būʿāt Sulaimānī.

Kabīruddīn, Muḥammad. 2008. *Bayāẓ-i Kabīr (ḥiṣṣah dom)*. Na'ī Dihlī: Sinṭral kaunsil fār rīsarc in yūnānī meḍīsīn.

Kabīruddīn, Muḥammad (ed.). 2012. *Kitāb al-Nabẓ*. Na'ī Dihlī: Idārah Kitāb al-Shifā.

Kasniyal, B. D. 2009. 'A Lifeline for the Musk Deer: A Four-acre Farm at Mehrori in Bageswar District of Uttarakhand is Successfully Breeding the Musk Deer'. *Dehradun Plus Online Edition*. 24 July. http://www.tribuneindia.com/2009/20090724/dplus.htm#4 (accessed 28 August 2018).

Ḳẖān, Muḥammad Ajmal. 2010. *Bayāẓ-i Ajmal: "Ḥakīm Ajmal Ḳẖān marḥūm"*. Na'ī Dihlī: Aiʿjāz pablishing hā'ūs.

Ḳẖān, Muḥammad Aʿẓ am. 2004. *Qarābādīn-i Aʿẓam (Fārsī)*. Na'ī Dihlī: Sinṭral kaunsil fār rīsarc in yūnānī meḍīsin.

Ḳẖān, R. A. 2002. *Ḥayāt-i Ajmal*. Dihlī: ʿĀlamī Urdū Markaz.

Kim, Jongyoung. 2007. 'Alternative Medicine's Encounter with Laboratory Science: The Scientific Construction of Korean Medicine in Global Age'. *Social Studies of Science* 37(6). 855–880.

King, Helen. 2013. 'Female Fluids in the Hippocratic Corpus? How Solid was the Humoral Body?' In Peregrine Horden & Elisabeth Hsu (eds.), *The Body in Balance: Humoral Medicines in Practice*, 25–52. New York: Berghahn.

Kleinman, Arthur. 1995. *Writing at the Margin: Discourse Between Anthropology and Medicine*. Berkeley: University of California Press.

Knorr Cetina, Karin. 1995. Laboratory Studies: The Cultural Approach to the Study of Science. In Sheila Jasanoff, Gerald E. Markle, James C. Peterson & Trevor Pinch (eds), *Handbook of Science and Technology Studies*, 140–166. London: SAGE Publications. https://methods.sagepub.com/book/handbook-of-science-and-technology-studies.

Krause, Kristine, Gabriele Alex & David Parkin. 2012. 'Medical Knowledge, Therapeutic Practice and Processes of Diversification'. Göttingen: MPI for the Study of Religious and Ethnic Diversity. http://hdl.handle.net/11858/00-001M-0000-000E-7D0B-3 (accessed 27 August 2018).

Kuhn, Thomas S. 2012 [1962]. *The Structure of Scientific Revolutions*. Chicago: University of Chicago Press.

Kuriyama, Shigehisa. 2002 [1999]. *The Expressiveness of the Body and the Divergence of Greek and Chinese Medicine*. New York: Zone Books.

Kurz, Susanne. 2014. 'Die Graeco-Islamische Medizin als globale Medizin ihrer Zeit: Das Medizinverständnis in indo-persischen Werken des 16. und 17. Jahrhunderts. https://omp.ub.rub.de/index.php/RUB/catalog/book/24 (accessed 27 August 2018).

Kurz, Susanne & Stefan Reichmuth. 2012. 'Zwischen Standardisierung und Literarisierung: Der Fallbericht in der graeco-islamische Medizin'. In Rudolf Behrens, Carsten Zelle & Maria Winter (eds.), *Der ärztliche Fallbericht: Epistemische Grundlagen und textuelle Strukturen dargestellter Beobachtung*, 227–258. Wiesbaden: Harrassowitz.

Laderman, Carol. 1992. 'A Welcoming Soil: Islamic Humoralism in the Malay Peninsula'. In Charles Leslie & Allan Young (eds.), *Paths to Asian Medical Knowledge*, 272–288. Berkeley: University of California Press.

Lambert, Helen. 2009. 'Evidentiary Truths? The Evidence of Anthropology through the Anthropology of Medical Evidence'. *Anthropology Today* 25(1). 16–20.

Lambert, Helen. 2012. 'Medical Pluralism and Medical Marginality: Bone Doctors and the Selective Legitimation of Therapeutic Expertise in India'. *Social Science & Medicine* (74). 1029–1036.

Langford, Jean M. 1999. 'Medical Mimesis: Healing Signs of a Cosmopolitan "Quack"'. *American Ethnologist* 26(1). 24–46.

Langford, Jean M. 2002. *Fluent Bodies: Ayurvedic Remedies for Postcolonial Imbalance*. Durham: Duke University Press.

Latif, Abdul. 2008. *Scope and Market Value of BUMS and BAMS: A Real Picture*. Aligarh: Aligarh Muslim University.

Laṭīf, 'A., Tajuddīn & S. A. Āfāq. 2004. *Kitāb-i 'Amal: 'Ilm al-Adviyah – I*. 'Aligaṛh: Ibn Sīnā Akāḍimī āf Meḍīval Meḍīsin ainḍ sā'īnz.

Latour, Bruno. 1993. *We Have Never Been Modern*. New York: Harvester Wheatsheaf.

Latour, Bruno & Steve Woolgar. 1986 [1979]. *Laboratory Life: The Construction of Scientific Facts*. Princeton: Princeton University Press.

Leong, Elaine & Alisha M. Rankin (eds.). 2011. *Secrets and Knowledge in Medicine and Science, 1500-1800*. Farham: Ashgate.

Leslie, Charles. 1974. 'The Modernization of Asian Medical Systems'. In John J. Poggie & Richard N. Lynch (eds.), *Rethinking Modernization: Anthropological Perspectives*, 69–108. London: Greenwood Press.

Leslie, Charles. 1976a. 'Introduction'. In Charles Leslie (ed.), *Asian Medical Systems: A Comparative Study*, 1–12. Berkeley: University of California Press.

Leslie, Charles. 1976b. 'The Ambiguities of Medical Revivalism in Modern India'. In Charles Leslie (ed.), *Asian Medical Systems: A Comparative Study*, 356–367. Berkeley: University of California Press.

Leslie, Charles. 1989. 'Indigenous Pharmaceuticals, the Capitalist World System, and Civilization'. *Kroeber Anthropological Society Papers* 69-70. 23–31.

Leslie, Charles. 1992. 'Interpretations of Ilnness: Syncretism in Modern Āyurveda'. In Charles Leslie & Allan Young (eds.), *Paths to Asian Medical Knowledge*, 177–208. Berkeley: University of California Press.

Leslie, Charles & Allan Young. 1992. 'Introduction'. In Charles Leslie & Allan Young (eds.), *Paths to Asian Medical Knowledge*, 1–18. Berkeley: University of California Press.

Lewis, Gilbert. 2007. 'On "Medical System" and Questions in Fieldwork'. In Roland Littlewood (ed.), *On Knowing and Not Knowing in the Anthropology of Medicine*, 28–38. Walnut Creek: Left Coast Press.

Liebeskind, Claudia. 1996. 'Unani Medicine in the Subcontinent'. In Jan van Alphen (ed.), *Oriental Medicine: An Illustrated Guide to the Asian Arts of Healing*, 39–65. Boston: Shambhala.

Liebeskind, Claudia. 2002. 'Arguing Science: Unani *Tibb*, Hakims and Biomedicine in India, 1900-50'. In Waltraud Ernst (ed.), *Plural Medicine, Tradition and Modernity, 1800-2000*, 58–75. London: Routledge.

Littlewood, Roland (ed.). 2007. *On Knowing and Not Knowing in the Anthropology of Medicine*. Walnut Creek: Left Coast Press.

Lock, Margaret & Vinh-Kim Nguyen. 2018. *An Anthropology of Biomedicine: Second Edition*. Hoboken: Wiley Blackwell.

Lynch, Michael. 2013. 'Ontography: Investigating the Production of Things, Deflating Ontology'. *Social Studies of Science* 43(3). 444–462.

Martin, Alfred. 1906. *Deutsches Badewesen in vergangenen Tagen: Nebst einem Beitrage zur Geschichte der Deutschen Wasserheilkunde*. Jena: Eugen Diederichs.

Martin, Emily. 2012. 'Grafting Together Medical Anthropology, Feminism, and Technoscience'. In Marcia C. Inhorn & Emily A. Wentzell (eds.), *Medical Anthropology at the Intersections: Histories, Activisms, and Futures*, 23–40. Durham: Duke University Press.

Matthews, D. J., Christopher Shackle & Shahrukh Husain. 2003. *Urdu Literature*. Islamabad: Alhamra.

Metcalf, Barbara Daly. 1982. *Islamic Revival in British India: Deoband, 1860 – 1900*. Princeton: Princeton University Press.

Metcalf, Barbara Daly. 1985. 'Nationalist Muslims in British India: The Case of Hakim Ajmal Khan'. *Modern Asian Studies* 19(1). 1–28.

Metcalf, Barbara Daly. 2004. *Islamic Contestations: Essays on Muslims in India and Pakistan*. New Delhi: Oxford University Press.

Ministry of AYUSH. 2014. AYUSH in India 2014. http://www.indianmedicine.nic.in/index2.asp?lang=1&slid=871&sublinkid=412 (accessed 24 July 2015).

Mol, Annemarie. 2002. *The Body Multiple: Ontology in Medical Practice*. Durham: Duke University Press.

Mol, Annemarie & Marc Berg. 1998. 'Differences in Medicine: An Introduction'. In Marc Berg & Annemarie Mol (eds.), *Differences in Medicine: Unraveling Practices, Techniques, and Bodies*, 1–12. Durham: Duke University Press.

Mol, Annemarie & John Law. 2002. 'Complexities: An Introduction'. In John Law & Annemarie Mol (eds.), *Complexities: Social Studies of Knowledge Practices*, 1–22. Durham: Duke University Press.

Mukharji, Projit Bihari. 2007. 'Structuring Plurality: Locality, Caste, Class and Ethnicity in Nineteenth-Century Bengal Dispensaries'. *Health and History* 9(1). 80–105.

Mukharji, Projit Bihari. 2011. *Nationalizing the Body: The Medical Market, Print and Daktari Medicine*. London: Anthem Press.

Mukharji, Projit Bihari. 2016. *Doctoring Traditions: Ayurveda, Small Technologies, and Braided Sciences*. Chicago: University of Chicago Press.

Müller, Irmgard. 2012. *Zur Rezeption der chinesischen Pulslehre in der westlichen Medizin*. Paper presented at the conference History, Culture and Science: Asian and European Perspectives on Complementary and Alternative Medicine, Ruhr-University Bochum.

n.n. 2012a. Six injured as police lathicharge protesting doctors in Lucknow. *India TV News*. 31 May (accessed 21 August 2015).

n.n. 2012b. 'Protesting Ayush Doctors Block Traffic'. *The Times of India*. 3 July. http://timesofindia.indiatimes.com/city/lucknow/Protesting-Ayush-doctors-block-traffic/articleshow/14620871.cms?prtpage=1 (accessed 27 August 2018).

n.n. 2012c. 'Ayush Doctors to Go on Strike from Tomorrow'. *The Times of India*. 19 July. http://timesofindia.indiatimes.com/city/mangaluru/Ayush-doctors-to-go-on-strike-from-tomorrow/articleshow/15038426.cms? (accessed 27 August 2018).

Naraindas, Harish. 2006. 'Of Spineless Babies and Folic Acid: Evidence and Efficacy in Biomedicine and Ayurvedic Medicine'. *Social Science & Medicine* 62(11). 2658–2669.

Naraindas, Harish. 2014a. 'My Vaidya and My Gynecologist: Agency, Authority, and Risk in Quest of a Child'. In Harish Naraindas, Johannes Quack & William S. Sax (eds.), *Asymmetrical Conversations: Contestations, Circumventions, and the Blurring of Therapeutic Boundaries*, 118–161. New York: Berghahn Books.

Naraindas, Harish. 2014b. 'Nosopolitics: Epistemic Mangling and the Creolization of Contemporary Ayurveda'. In Martin Dinges (ed.), *Medical Pluralism and Homeopathy in India and Germany (1810-2010)*, 105–136. Stuttgart: Franz Steiner Verlag.

Naraindas, Harish. 2014c. 'Of Shastric "Yogams" and Polyherbals: Exogenous Logics and the Creolisation of the Contemporary Ayurvedic Formulary'. *Asian Medicine* 9. 12–48.

Naraindas, Harish, Johannes Quack & William S. Sax. 2014. 'Introduction: Entangled Epistemes'. In Harish Naraindas, Johannes Quack & William S. Sax (eds.), *Asymmetrical Conversations: Contestations, Circumventions, and the Blurring of Therapeutic Boundaries*, 1–25. New York: Berghahn Books.

Nichter, Mark. 1996. 'Pharmaceutcials, the Commodification of Health, and the Health Care-Medicine Use Transition'. In Mark Nichter & Mimi Nichter (eds.), *Anthropology and International Health: Asian Case Studies*, 265–326. Amsterdam: Gordon and Breach Publishers.

Nichter, Mark & Nancy Vukovic. 1994. 'Agenda for and Anthropology of Pharmaceutical Practice'. *Social Science & Medicine* 39. 1509–1525.

Nigramī, Ḥakīm Sayyid Muḥammad Ḥasān. 2009 [1989]. *Tārīḵẖ-i Ṭibb: (Ibtidā tā ʿahad ḥāẓar)*. Na'ī Dihlī: Qaumī kaunsil barā'e farogẖ urdū zabān.

Obeyesekere, Gananath. 1992. 'Science, Experimentation, and Clinical Practice in Āyurveda'. In Charles Leslie & Allan Young (eds.), *Paths to Asian Medical Knowledge*, 160–176. Berkeley: University of California Press.

Oesterheld, Christina. 2002. 'Problems of Teaching Urdu in Germany: A Foreigner's Reflections on the Status of Urdu'. *Anual of Urdu Studies* 17. 125–137.

Pandey, Gyanendra. 2012. *The Construction of Communalism in Colonial North India*. Oxford: Oxford University Press.

Parkin, David. 2000. 'Islam among the Humours: Destiny and Agency among the Swahili'. In Ivan Karp & D. A. Masolo (eds.), *African Philosophy as Cultural Inquiry*, 50–65. Bloomington: Indiana University Press.

Parkin, David. 2007. 'In Touch without Touching: Islam and Healing'. In Roland Littlewood (ed.), *On Knowing and Not Knowing in the Anthropology of Medicine*, 194–219. Walnut Creek: Left Coast Press.

Petchesky, Rosalind P. 1987. 'Fetal Images: The Power of Visual Culture in the Politics of Reproduction'. *Feminist Studies* 13(2). 263–292.

Pordié, Laurent (ed.). 2008a. *Tibetan Medicine in the Contemporary World: Global Politics of Medical Knowledge and Practice*. London: Routledge.

Pordié, Laurent. 2008b. 'Tibetan Medicine Today: Neo-Traditionalism as an Analytical Lens and a Political Tool'. In Laurent Pordié (ed.), *Tibetan Medicine in the Contemporary World: Global Politics of Medical Knowledge and Practice*, 3–32. London: Routledge.

Pordié, Laurent. 2010. 'The Politics of Therapeutic Evaluation in Asian Medicine'. *Economic & Political Weekly* XLV(18). 57–64.

Pordié, Laurent. 2011. 'Asian Therapeutic Knowledge and Globalization'. *Revue d'anthropologie des connaissances* 5(1). a-j.

Pordié, Laurent. 2014a. 'Learning Institutions in South Asian Medicine'. *Culture, Medicine and Psychiatry* 38. 335–339.

Pordié, Laurent. 2014b. 'Pervious Drugs: Making the Pharmaceutical Object in Techno-Ayurveda'. *Asian Medicine* 9. 49–76.

Pordié, Laurent. 2015. 'Hangover Free! The Social and Material Trajectories of PartySmart'. *Anthropology & Medicine* 22(1). 1–15.

Pordié, Laurent & Calum Blaikie. 2014. 'Knowledge and Skill in Motion: Layers of Tibetan Medical Education in India'. *Culture, Medicine and Psychiatry* 38. 340–368.

Pordié, Laurent & Jean-Paul Gaudillière. 2014a. 'Introduction: Industrial Ayurveda'. *Asian Medicine* 9. 1–11.

Pordié, Laurent & Jean-Paul Gaudillière. 2014b. 'The Reformulation Regime in Drug Discovery: Revisiting Polyherbals and Property Rights in the Ayurvedic Industry'. *East Asian Science, Technology and Society: An International Journal* 8. 57–79.

Pordié, Laurent & Anita Hardon. 2015. 'Drugs' Stories and Itineraries: On the Making of Asian Industrial Medicines'. *Anthropology & Medicine* 22(1). 1–6.

Pormann, Peter E. & Emilie Savage-Smith. 2007. *Medieval Islamic Medicine*. Edinburgh: Edinburgh University Press.

Preckel, Claudia. 2012. 'Healing the People and the Princess: Hospitals, Ḥakīms and Doctors in Bhopal'. In Fabrizio Speziale (ed.), *Hospitals in Iran and India: 1500 – 1950s*, 191–214. Leiden: Brill.

Press Information Bureau. 2007. *AYUSH Practitioners Prescribing Allopathic Medicines*. http://pib.nic.in/newsite/erelease.aspx?relid=30117 (Accessed 23 April 2020).

Priya, Ritu. 2013. 'The Status and Role of AYUSH and Local Health Traditions in Public Health'. *IIAS Newsletter* 65. 24–25.

Pugh, Judy F. 2003. 'Concepts of Arthritis in India's Medical Traditions: Ayurvedic and Unani Perspectives'. *Social Science & Medicine* 56(2). 415–424.

Punwani, Jyoti. 2012. 'Police Conduct during Communal Riots: Evidence from 1992-93 Mumbai Riots and Its Implications'. In Abdul Shaban (ed.), *The Lives of Muslims in India: Politics, Exclusion and Violence*, 187–207. New Delhi: Routledge India.

Qadīr, Ashhar. 2004a. *Ṭibbī Ṣaḥā'if*. Dihlī: Ejūkeshanal Pablishing Hā'ūs.

Qadīr, Ashhar. 2004b. Urdū Zabān ke Farog ẖ maiṉ Ṭibb-i Yūnānī kā Kirdār, Ẕary'ah-i Ta'līm ke Ḥavāle se. In Alṭaf Aḥmad 'Aẕmī (ed.), *Ṭibb-i Yūnānī aur Urdū Zabān o Adab*, 447–456. Na'ī Dilhī: Jami'ah Hamdard.

Qadīr, Ashhar. 2011 [2001]. *Tārīḵẖ-i Ṭibb o Aḵẖlāqyāt*. Dihlī: Bhārat Āfseṭ.

Quaiser, Neshat. 2001. 'Politics Culture and Colonialism: Unani's Debate with Doctory'. In Biswamoy Pati & Mark Harrison (eds.), *Health, Medicine and Empire: Perspectives on Colonial India*, 317–355. Hyderabad: Orient Longman.

Quaiser, Neshat. 2010. 'Science, Institution, Colonialism: Tibbiya College of Delhi, 1889-1947'. In Uma Dasgupta (ed.), *Science and Modern India: An Institutional History – c. 1784-1947*, 523–562. Delhi: Pearson Longman.

Quaiser, Neshat. 2012a. 'Tension, Placation, Complaint: Unani and Post-Colonial Medical Communalism'. In Venkatesh Sujatha & Leena Abraham (eds.), *Medical Pluralism in Contemporary India*, 130–162. New Delhi: Orient Blackswan.

Quaiser, Neshat. 2012b. 'Unani Medical Culture. Memory, Representation, and the Literal Critical Anticolonial Public Sphere'. In Poonam Bala (ed.), *Contesting Colonial Authority. Medicine and Indigenous Responses in Nineteenth- and Twentieth-Century India*, 115–135. Lanham: Lexington Books.

Quaiser, Neshat. 2013. 'Essentialising the Body'. *IIAS Newsletter* 65. 30–31. https://iias.asia/sites/default/files/IIAS_NL65_3031.pdf (accessed 27 August 2018).

Rahman, Fazlur. 1987. *Health and Medicine in the Islamic Tradition*. New York: Crossroad.

Rahman, T. 2006. 'Urdu as Islamic Language'. *The Annual of Urdu Studies* 26. 101–119.

Reddy, Sita. 2002. 'Asian Medicine in America: The Ayurvedic Case'. *The Annals of the American Academy of Political and Social Science* 583(1). 97–121.

Redfield, Robert. 1960 [1956]. *The Little Community and Peasant Society and Culture*. Chicago: The University of Chicago Press.

Reichmuth, Stefan. 2016. 'Wissen, Praxis und pluraler kultureller Kontext der graeco-islamischen Medizin (*yūnānī ṭibb*/Unani Medicine) in Nordindien'. In Susanne Kurz & Claudia Preckel (eds.), *Muslim Bodies: Körper, Medizin und Sexualität in muslimischen Gesellschaften*, 357–406. Berlin: LIT.

Rex Remedies. 2014. 'Awards'. http://www.rexremedies.com/awards.html (accessed 27 August 2018).

Roger, Delphine. 1991. 'Food Practices and Traditional Medicine among the Muslims of Hyderabad'. Pondicherry: French Institute Pondicherry. http://www.ifpindia.org/sites/default/files/bookstore/remarks-pdf/PPSS_008.pdf (accessed 27 August 2018).

Saradamma, R. D., N. Higginbotham & M. Nichter. 2000. 'Social Factors Influencing the Acquisition of Antibiotics without Prescription in Kerala State, South India'. *Social Science & Medicine* 50(6). 891–903.

Savage-Smith, Emilie. 2013. 'Where the Four Humours Fundamental to Medieval Islamic Medical Practice?' In Peregrine Horden & Elisabeth Hsu (eds.), *The Body in Balance: Humoral Medicines in Practice*, 89–106. New York: Berghahn.

Savage-Smith, Emilie. 2014. 'The Universality and Neutrality of Science'. In Michael G. Morony (ed.), *Universality in Islamic Thought: Rationalism, Science and Religious Belief*, 157–192. London: I.B. Tauris.

Sax, William S. 2013. 'The Reality of 21st Century Islamic Healing – An Interview with a Muslim Healer'. *Curare* 26(3). 168–171.

Schmidt Stiedenroth, Kira. 2019a. 'Beyond Evidence: Eminence and Therapeutic Success in Unani (Greco-Islamic) Medicine'. *Asian Medicine* 14(2). 209-232.

Schmidt Stiedenroth, Kira. 2019b. 'Reviving "A Forgotten Sunna": Hijamah (Cupping Therapy), Prophetic Medicine, and the Re-Islamization of Unani Medicine in Contemporary India'. *Contemporary Islam* 13(2). 183–200.

Schrempf, Mona (ed.). 2007. *Soundings in Tibetan Medicine: Anthropological and Historical Perspectives*. Leiden: Brill.

Schwabl, Herbert. 2009. 'It is Modern to Be Traditional: Tradition and Tibetan Medicine in the European Context'. *Asian Medicine* 5. 373–384.

Scott, Joan W. 1991. 'The Evidence of Experience'. *Critical Inquiry* 17(4). 773–797.

Shaban, Abdul. 2012a. 'Introduction'. In Abdul Shaban (ed.), *The Lives of Muslims in India: Politics, Exclusion and Violence*, 1–24. New Delhi: Routledge India.

Shaban, Abdul (ed.). 2012b. *The Lives of Muslims in India: Politics, Exclusion and Violence*. New Delhi: Routledge India.

Sheehan, Helen E. 1983. 'Organization, Practice and Patronage of Ayurvedic and Unani Medical Systems in Contemporary Hyderabad'. PhD Thesis, University of Pennsylvania.

Sheehan, Helen E. & S. J. Hussain. 2002. 'Unani Tibb: History, Theory, and Contemporary Practice in South Asia'. *The Annals of the American Academy of Political and Social Science* 583(1). 122–135.

Shelar, Jyoti. 2015. 'IMA Warns Docs against Hiring Ayurveda, Homoeopathy Practitioners'. *Mumbai Mirror*. 3 January. https://mumbaimirror.indiatimes.com/mumbai/other/ima-warns-docs-against-hiring-ayurveda-homoeopathy-practitioners/articleshow/45735793.cms (accessed 27 August 2018).

Sieler, Roman. 2013. 'From Lineage Transmission to Transnational Distance Education: The Case of Siddha Varmam Medicine'. *European Journal of Transnational Studies* 5(1). 112–143.

Sieler, Roman. 2014. 'Patient Agency Revisited: "Healing the Hidden" in South India'. *Medical Anthropology Quarterly* 28(3). 323–341.

Sieler, Roman. 2015. *Lethal Spots, Vital Secrets: Medicine and Martial Arts in South India*. New York: Oxford University Press.

Sivaramakrishnan, Kavita. 2006. *Old Potions, New Bottles: Recasting Indigenous Medicine in Colonial Punjab (1850-1945)*. Hyderabad: Orient Longman.

Smith, Frederick M. & Dagmar Wujastyk. 2008. 'Introduction'. In Dagmar Wujastyk & Frederick M. Smith (eds.), *Modern and Global Ayurveda: Pluralism and Paradigms*, 1–28. Albany: State University of New York Press.

Solomon, Harris. 2016. *Metabolic Living: Food, Fat and the Absorption of Illness in India*. Durham and London: Duke University Press.

Speziale, Fabrizio. 2005. 'Linguistic Startegies of De-Islamization and Colonial Science: Indo-Muslim Physicians and the Yûnânî Denomination'. *IIAS Newsletter* (37). 18.

Speziale, Fabrizio. 2010a. 'Muslim or Greek? Past and Present of Yunani Medicine in the Deccan'. In Rais Akhtar & Nilofar Izhar (eds.), *Global Medical Geography: In Honour of Prof. Yola Verhasselt*, 305–332. Jaipur: Rawat Publications.

Speziale, Fabrizio. 2010b. *Soufisme, religion et médecine en Islam indien*. Paris: Éd. Karthala.

Speziale, Fabrizio. 2011. 'India – Indo-Muslim Physicians'. In *Encyclopaedia Iranica (online edition)*. http://www.iranicaonline.org/articles/india-xxxiii-indo-muslim-physicians (accessed 11 January 2016).

Speziale, Fabrizio. 2012a. 'Introduction'. In Fabrizio Speziale (ed.), *Hospitals in Iran and India: 1500 – 1950s*, 1–26. Leiden: Brill.

Speziale, Fabrizio. 2012b. 'Tradition et réforme du Dār al-šifā au Deccan'. In Fabrizio Speziale (ed.), *Hospitals in Iran and India: 1500 – 1950s*, 159–189. Leiden: Brill.

Speziale, Fabrizio. 2014a. 'A 14th Century Revision of the Avicennian and Ayurvedic Humoral Pathology: The Hybrid Model by Šihāb al-Dīn Nāgawrī'. *Oriens* 42. 514–532.

Speziale, Fabrizio. 2014b. 'The Persian Translation of the Tridoṣa: Lexical Analogies and Conceptual Incongruities'. *Asiatische Studien – Études Asiatiques* 68(3). 783–796.

Speziale, Fabrizio. 2018. *Culture persane et médecine ayurvédique en Asie du Sud*. Leiden: Brill.

Spivak, Gayatri Chakravorty. 1988. 'Can the Subaltern Speak?' In Cary Nelson & Lawrence Grossberg (eds.), *Marxism and the Interpretation of Culture*, 271–313. Chicago: University of Illinois Press.

Stolberg, Michael. 2009. *Die Harnschau: Eine Kultur- und Alltagsgeschichte*. Köln: Böhlau.

Storey, Charles A. 1971. *Persian Literature: A Bio-Bibliographical Survey*. Volume II, Part 2 E. Medicine. London: The Royal Asiatic Society of Great Britain and Ireland.

Sujatha, V. 2011. 'Innovation within and between Traditions: Dilemma of Traditional Medicine in Contemporary India'. *Science, Technology and Society* 16(2). 191–213.

Swartz, Marc J. 1997. 'Illness and Morality in the Mombasa Swahili Community: A Metaphorical Model in an Islamic Culture'. *Culture, Medicine and Psychiatry* 21(1). 89–114.

Taylor, Carl E. 1976. 'The Place of Indigenous Medical Practitioners in the Modernization of Health Services'. In Charles Leslie (ed.), *Asian Medical Systems: A Comparative Study*, 285–299. Berkeley: University of California Press.

1940. *The Drugs and Cosmetics Act, 1940*.

1970. *The Indian Medicine Central Council Act, 1970*.

1972. *The Indian Wildlife (Protection) Act, 1972*.

Tritton, A. S. 1971. 'Man, nafs, rū, 'aql'. *Bulletin of the School of Oriental and African Studies* 34(3). 491–495.

Ullmann, Manfred. 1997 [1978]. *Islamic Medicine*. Edinburgh: Edinburg University Press.

Unschuld, Paul U. 1992. 'Epistemological Issues and Changing Legitimation: Traditional Chinese Medicine in the Twentieth Century'. In Charles Leslie & Allan Young (eds.), *Paths to Asian Medical Knowledge*, 44–61. Berkeley: University of California Press.

'Usmānī, Syed. 1987. *Tazkirah Ḵẖāndān-i 'Usmānī*. Allāhābād: 'Usmānyah Akeḍimī.

van der Geest, Sjaak & Susan Reynolds Whyte. 1988. *The Context of Medicines in Developing Countries: Studies in Pharmaceutical Anthropology*. Dordrecht: Kluwer.

van der Geest, Sjaak & Susan Reynolds Whyte. 1989. 'The Charm of Medicines: Metaphors and Metonyms'. *Medical Anthropology Quarterly* 3(4). 345–367.

Vohora, S. B. & J. W. Dobrowolski. 1990. *New Horizons of Health Aspects of Elements*. New Delhi: Jamia Hamdard.

Vohora, S. B. & M.S.Y. Khan (eds.). 1983. *Proceedings of the First International Conference on Elements in Health and Disease New Delhi, 6-10 January 1983*. Institute of History of Medicine and Medical Research.

Voswinckel, Peter. 1993. *Der schwarze Urin: Vom Schrecknis zum Laborparameter*. Urina Nigra; Alkaptonurie; Hämoglobinurie; Myoglobinurie; Porphyrinurie; Melanurie. Berlin: Blackwell Wissenschaft.

Watson-Verran, Helen & David Turnbull. 1995. Science and Other Indigenous Knowledge Systems. In Sheila Jasanoff, Gerald E. Markle, James C. Peterson & Trevor Pinch (eds), *Handbook of Science and Technology Studies*, 115–139. London: SAGE Publications.

Weiss, Richard Scott. 2009. *Recipes for Immortality: Medicine, Religion, and Community in South India*. Oxford: Oxford University Press.

Weisser, U. 2011 [1987]. 'AVICENNA xiii: The Influence of Avicenna on Medical Studies in the West'. In *Encyclopædia Iranica (online edition)*, 107–110. http://www.iranicaonline.org/articles/avicenna-xiii (accessed 5 January 2016).

Welch, Claudia. 2008. 'An Overview of the Education and Practice of Global Ayurveda'. In Dagmar Wujastyk & Frederick M. Smith (eds.), *Modern and Global Ayurveda: Pluralism and Paradigms*, 129–138. Albany: State University of New York Press.

WHO. 1978a. 'Declaration of Alma-Ata'. International Conference on Primary Health Care, Alma-Ata, USSR, 6-12 September 1978. World Health Organization. http://www.who.int/publications/almaata_declaration_en.pdf (accessed 20 February 2015).

WHO. 1978b. 'The Promotion and Development of Traditional Medicine'. Report of a WHO meeting. http://apps.who.int/medicinedocs/documents/s7147e/s7147e.pdf (accessed 23 July 2015).

WHO. 2013. 'Silent Killer, Global Public Health Crisis'. http://www.who.int/campaigns/world-health-day/2013/en/ (accessed 27 August 2018).

Whyte, Susan Reynolds, Sjaak van der Geest & Anita Hardon. 2002. *Social Lives of Medicines*. Cambridge: Cambridge University Press.

Wujastyk, Dagmar & Frederick M. Smith (eds.). 2008. *Modern and Global Ayurveda: Pluralism and Paradigms*. Albany: State University of New York Press.

Wujastyk, Dominik. 2003. *The Roots of Ayurveda: Selections from Sanskrit Medical Writings*. London: Penguin Books.

Wujastyk, Dominik. 2008. 'The Evolution of Indian Government Policy on Ayurveda in the Twentieth Century'. In Dagmar Wujastyk & Frederick M. Smith (eds.), *Modern and Global Ayurveda: Pluralism and Paradigms*, 43–76. Albany: State University of New York Press.

Ẓillurraḥmān, Ḥakīm Syed. 1995. *Dillī aur Ṭibb-i Yūnānī*. Dillī: Urdū Akādimī Dillī.

Ẓillurraḥmān, Ḥakīm Syed. 2004. *Ḥakīm Ajmal Ḵẖān*. Na'ī Dihlī: Neshanal buk ṭrasṭ, Inḍyā.

Ẓillurraḥmān, Ḥakīm Syed. 2009 [1978]. *Tazkirah Ḵẖāndān-i 'Azīzī*. 'Alīgaṛh: Ibn Sīnā Akāḍimī.

Zimmerman, Francis. 1992. 'Gentle Purge: The Flower Power of Ayurveda'. In Charles Leslie & Allan Young (eds.), *Paths to Asian Medical Knowledge*, 209–223. Berkeley: University of California Press.

Zimmermann, Francis. 2011 [1982]. *The Jungle and the Aroma of Meats: An Ecological Theme in Hindu Medicine*. Delhi: Motilal Banarsidass.

Zysk, Kenneth G. 2001. 'New Age Ayurveda or What Happens to Indian Medicine When It Comes to America'. *Traditional South Asian Medicine* 6. 10–26.

Index

People

Places

Subjects

For Product Safety Concerns and Information please contact our EU representative GPSR@taylorandfrancis.com
Taylor & Francis Verlag GmbH, Kaufingerstraße 24, 80331 München, Germany

www.ingramcontent.com/pod-product-compliance
Ingram Content Group UK Ltd.
Pitfield, Milton Keynes, MK11 3LW, UK
UKHW010957180926
475701UK00004B/408
9781041190011